Florian Steger, Marcin Orzechowski,
Giovanni Rubeis and Maximilian Schochow (Hg.)

# Migration and Medicine



ANGEWANDTE ETHIK

ANGEWANDTE ETHIK

Herausgegeben von
Nikolaus Knoepffler, Peter Kunzmann, Reinhard Merkel,
Ingo Pies, Anne Siegetsleitner und Florian Steger



Medizin
Band 4

Florian Steger
Marcin Orzechowski
Giovanni Rubeis
Maximilian Schochow (Eds.)

# Migration and Medicine

Verlag Karl Alber Freiburg / München

Florian Steger, Marcin Orzechowski, Giovanni Rubeis and Maximilian Schochow (Eds.)

# Migration and Medicine

In the summer of 2015, a strong migration movement towards Europe set in. This led to ethical, legal and societal challenges in the medical care of the refugees. These included cultural conflicts in medical practice and deficits in the institutional handling of cultural diversity. The book analyzes different challenges and offers possible solutions.

The Editors:

Professor Dr. Florian Steger is director of the Institute of the History, Philosophy and Ethics of Medicine at Ulm University.

Dr. Marcin Orzechowski is scientific assistant at the Institute of the History, Philosophy and Ethics of Medicine at Ulm University.

Dr. Giovanni Rubeis is research associate at the Institute of the History and Ethics of Medicine at Ruprecht-Karls-University Heidelberg.

PD Dr. Maximilian Schochow is scientific assistant at the Institute of the History, Philosophy and Ethics of Medicine at Ulm University.

Gedruckt mit freundlicher Unterstützung des Bundesministeriums für Bildung und Forschung (BMBF), www.bmbf.de

Bundesministerium
für Bildung
und Forschung

MIX
Papier aus verantwortungsvollen Quellen
FSC
www.fsc.org
FSC® C083411

Originalausgabe


www.verlag-alber.de

Satz: SatzWeise, Bad Wünnenberg
Herstellung: CPI books GmbH, Leck

Printed in Germany

ISBN 978-3-495-49134-8

# Content

# Preface

From 11$^{th}$ to 15$^{th}$ March 2019 the symposium »Migration as a challenge for medicine. A comparison of ethical, legal and social aspects in Germany, Croatia and Austria« took place at the Institute of the History, Philosophy and Ethics of Medicine of Ulm University. The symposium was financed by the German Federal Ministry of Education and Research (BMBF). The aim of this international symposium was to create a scientific platform for presenting and discussing the challenges for healthcare related to migration from an ethical, legal and social point of view. On this basis, the symposium should serve for development of country-specific solutions for medical care.

For this purpose, junior researchers from different fields met in Ulm together with internationally recognized experts. While the contributions of the young scientists were discussed internally, the lectures of the experts were addressed to a broad public. The contributions of the authors published in this volume are based on the revised presentations provided during the symposium. All articles were peer-reviewed.

The organization of the symposium and the publication of this volume would not have been possible without generous support. We thank the Federal Ministry of Education and Research for the approval of the project. We would like to thank the staff of Deutsches Zentrum für Luft- und Raumfahrt e. V. (DLR), who accompanied and supported the work and thus the implementation of the symposium. We thank all participants and experts of the symposium as well as the authors for the provision of their contributions to the volume. We would also like to thank the staff of the Ulm Institute of the History, Philosophy and Ethics of Medicine for their energetic support in this project.

Ulm, October 2019

Florian Steger, Marcin Orzechowski,
Giovanni Rubeis and Maximilian Schochow

*Florian Steger, Marcin Orzechowski, Giovanni Rubeis and Maximilian Schochow*

# Introduction

International migration is one of the most urgent challenges for public health and healthcare. The number of international migrants worldwide has continued to grow rapidly in recent years, reaching 258 million in 2017, up from 173 million in 2000. That Europe is one of the most important destinations can be supported by current statistical data.[1] According to the Statistical Office of the European Union – Eurostat, a total of 4.4 million people immigrated to one of the member states of the European Union in 2017.[2] Among these, were estimated 2 million citizens of non-EU countries. The number of people residing in an EU Member State with citizenship of a non-member country on 1 January 2018 was 22.3 million, representing 4.4 % of the EU-28 population. Especially since the beginning of the increased migration movement towards the European Union in the summer of 2015, migration constitutes one of the most pressing issues for both transit and destination countries in this region. These issues include several aspects: from humanitarian challenges for provision of appropriate protection and accommodation, through legal questions of asylum and citizenship, to cultural and social questions of integration and cohabitation. Among these topics, medical care for migrants remains one of the most essential concerns. Deprived, in many cases, of adequate healthcare in their countries of origin, susceptible to illness and physical as well as psychological abuse or tor-

---

[1] United Nations: International Migration Report. https://un.org/en/development/desa/population/migration/publications/migrationreport/docs/MigrationReport2017_Highlights.pdf (accessed 9/24/2019).

[2] Eurostat: Migration and migrant population statistics. https://ec.europa.eu/eurostat/statistics-explained/index.php/Migration_and_migrant_population_statistics (accessed 9/24/2019).

ment en route, migrants can place substantive challenges on host societies with regard to healthcare.[3]

Such challenges comprise many aspects – clinical, ethical, legal, and societal. Among the most visible are clinical factors such as the frequency of certain infectious diseases. In general, migrants in Europe are susceptible to similar diseases as the host societies. However, due to the difficult living conditions during flight, possibly incomplete vaccination, the sometimes higher prevalence of some diseases in the countries of origin, and the limited space in mass housing, migrants can be particularly vulnerable to infectious diseases.[4] Reports show increased prevalence of tuberculosis, HIV and hepatitis B, respiratory infections and gastroenteritis, chickenpox, measles, mumps, rotavirus and norovirus infections among migrants.[5] Also occurring are cases of tropical diseases such as malaria.[6] Therefore, first and foremost, migrants are often in need of a rapid and adequate medical care. Yet, provision of such care in timely manner can encounter many obstacles of which not least important are financial, cultural, and language barriers.

In general, migrants do not constitute an acute healthcare emergency for the host society.[7] Nevertheless, the healthcare services are required not only for infectious diseases but also for other conditions. Non-infectious diseases, such as diabetes mellitus, cardiovascular diseases, or chronic respiratory diseases create a need for long-term and complex treatment. Also, in many cases, migrants are in dire need of psychotherapeutic or psychosocial support. Numerous migrants and asylum-seeking persons experienced highly traumatizing events before their exodus from countries of origin. They were subjected to atrocities of war, torture or political persecution. In addition, severe conditions during flight leave distinctive marks on their psychic

[3] Julian Bion, Elie Azoulay: The ethics of migration and critical illness. In: Intensive Care Medicine 42 (2016), pp. 256–257.

[4] Sotirios Tsiodras: Irregular migrants: a critical care or a public health emergency. In: Intensive Care Medicine 42 (2015), pp. 252–255.

[5] Tanja Artelt, Martin Kaase, Simone Scheithauer: Infektiologische Herausforderungen nach Migration. Besonderheiten bei der Betreuung weiblicher Flüchtlinge. In: Der Gynäkologe 50 (2017), pp. 134–138.

[6] Jenny Höcker, Florian Fischer, Alexander Krämer, Luise Prüfer-Krämer: Ambulante Versorgung von Geflüchteten durch Tropenmediziner. In: Flugmedizin, Tropenmedizin, Reisemedizin 24 (2017), pp. 181–184.

[7] August Stich: Häufige Infektionskrankheiten bei Migranten. In: Der Internist 57 (2016), pp. 409–415.

health. Narratives of migrant often recount cases of sexual assaults, loss of family, threats to own life or experiences of death or suffering of others. These experiences increase the risk of trauma-related disorders like post-traumatic stress disorder (PTSD), depression, anxiety disorders, or chronic pain.[8]

In addition to clinical challenges, ethical challenges must be considered. One of the primary considerations is the language barrier, which, in many cases, complicates the patient-doctor-conversation.[9] Functioning communication between patient and physician is the essential condition for informed consent and thus highly relevant from the ethical point of view. In addition, different cultural conceptions of self-determination can complicate the treatment situation. Informed consent as a prerequisite for a self-determined decision is often replaced by a model of decision-making called broader consent. Accordingly, the patient does not make the decision to consent to treatment alone but with the help of family members. In addition, practitioners are often confronted with disease concepts that differ from those of Western-focused medicine. Finally, deficits in diversity management, that is the institutional handling of cultural diversity, can be identified in the healthcare systems of many European countries.[10] These deficits often result from structural conditions, such as a lack of interpreters.[11] In addition, it is unclear to what extent practitioners are familiar with the subject of diversity through medical education and whether they acquire intercultural skills. This includes the knowledge of different disease etiologies and a foreign cultural understanding of

---

[8] Laura Frank, Rahsan Yesil-Jürgens, Oliver Razum, Kayvan Bozorgmehr, Liane Schenk, Andreas Gilsdorf, Alexander Rommel, Thomas Lampert: Gesundheit und gesundheitliche Versorgung von Asylsuchenden und Flüchtlingen in Deutschland. In: Journal of Health Monitoring 2 (2017), pp. 24–47.

[9] Bernd Rechel, Philipa Mladovsky, David Ingleby, Johan P. Mackenbach, Martin McKee: Migration and health in an increasingly diverse Europe. In: The Lancet 381 (2013), pp. 1235–1245.

[10] Thomas Köllen: Diversity Management in the European Health Care Sector: Trends, Challenges, and Opportunities. In: Sebastian Gurtner, Katja Soyez (Eds.): Challenges and Opportunities in Health Care Management. Cham, Heidelberg, New York 2015, pp. 27–45.

[11] Tim Peters, Tatjana Grützmann, Walter Bruchhausen, Michael Coors, Fabian Jacobs, Lukas Kaelin, Michael Knipper, Frank Kressing, Gerald Neitzke: Grundsätze zum Umgang mit Interkulturalität in Einrichtungen des Gesundheitswesens. Positionspapier der Arbeitsgruppe Interkulturalität in der medizinischen Praxis in der Akademie für Ethik in der Medizin. In: Ethik in der Medizin 26 (2014), pp. 65–75.

illness. The confrontation with these cultural challenges very often takes place against the background of different social and legal contexts and requirements. Thus, culturally sensible contact with patients with migration background requires adjusting to specific needs of migrants and foreign patients combined with culturally sensible medical analysis.

From the legal point of view, one of most fundamental barriers for migrants in accessing health services in Europe are inadequate legal entitlements and, where entitlements exist, mechanisms for ensuring their implementation in practice.[12] Numerous international treaties describe access to health services as a basic human right. Already in 1946, the constitution of the World Health Organization proclaimed the right to health.[13] In the following decades, this right has been recognized by several international documents such as the International Covenant on Economic, Social and Cultural Rights (ICESCR) of 1966[14], the Convention on the Rights of the Child of 1989[15] or the International Convention on the Protection of the Rights of All Migrant Workers and Members of their Families of 1990.[16] Also on the level of European Institutions, the issue of access to healthcare for migrants receives particular attention. Central European documents, such as the European Convention for the Protection of Human Rights and Fundamental Freedoms recognize the right to physical and mental health.[17] Especially the European Social Charter or the Charter of Fundamental Rights sets out right of everyone to access preventive healthcare and to benefit from medical treatment.

However, within the area of provision of health care for asylum seekers, the protection of international regulations is still not met in practice. In order to improve the situation, the Council of the Eur-

---

[12] Rechel et al.: Migration and health (Note 8).

[13] World Health Organization: WHO Constitution. Geneva 1946.

[14] International Covenant on Economic, Social and Cultural Rights, adopted and opened for signature, ratification and accession by General Assembly resolution 2200A (XXI) of 16 December 1966, entry into force 3 January 1976.

[15] United Nations: Convention on the Rights of the Child. https://www.ohchr.org/Documents/ProfessionalInterest/crc.pdf (accessed 9/24/2019).

[16] United Nations: International Convention on the Protection of the Rights of All Migrant Workers and Members of Their Families. https://www.ohchr.org/Documents/ProfessionalInterest/cmw.pdf (accessed 9/24/2019).

[17] European Court of Human Rights, Council of Europe: European Convention on Human Rights. https://www.echr.coe.int/Documents/Convention_ENG.pdf (accessed 9/24/2019).

opean Union outlined in 2003 the minimum standards for the reception of asylum-seekers. These include emergency care, essential treatment of illness, and necessary medical or other assistance for applicants with special needs.[18] Despite this, these minimum standards are still not met in many European Union Member States. Huge differences exist within the European Union when it comes to national asylum policy regimes, with consequences for access to healthcare and other social services.[19]

In Germany, medical care for asylum-seekers is regulated in the Asylum Seekers' Benefit Act (Asylbewerberleistungsgesetz – AsylLG).[20] According to §4, section 1, asylum-seekers have an entitlement to healthcare in case of acute and treatable diseases and pain. Similarly, chronic diseases, which if not treated, can effect a decrease of health, can also be covered. However, such limitations of the entitlement for treatment in case of illness for asylum-seekers by the §4 and 6 of the AsylbLG and their implementation in practice are often criticized.[21] An important point of criticism is that asylum seekers without an electronic health card have to apply for a doctor's visit beforehand to the competent authority, for example the social welfare office, in order to receive a doctor's certificate. An application for treatment is often granted or denied at the discretion of non-specialist personnel.[22] Introduction of an electronic health card, which is issued to all asylum-seekers after 15 months of residence in Germany, should improve the provision of medical care for persons that are affected by a long process of asylum granting. However, even with such a card, asylum-seekers have a limited access to health service. Some benefits that are offered to native population, for example arti-

---

[18] The Council of the European Union: COUNCIL DIRECTIVE 2003/9/EC of 27 January 2003 laying down minimum standards for the reception of asylum seekers. https://eur-lex.europa.eu/LexUriServ/LexUriServ.do?uri=OJ:L:2003:031:0018:0025:EN:PDF (accessed 9/24/2019).

[19] Rechel et al.: Migration and health (Note 8).

[20] Bundesministerium der Justiz und für Verbraucherschutz: Asylbewerberleistungsgesetz (AsylbLG). https://www.gesetze-im-internet.de/asylblg/BJNR107410993.html (accessed 9/24/2019).

[21] Frank et al.: Gesundheit und gesundheitliche Versorgung (Note 7); Gisela Klinkhammer, Heike Korzilius: Asylleistungen in Deutschland: Flüchtlinge sind Patienten dritter Klasse. In: Deutsches Ärzteblatt 111: A540–A543.

[22] Oliver Razum, Judith Wenner, Kayvan Bozorgmehr: Wenn Zufall über den Zugang zur Gesundheitsversorgung bestimmt: Geflüchtete in Deutschland. In: Das Gesundheitswesen 78 (2016), pp. 711–714.

ficial insemination, are not covered by statutory health insurance. Although the financial benefits of introduction of electronic health card for asylum-seekers in form of economization of administrative processes are visible, such forms of access discrimination lead to further criticism of this procedure. Furthermore, studies show that per capita healthcare spending per year for asylum seekers with limited access was higher than for asylum seekers with full entitlement to benefits.[23] Therefore, further removal of barriers to access to healthcare is to be evaluated positively, not only from the humanitarian but also from the economic point of view.

The questions of access to healthcare in destination countries closely tie together the legal regulations of access to medical services with societal acceptance of migrants. In many European countries, migration is regarded as a problem or even a threat. Increased migration provides nationalist and populist movements with an image of cultural »aliens« that raise claims to medical care. At the center of discussion are issues of providing adequate medical care for migrants. This topic is often critically viewed from the economic perspective. Such a provision of medical care could put a pressure on limited resources available for healthcare, especially in countries that are most susceptible to immigration.[24] Here emerges the question of just allocation of the resources in a society. On the one hand, basic human rights would require that all migrants receive sanctuary and access to protection, including medical health. On the other hand, some argue that only permanent residency or citizenship should provide full social benefits. Inclusion of individuals perceived as ›outsiders‹ that did not yet contribute to the national income in these benefits could lead to implosion of the social system and to limitation of access to healthcare for all. Special challenge in this regard concerns physicians and their responsibility in determining access to healthcare. They are often confronted with the question of the best use of scarce resources. Yet, it is primarily a societal and political task to determine the entitlement to medical care. In a situation of rising numbers of migrants,

---

23 Kayvan Bozorgmehr, Oliver Razum: Effect of Restricting Access to Health Care on Health Expenditures among Asylum-Seekers and Refugees: A Quasi-Experimental Study in Germany, 1994–2013. In: PLoS One 10 (2015), doi: 10.1371/journal.pone.0131483.

24 Garyphallia Poulakou, Matteo Bassetti, Jean-François Timsit: Critically ill migrants with infection: diagnostic considerations for intensive care physicians in Europe. In: Intensive Care Medicine 42 (2016), pp. 245–248.

this question will be more and more imperative and will require a wide societal debate.

Further societal challenges related to migration and health concern the issues of integration and assimilation of migrants with the aim of providing them access to healthcare. Not migration itself but rather causes and circumstances of migration as well as life and working environments can lead to deteriorating health. People with migration background often have a lower socio-economic status, work in health-damaging conditions, are unemployed or live in unfavorable living conditions.[25] Each one of these factors can have a deteriorating result on the healthcare situation but they are especially dangerous if they coincide. Therefore, political and social objectives here should aim at providing strategies to improve the socio-economic position of migrants. Political measures to reduce social inequality can contribute to improvement of migrant's health. Furthermore, marginalization and xenophobia can also directly influence health of migrants.[26] Consequently, integration of newcomers into society and prevention of building of parallel societies can yield positive effects on the health of people with migration background.

The issues of migration pose a challenge for medicine in several contexts: ethical, legal, and societal. Improvement of contemporary strategies in this area requires international and national initiatives that aim at amelioration of current situation and provision of appropriate solutions. Basis for development of such solutions is, above all, a multifaceted consideration of various perspectives that include viewpoints of both migrants and host population. Articles of authors complied in this publication present an impulse for such a debate from ethical, legal and societal point of view. The following passages shortly describe individual contributions to the volume.

---

[25] Oliver Razum, Hajo Zeeb, Uta Meesmann, Liane Schenk, Maren Bredehorst, Patrick Brzoska, Tanja Dercks, Susanne Glodny, Björn Menkhaus, Ramazan Salman, Anke-Christine Saß, Ralf Ulrich: Schwerpunktbericht der Gesundheitsberichterstattung des Bundes: Migration und Gesundheit. Berlin 2008.

[26] Ulrike Igel, Elmar Brähler, Gesine Grande: Der Einfluss von Diskriminierungserfahrungen auf die Gesundheit von MigrantInnen. In: Psychiatrische Praxis 37 (2010), pp. 183–190; Saffron Karlsen, James Y. Nazroo: Relation between Racial Discrimination, Social Class, and Health among Ethnic Minority Groups. In: American Journal of Public Health 92 (2002), pp. 624–631.

In the first section of this book, authors offer their deliberations on challenges for provision of adequate and high-quality healthcare for migrants and refugees. Migrants certainly belong to vulnerable groups within society; yet, the very concept of vulnerability often cannot be precisely defined. In addition, migrants repeatedly encounter barriers in current healthcare systems that lead to exclusion or discontinuation of therapy. In this context, the provision of culturally sensitive healthcare, establishment of appropriate structures, and removal of language barriers are the main recommendations.

The section begins with Giovanni Rubeis' contribution »Mental healthcare in migrants from the perspective of public health ethics: clinical factors, cultural diversity, and access barriers«. In his contribution, Rubeis analyses various factors affecting psychiatric and psychotherapeutic treatment of migrants. According to Rubeis, clinical factors, cultural diversity, and accessibility barriers play here a dominant role. Clinical factors include the high prevalence of mental health and related care needs among refugees, the high prevalence of vulnerable patients such as minors and female refugees, and the often inadequate therapies resulting from a lack of awareness of individual patient needs. The question of cultural diversity concentrates on the cultural competences of the practitioners. In addition, further issues constitute the questions of the different types of access barriers that should be analyzed with regard to healthcare offers. In his analysis, Rubeis considers these factors in the context of existing principles such as self-determination, patient well-being, benevolence, and distributive justice, and provides recommendations for clinical practice.

The examination of the topic of psychiatric and psychotherapeutic care for migrants is continued in Vera Vogel's contribution »Healthcare for refugees suffering from psychiatric disorders: an overview of the current care provision in Germany«. Faced with rising number of migrants arriving in Germany, the public health system is increasingly confronted with the question of provision of effective care in treatment of trauma-related mental disorders. The author aims to provide an analysis of the current supply situation in Germany by providing an overview of existing care services for mentally ill refugees, while also revealing the specific challenges in this area. Particular attention is paid to trauma disorders, among which refugees are more likely to suffer, as well as to the difficulties encountered in diagnosis, therapy, and estimation of the prevalence of these diseases. Vogel describes the current care system using four criteria of accessibility, availability, affordability, and acceptance, simultaneously pointing out some of the most significant difficulties in the process of diagnosis, therapy, and prevalence rate estimation. Moreover, she provides an overview of the field of transcultural psychiatry, which constitutes the essential basis for the effective treatment of refugees suffering from mental illness.

Issues of informed consent and the principle of self-determination constitute some of the most important challenges in the provision of healthcare for migrants and refugees. Both issues are increasingly subjects of scientific controversy, especially due to the problematic notion of self-determination for patients with a non-Western background. In community-based cultures characterized by different family dynamics and different perceptions of the relationship between physicians and their patients, there are a number of ethical and legal challenges facing contemporary moral philosophers, bioethicists and lawyers within the framework of multicultural societies. Starting with a brief overview of the most influential theoretical foundation of informed consent, Ivana Tucak describes in her essay »Cultural differences and informed consent« the cultural challenges for this principle in today's culturally diverse societies. Especially she examines the justifiability of the recent critique of perception of patient's autonomy. Based on this, Tucak explores the regulation of informed consent in the Republic of Croatia in order to determine whether the Croatian legal system can accommodate cultural challenges resulting from the changing cultural outlook of modern societies.

The question of the physician-patient relationship in culturally diverse setups remains in focus in Pranab Rudra's contribution »Physician-patient relationship models in Bangladesh and Germany«. Beginning with the description of differences in healthcare systems in both countries, Rudra moves to examine various models of information provision and self-determination within the framework of medical contact between patient and physician. In such a situation, several factors can influence the quality of provided medical service. Factors that affect contact with medical professionals for Bangladeshi migrants in Germany are mostly culturally conditioned and include cultural backgrounds relating to sex and gender as well as religious beliefs. Moreover, the paternalistic model of patient-physician relationship that is still dominant in Bangladesh can to a significant degree influence decision making process in a clinical situation. In order to improve the situation, development of good relationship with the patient and experience in treating patients with culturally different background are of the utmost importance. Here, a four-step model of cross-cultural care can lead to significant betterment of the existing situation.

In her contribution entitled »Understanding vulnerability and deliberations on justice – the case of health care for refugees and asylum seekers in Germany«, Silvia Agbih endeavors to develop an understanding of human vulnerability and its importance, especially in care for refugees. According to Agbih, both the concept of vulnerability and its use carry with them a certain ambiguity. Using the taxonomy of vulnerability of refuges and asylum seekers in Germany, she concludes that that navigating the positive and negative effects of using vulnerability as a guideline for the practical necessity of distributing resources remains a challenging task. Assessing the current situation in Germany as a destination country shows many pathogenic sources of vulnerability. However, a complete forego of this concept could negatively affect the situation of refugees or asylum seekers. The restrictions and derogations of healthcare in Germany for refugees in entitlement, access, and quality of care increase vulnerability to an extent that health and well-being are at stake.

Ivana Zagorac' essay »The power of empathy in the treatment of vulnerable subjects« follows these reflections. Her main question is whether empathy can be re-modelled in order to improve attitudes toward migrants, which would further result in the increased level of the acceptance of migrants. To this end, Zagorac examines the challenges that arise from using empathy as an aid in improving attitudes towards vulnerable groups. One of these challenges is the lack of a clear and generally accepted definition of empathy. In the discussions on vulnerability, often used terms are duties and obligation, but also empathy and compassion. Therefore, both scientific community and policy makers are still unsure about many aspects of the very concept of vulnerability and what it entails. Zagorac reaches the conclusion that the careful implementation of perspective-taking exercises in anti-prejudice and anti-stigmatization programs has a great potential for inducing a positive change in attitudes toward the vulnerable.

Language barriers and the experience of migration pose significant challenge for medicine and communication in clinical situation. In her contribution entitled »Narration without borders. Migration, narrative medicine, and témoignage in the public work of Médecins

Sans Frontières (Doctors Without Borders)«, Katharina Fürholzer argues that language barriers can lead to hierarchical communication structures, where patients are rather talked about than encouraged to find their own voice. The humanitarian NGO Médecins Sans Frontières provides a different approach to this issue. This organization has published a series of reports after missions in regions of crisis to raise public awareness of the hardship their patients face. In her essay, Fürholzer examines several patients' stories and appeals for provision of a platform for migrants to speak out as experts of their own stories. The focus on patients' personal narratives could result in better communication and quality of medical care, and can lead to strengthening patient autonomy.

Ethical reflections are often closely tied to legal questions. Not only personal, cultural or language barriers define the accessibility to healthcare but, in many cases, legal barriers have a decisive effect. Implications of migration influence legislation and jurisprudence, both on the international and national level. Over the past century, international organizations moved the migration and health agenda forward through various instruments. Yet, these guidelines are seldom transferred into the national legislations. Thereby a particular field of tension is visible in this area.

This is the focus point of the second thematic section of this volume. It opens with the contribution from Pedro A. Villarreal »Differential treatment in the international health regulations: towards a nuanced perspective«. In his essay, Villarreal analyzes International Health Regulations (IHR) adopted in 2005 by the World Health Organization (WHO)'s Member States, which aims at the protection against the trans-border spread of communicable diseases. Beginning with an overview of the concept of differential treatment in international law, the author then moves to describing the obligations established by the IHR and appraisal of the data from the WHO with regard to the fulfillment of surveillance and response requirements. It becomes visible that challenges posed by disparities in economic development between countries influence obligations to the international law in the field of the protection against epidemics. Therefore, Villarreal calls for more nuanced perspectives towards assessing pandemic preparedness and response.

The impact of the international law on human right to health on the German legal system stands in the center of Katarina Weilert's essay »The human right to health in public international law with particular reference to asylum-seekers, refugees, and migrants and its reception in German law«. Weilert argues that although, the human right to health is guaranteed in various international legal documents, the precise content of the right to health depends on the health system of the particular state. As the costs for a high-quality health system present a challenge even for developed countries, the idea of unlimited access to free healthcare is untenable. This is especially true if one considers various healthcare systems in different countries. Yet, as Weilert stresses, the access to basic healthcare is a condition for a life in dignity. Therefore, while it may be well justified for a country to make free access to health services dependent on the duration of the person's stay, a state cannot exclude any person from such care merely because of his or her nationality or legal status.

Legal and social questions concerning medical care for migrants overlap in many aspects. On the one hand, the legal framework defines what is allowed in a healthcare or how the medical system should work. On the other hand, cultural appreciation and recognition creates a social dimension of practical provision of medical service for migrants. Understanding issues of culture, ethnicity, and identity is crucial for achieving equity in health. Lack of such understanding can result in higher morbidity due to the effect of immigration laws and legal status, the deleterious interaction of multiple adverse structural factors, including xenophobia, marginalization, poverty, communication problems, and poor access to healthcare.

The contribution of Frank Kressing and Maximilian Schochow »Aspects of migration, culture and health care in Germany's past and present« opens the section of the volume that focuses on societal considerations regarding medicine and migration. Beginning with the historical outlook of Germany as a country characterized by migration movements, the authors move to considerations relating to different concepts of culture in the past and present. In this context, they elaborate a concept of diversity that should not only cover cultural or religious diversity but patients' diversity in a broader sense, comprising i.e., sex, gender, age, socio-economic status. Therefore, Kressing and Schochow advocate a careful usage of the term »culture«, transgressing the established notion of fixed ethnic, cultural, and linguistic identities. On the basis of their considerations, authors offer suggestions for the improvement of cultural sensitive healthcare in hospitals in Germany, for example through strengthening these aspects in medical education of students with the goal of high quality of healthcare.

The essay of Tamara Schwertel »Difficulties in the trajectories: an investigation of care structures for refugees suffering from tuberculosis in Germany« focusses especially on the treatment of refugees suffering from tuberculosis. In media reports and national discourses, migrants are often characterized as disease carriers and a potential danger to the native population. This leads to stigmatization by medical personnel and racial prejudice towards migrants that can result in discontinuation of treatment. In her research based on interviews with affected individuals, Schwertel provides a qualitative analysis of these challenges and the strategies to avoid them. On the one hand, anticipatory actions can increase speed and effectiveness of the treatment of migrants. On the other hand, a lack of understanding for refugee patients is visible. Compliance issues are reduced to language or cultural barriers and are less often localized in the organization of treatment. Therefore, the development of new organizational structures is necessary to counteract inadequately sensitized personnel, communication difficulties, and time lost in treatment.

In his essay »The challenges of the migration crisis in Croatia – the Primorje-Gorski Kotar county and the city of Rijeka example«, Robert Doričić shows a practical example of support for medical treatment of refugees in Croatia. In response to a large number of migrants arriving in Croatia through the so-called Western Balkan route towards Western Europe, the Croatian government established a network of aid agencies. This network shows an example of a system of measures and institutions responsible for the acceptance, registration, and provision of healthcare for migrants. On the example of an exercise held in the city of Rijeka in autumn of 2017, Doričić examines the effectiveness of the system in the crisis situation of managing a large number of refugees. The results show a high degree of preparedness for a humanitarian response but also negative reactions in local media related to the general social acceptance of migrants in Croatia.

In their chapter »Challenges faced by refugees to access healthcare in Germany«, Prerna Thaker and Ravi Rao investigate barriers for migrant populations to use health services. Based on a systematic review of the literature on the topic, the authors identify three barriers that restrict access to healthcare in Germany: interpersonal barriers, organizational barriers, and policy barriers. Thaker and Rao argue that a flexible response is required in order to meet medical needs of newly arrived refugees. Such a response could include a digital documentation in form of a uniform health book, courses for migrants introducing them to the basic framework of medical assistance in Germany as well as training for the medical staff in cultural sensitivity and communication with patients.

The issue of societal acceptance and integration may have significant repercussions on migrants' social well-being and, in consequence, on their physical and mental health. Tarek Mahjoub's essay »What it takes to fit in: an opinion piece on the integration of adolescent refugee migrants in Germany« is based on this initial reflection. Mahjoub studies factors that help migrants to adapt to living in a host community. He investigates the impact of language barriers, the family environment, and the school system on the development of migrant children and their adaptation to living in a culturally different society. The author reaches the conclusion that integration is not the responsibility of the migrants alone; the host communities are also responsible for facilitating inclusion by providing opportunities of language and culture learning programs, education, and career building. Therefore, proper integration will require welcoming and realistic local policies that include vocational training programs, overcoming segregation of migrants in restricted areas, and social events that include members of migrant populations.

The importance of local programs for understanding cultural diversity and multiculturality is further highlighted in the contribution of Iva Rinčić and Amir Muzur »Migrants' health and European culture: strengthening ties for better understanding. The case of Rijeka 2020 European Capital of Culture«. The authors argue that migrants' health is a challenging concept, formed of objective and subjective dimensions. Thus, it is often neglected, remaining on the margins of mainstream migration related research, professional interest, and societal as well as political initiatives. The case in point is the approach of the program »European Capital of Culture 2020« which was awarded to Rijeka in Croatia. According to Rinčić and Muzur, this program exemplifies an inadequate approach to the issues of migration, culture, and health. The authors assert that even though Rijeka has historically been the scene of major migration movements, the city missed the opportunity to reveal the complexness of the problems of migrants' health and culture, ceding instead to the more popular aspects of migrant cuisine and music.

Wielant Machleidt in his essay »The importance of strangeness experiences for ego-constitution and society« addresses the essential questions of xenophobia and acceptance of migrants in host societies. According to the author, the postmodern project of global migration and cultural change has proven as vulnerable for worldwide fears of strangers, hate, and populism. Because migration means transgression of national and cultural borders and coping with the experience of strangeness, people with lack of basic trust develop aversive feelings towards strangers resulting in xenophobia. This significantly affects the mental health of migrants. A positive attitude toward strangers requires a certain cultural adolescence from both migrants and the native population. Such a developmental step can contribute to the management of foreign experiences and the growth of tolerance in multi-cultural societies. Machleidt concludes that mutual trust through intercultural communication prevents social exclusion and separation processes and paves the way for social integration.

The contributions to this book make the ethical, legal, and social challenges of migration and medicine apparent. Ethical challenges result, among other things, from institutional and structural deficits, for example from a lack of interpreters or trained specialist staff. Questions of the vulnerability of individual groups as well as the relationship between patients and physicians are crucial to this discussion. These topics require specific solutions, which should be developed jointly by all affected groups. For example, different cultural understandings of self-determination may result in the replacement of informed consent by other models of decision-making in the medical setting. Therefore, both on the side of migrants and on the side of the medical professionals, there is a need for information about perspective of the respective counterpart. In addition, the legal challenges of access to healthcare need to receive more attention. For this, it is necessary to describe and analyze the country-specific legal and structural deficits. On this basis, guidelines valid throughout Europe can then be developed. The examination of the social challenges makes it clear that readiness for solidarity with refugees is a central issue. Processes of gradual tightening of the legal regulations on the medical care of migrants are observable in several European countries. This development results from an increasingly critical attitude towards migrants in large parts of societies. With the rise of populist movements in Europe, fundamental become the issues of xenophobia but also of legal and societal status of migrants, which often have influence on health of migrating individuals. Therefore, it is of crucial importance to address the issues of migration and healthcare both in social as well as scientific debates. This volume aims at providing such voice.

# I. Ethical Aspects

*Giovanni Rubeis*

# Mental healthcare in migrants from the perspective of public health ethics: clinical factors, cultural diversity, and access barriers

Abstract
Ethical issues in mental healthcare for refugees entail clinical factors, cultural diversity, and questions of access to mental health services. Clinical factors include the high prevalence of mental disorders and thus high mental health need within the refugee population, the high prevalence of vulnerable patients like minors and women, and the often inappropriate therapeutic measures, which result from a lack of awareness towards individual patient's needs. Cultural diversity the question of cultural competence on behalf of mental health professionals arises. Finally, the different kinds of access barriers refugees seeking mental health services have to be analyzed. In my analysis I will frame those issues within the network of existing principles like autonomy, patient well-being, beneficence, and equity, and give recommendation for mental health practice.

## 1. Introduction

According to the recent UNHCR Global Trends report, 70.8 million people worldwide were forcibly displaced as a result of persecution, conflict, violence, or human rights violations by the end of 2018.[1] This is the highest number of displaced persons ever recorded. In the view of many Europeans, the so-called migration crisis had its peak in 2015, when a high number of people migrated to Europe, primarily as a reaction to wars in the Middle East and Africa, poverty, draught, and climate change. After the Austrian government closed the so-called Balkan Route in 2016 and the EU and the Turkish government found an agreement forcing migrants back to Turkey the same year, the influx of migrants into the EU was significantly reduced. However,

[1] The UNHCR: Global Trends. Forced Displacement in 2018. https://www.unhcr.org/statistics/unhcrstats/5d08d7ee7/unhcr-global-trends-2018.html (accessed 9/24/2019).

as the recent UNHCR Global Trends report shows, the global migration movement is far from over. Also, there are thousands of refugees living in Europe without a clear legal status, which often means living in special facilities without the possibility to work or participate in social life. The high numbers of people in the process of migration as well as people that have already arrived in Europe also means great challenges when it comes to public health. That these public health challenges are associated with ethical implications has been noted before.[2] To regard migration as an issue of public health ethics means taking into account socioeconomic and political aspects as well as clinical factors. Therefore, questions of social justice and health equity, mostly in terms of access to health services, are of relevance in this context. This approach is also suitable for analyzing the challenges of mental healthcare in refugees. An analysis of this topic is of crucial importance since the empirical evidence shows high mental health needs in refugees.[3]

Some preliminary remarks on the question of methodology are necessary at this point. I will use the term refugee as signifying people who are forcibly displaced due to human rights violations, persecution, violence, climate factors, or population growth. The distinctions between asylum seekers, migrants, and refugees are complex and mostly of interest in the legal context, since the legal status defines the entitlements and rights ascribed to a person.[4] For the ethical *prima facie* analysis that is conducted in this article, these distinctions are of minor importance, especially since they vary from country to country, thus making them somewhat arbitrary. Important for this analysis are the aspects of forced relocation and flight due to their effects on mental health. Whether for example climate change is ac-

---

[2] Verena Wild, Angela Dawson: Migration: a core public health ethics issue. In: Public Health 158 (2018), pp. 66–70.

[3] Emily Satinsky, Daniela C. Fuhr, Aniek Woodward, Egbert Sondorp, Bayard Roberts: Mental health care utilisation and access among refugees and asylum seekers in Europe: A systematic review. In: Health Policy 2019, doi: /10.1016/j.healthpol.2019.02.007; Malek Bajbouj, Jihad Alabdullah, Salah Ahmad, S. Schidem, Henrike Zellmann, Frank Schneider, Isabella Heuser: Psychosoziale Versorgung von Flüchtlingen in Deutschland Erkenntnisse aus der Not- und Entwicklungshilfe. In: Der Nervenarzt 89 (2018), pp. 1–7.

[4] Judith Wenner, Yudot Namer, Oliver Razum: Migrants, Refugees, Asylum Seekers: Use and Misuse of Labels in Public Health Research. In: Alexander Krämer, Florian Fischer (Eds.): Refugee Migration and Health. Challenges for Germany and Europe. Migration, Minorities and Modernity, Vol. 4. Cham 2019, pp. 49–62.

cepted as cause for forced relocation in several countries while it is not accepted in others, does not change the fact that leaving one's home country due to hazardous conditions may affect a person's mental health. Although I focus on people who are forcibly displaced, some insights provided in this article may also be transferred to other groups of migrants.

In my ethical analysis, I will not use any specific ethical concept or theory. Instead of such a top down-approach, I aim to detect and to highlight issues within mental healthcare for refugees that have ethical implications, and try to frame them within the network of existing principles and values. These are mainly patient autonomy, patient well-being, beneficence, and equity, which are well-accepted within the medical community and need no further introduction or theoretical foundation. This methodological approach is often referred to as clinical pragmatism,[5] although I will not refer to any specific author or theory that bears this label. Clinical pragmatism is a method rather than a theory, and I will use this method to analyze the ethical issues of mental healthcare for refugees bottom-up.

The ethical aspects of refugee mental healthcare are multifaceted and complex, encompassing different factors and issues. First, clinical factors have to be taken into consideration. Among migrants, a high prevalence of mental disorders has been noted, whereby affective disorders and trauma-related issues are especially prominent.[6] Another epidemiological issue is the high prevalence of vulnerable patients, first and foremost minors and women.[7] Furthermore, studies show that therapeutic measures are often ill suited or inappropriate because they do not apply to the individual patient's needs.

Second, cultural diversity is a main issue. Concepts of mental health and illness as well as the attitude towards mental health treatment often differ between different cultural backgrounds.[8] These aspects may lead to a reduced effectiveness of mental health treatment.

Third, questions of access to mental health services arise. The

---

[5] John D. Arras: Freestanding Pragmatism in Law and Bioethics. In: Theoretical Medicine and Bioethics 22 (2001), pp. 69–85.

[6] Satinsky et al.: Mental health care utilization (Note 3).

[7] Bajbouj et al.: Psychosoziale Versorgung von Flüchtlingen (Note 3); Frank Schneider, Malek Bajbouj, Andreas Heinz: Psychische Versorgung von Flüchtlingen in Deutschland. Modell für ein gestuftes Vorgehen. In: Der Nervenarzt 88 (2017), pp. 10–17.

[8] Lavan Kandiah: Refugee Mental Health – A Review of Literature on Treatment,

access to and the availability of mental health services is often insufficient or restricted by legal regulations. In addition, psychosocial and cultural factors as well as individual attitudes can create access barriers.

In the following, I will analyze these three topics from an ethical point of view. After the analysis follow recommendations for mental health practice.

## 2. Clinical factors

### *2.1 Prevalence of disorders*

The prevalence of mental disorders among migrants is noticeably high. Studies show that up to 40 % of migrants suffer from some kind of mental health issue, most frequently affective disorders like post-traumatic stress.[9] It is estimated that 80 % of refugees have been exposed to traumatic experiences.[10] Especially the accumulation of extreme stressors and adverse conditions affect refugees on the individual, family, and community level.[11] From an ethical perspective, the high prevalence of mental health issues among refugees calls for an easy accessible treatment. However, since the legal status of refugees often sets them apart from members of the host population, they are not considered as being entitled to the complete spectrum of mental health services.[12] That means that many mental health issues may remain untreated, thus creating a treatment gap. Furthermore, the high prevalence of mental health disorders may also be an obstacle for integration. Psychopathological symptoms may lead to an impair-

---

Practices and Recommendations. In: Journal of Ethics in Mental Health 10 (2018), pp. 1–19.

[9] Bajbouj et al.: Psychosoziale Versorgung von Flüchtlingen (Note 3).

[10] Ekaterini Georgiadou, Eva Morawa, Yesim Erim: High Manifestations of Mental Distress in Arabic Asylum Seekers Accommodated in Collective Centers for Refugees in Germany. In: International Journal of Environmental Research and Public Health 14 (2017), doi: 10.3390/ijerph14060612.

[11] Tobias Hecker, Frank Neuner: Mental Health Enables Integration: Re-thinking Treatment Approaches for Refugees. In: Krämer, Fischer: Refugee Migration and Health (Note 4), pp. 63–72.

[12] Sandra Kramer, Erik Olsman, Mariëtte H. H. Hoogsteder, Loes H. M. Van Willigen: Sleepless Nights because of Ethical Dilemmas in Mental Health Care for Asylum Seekers. In: Journal of Refugee Studies 31 (2017), pp. 466–487.

ment of psychosocial functioning, thus influencing the ability to cope with the tasks of everyday life.[13] This may lead to a reduced ability to take part in crucial activities such as language courses or administrative procedures. Thus, families and whole community can be affected by an individual's impaired functioning due to mental health issues.

### 2.2 *Vulnerable groups*

Vulnerable groups within the refugee population are especially women and minors, with the latter making up about half of the refugee population worldwide.[14] Women and minors are vulnerable for two reasons:[15] First, since they mostly come from male-dominated societies, the lack of male company means a security risk. Second, women and minors are more likely to become victims of violence or other forms of traumatization. As a result, it has been noted that female refugees are more frequently affected by mental health issues.[16] When it comes to minors, traumatizing experiences can cause severe mental as well as physical changes and affect their mental development, especially when experienced over a longer period.[17] Especially unguarded minors are at risk of being affected by trauma or other causes for mental disorders.[18] As a positive aspect, it has been noted that refugee youth show resources that may be used for their own benefit, namely high resilience and community support.[19] As with refugees in general, these vulnerable groups do not always receive the treatment they need. Especially when it comes to minors, considerable discrepancies between various European countries in terms of

---

[13] Hecker, Neuner: Mental Health Enables Integration (Note 11).

[14] UNHCR: Global Trends (Note 1).

[15] Schneider, Bajbouj, Heinz: Psychische Versorgung von Flüchtlingen (Note 7).

[16] Matthew Hodes, Melisa Mendoza Vasquez, Dimitris Anagnostopoulos, Kalliopi Triantafyllou, Dalia Abdelhady, Karin Weiss, Roman Koposov, Fusun Cuhadaroglu, Johannes Hebebrand, Norbert Skokauskas: Refugees in Europe: national overviews from key countries with a special focus on child and adolescent mental health. In: European Child & Adolescent Psychiatry 27 (2018), pp. 389–399.

[17] Schneider, Bajbouj, Heinz: Psychische Versorgung von Flüchtlingen (Note 7).

[18] Bajbouj et al.: Psychosoziale Versorgung von Flüchtlingen (Note 3).

[19] E. Anne Marshall, Deborah L. Begoray: Mental health literacy for refugee youth: A cultural approach. In: Orkan Okan, Ullrich Bauer, Diane Levin-Zamir, Paulo Pinheiro, Kristine Sørensen (Eds.): International Handbook of Health Literacy. Research, Practice and Policy across the Life-Span. Bristol 2019, pp. 261–274.

providing mental health services have been noted.[20] This is mostly due to the varying restrictiveness of national migration policies which also affects the accessibility and provision of mental health services for minors.

## 2.3 *Therapeutic factors*

Empirical evidence shows that there is a strong focus on pre-migration stressors in the treatment of refugees.[21] Pre-migration stressors are mainly combat, discrimination and prosecution due to ethnicity, gender, or political reasons, forced relocation, imprisonment, loss of family members, and torture. Also, the flight experience itself can be regarded as a major stressor.[22] This entails the hardship and dangers of the flight as well as the constant fear of being discovered and sent back. Therefore, the migration process itself with its hardships and dangers as well as stress can be seen as a straining experience. Furthermore, the flight is often a matter of human trafficking, which in many cases also means forced labor or sexual exploitation. The intensity of these experiences contributes to the view that therapy should aim for pre- and peri-migration stressors. Although these stressors are important for the treatment process, studies suggest that post-migration stressors linked to socioeconomic and socio-political factors might have a more severe impact.[23] Post-migration stressors entail denied or restricted access to health services, difficulties in acculturation, housing, learning a new language, long-term effects related to post-traumatic experiences, social isolation and loss of community, and unemployment.[24] Furthermore, cultural and language barriers as well as visible indicators of belonging to a minority group

---

[20] Hodes et al.: Refugees in Europe (Note 16).

[21] Kandiah: Refugee Mental Health (Note 8).

[22] Johannes Hebebrand, Dimitris Anagnostopoulos, Stephan Eliez, Henk Linse, Milica Pejovic-Milovancevic, Henrikje Klasen: A first assessment of the needs of young refugees arriving in Europe: what mental health professionals need to know. In: European Child and Adolescent Psychiatry 25 (2016), pp. 1–6.

[23] Poppy James, Aarti Iyer, Thomas L. Webb: The impact of post-migration stressors on refugees' emotional distress and health: A longitudinal analysis. In: European Journal of Social Psychology 2019, doi.org/10.1002/ejsp.2589; Kandiah: Refugee Mental Health (Note 8).

[24] Kandiah: Refugee Mental Health (Note 8).

like skin color can lead to stigma and social isolation.[25] The emotional distress caused by these factors can lead to anxiety and depression or aggravate already existing mental health issues. It is important to note that since the therapeutic focus is on pre- and peri-migration stressors, the clinical view often differs from the patient's view: Refugees often consider present factors such as problems with acculturation, financial security, or issues of identity as more stressful than their pre-migration or flight experiences.[26] From a clinical as well as from an ethical point of view, social support is a crucial aspect in this regard.[27] Social support means the availability of resources that are provided by a social network, i. e. family, friends, or other groups. The loss of these resources, which may be caused by the resettlement, can create feelings of stigma, vulnerability, and weakness, which often hold back persons from using mental healthcare services. Thus, an approach that strengthens social support can be beneficial for the patient from a clinical as well as an ethical perspective. Not only can such an approach lead to symptom reduction, but also strengthen the patient's sense of agency, thus empowering their autonomy. At the moment, the state of the art is the matched care approach, which implies the provision of mental health services depending on the location where the patient requests a service, the available resources, and the preferences of the patient.[28] This approach is less effective when it comes to using resources and sees refugees primarily as people in need without the capability for self-help. The alternative is the so-called stepped-and-collaborative-care-Modell (SCCM).[29] Following this approach, mental health professionals should start with interventions that use resources, which are readily available, and only if this proves insufficient, use more resource-intensive interventions. The crucial aspect is to activate available resources and focus on the agency and collaboration of refugees instead of treating them as needful victims.[30] Since these people survived their ordeal and showed a great measure of resilience, it is much more appropriate to build upon

25 James, Iyer, Webb: The impact (Note 23).
26 Kandiah: Refugee Mental Health (Note 8).
27 James, Iyer, Webb: The impact (Note 23).
28 Schneider, Bajbouj, Heinz: Psychische Versorgung von Flüchtlingen (Note 7).
29 Schneider, Bajbouj, Heinz: Psychische Versorgung von Flüchtlingen (Note 7).
30 Bajbouj et al.: Psychosoziale Versorgung von Flüchtlingen (Note 3); Kandiah: Refugee Mental Health (Note 8).

their strengths and resources.[31] Refugees as cultural mediators within mental health services could mitigate the stress of acculturation, make structures of mental healthcare more accessible to others, and thus facilitate faster integration. This approach requests preventive measures, early diagnosis, and easy accessibility as well as culturally sensitive interventions.[32] These elements may best be provided in a community setting. This means that the family or broader community looks out for signs like violent behavior or alcoholism. Religion can also be seen as a crucial factor. Often spiritual guidance is a resource provided within the community that can be used for facilitating better access to mental health services.[33]

## 3. Cultural Diversity

### *3.1. Concepts of mental health and illness*

Refugees bring with them different experiences, but also different perspectives, priorities, and values.[34] One of the main challenges in mental healthcare for refugees is the so-called cultural gap. This term refers to the mismatch between western models of mental health as well as treatment and cultural conceptions the refugees bring with them.[35] On the one hand, concepts of illness, e.g. trauma and depression, may not be familiar among refugee groups. On the other hand, refugees may present with symptoms or types of distress that are unknown among Western practitioners. These phenomena, hitherto known as culture-bound syndromes, have been recently relabeled as cultural concepts of distress, which signifies a more inclusive and less static view of cultural factors.[36] One example for such a concept is *buufis,* a term used by Somali refugees to describe a certain feeling of distress that derives from an obsession with the desire to leave

---

31 Kandiah: Refugee Mental Health (Note 8).

32 Schneider, Bajbouj, Heinz: Psychische Versorgung von Flüchtlingen (Note 7).

33 Kandiah: Refugee Mental Health (Note 8).

34 Kandiah: Refugee Mental Health (Note 8).

35 Kandiah: Refugee Mental Health (Note 8).

36 Bonnie N. Kaiser, Lesley Jo Weaver: Culture-bound syndromes, idioms of distress, and cultural concepts of distress: New directions for an old concept in psychological anthropology. In: Transcultural Psychiatry 56 (2019), pp. 589–598.

one's home country due to dire living conditions.[37] *Buufis* could be interpreted as a form of anxiety, but more severe cases could also be understood as forms of paranoia. What this shows is that prefixed concepts of mental illness are in many cases not helpful when treating people with a different cultural background. Also, it is doubtful whether it would be possible to classify concepts of mental illness from different cultures in a way that for example the DSM works. This would assume that other concepts of illness are structured in the same way as in Western countries, defined by clear symptoms, and understood within the scientific, biomedical framework. A much more fruitful approach could be to take the individual patient's illness narratives into account. Important in this regard is the conceptualization of the individual patient's experience in terms of idioms of distress.[38] Patients use these idioms to express their individual feelings of distress and suffering apart from clear-cut classification of mental disorders. Individual illness narratives may help the patient to explain their situation as well as the practitioner to understand the patient's distress and treat them accordingly. That means that a patient-centered, narrative approach to treatment is crucial in order to bridge the cultural gap. This is also important from an ethical point of view, since listening to the patient's narrative strengthens their position within the therapeutic alliance and empowers agency on behalf of the patient.

### *3.2 Attitude towards mental health treatment*

The cultural gap can manifest in refugee's attitudes towards mental health practice. Stigma is a crucial factor here:[39] In some cultural contexts, mental health issues and treatment are often associated with weakness or low social status. A patient who undergoes mental health treatment is thus in risk of becoming a social pariah. Even opening to others about mental health issues may be a taboo.[40] As Zolezzi et al.[41]

---

[37] Hyojin Im, Aidan Ferguson, Margaret Hunter: Cultural translation of refugee trauma: Cultural idioms of distress among Somali refugees in displacement. In: Transcultural Psychiatry 54 (2017), pp. 626–652.

[38] Kaiser, Weaver: Culture-bound syndromes (Note 36).

[39] Kandiah: Refugee Mental Health (Note 8).

[40] Kandiah: Refugee Mental Health (Note 8).

[41] Monica Zolezzi, Maha Alamri, Shahd Shaar, Daniel Rainkie: Stigma associated

have shown for people in Arab countries or with Arab heritage, stigmatizing attitudes, action, and beliefs towards mental treatment are highly prevalent. Feelings of shame and fears of harming the family's reputation are among the main reasons that prevent these people from utilizing mental healthcare services. In many cases, faith healers or other forms of religious or spiritual guidance are preferred to mental health treatment. Another aspect is the sometimes different understanding of treatment in refugees. The Western model of individual treatment is often seen as inappropriate given the family- and community-focused background of many refugee groups.[42] This constitutes an ethical dilemma for practitioners trained in the Western model of mental healthcare, since patient autonomy is a key principle in this respect. According to the Western point of view, autonomy means the self-determined deliberation and decision of the individual. However, family and other forms of community may be essential to a patient's deliberation and decision-making process. Although this aspect constitutes a dilemma, it can also be seen as a resource: Family and community support, social connectivity, and collective group identity can be used as a framework for group, family, and community interventions.[43] Thus, a family- or community-based approach does not necessarily contradict patient autonomy, but can be seen as a form of empowerment, since it enables the patient to make use of their own resources.

### *3.3 Diversity as a challenge for practitioners*

The cultural gap opens mostly due to a lack of cultural competence as well as knowledge regarding cultural coping mechanisms on behalf of many mental healthcare professionals.[44] Meeting the needs of refugees implies possessing the skills to deal with the diversity of experiences and cultural backgrounds. Thus, the main challenge for practitioners faced with treating refugees is cultural competence, which

---

with mental illness and its treatment in the Arab culture: A systematic review. In: International Journal of Social Psychiatry 64 (2018), pp. 597–609.

[42] Fred Bemak, Rita Chi-Ying Chung: Refugee Trauma: Culturally Responsive Counseling Interventions. In: Journal of Counseling & Development 95 (2017), pp. 299–308.

[43] Bemak, Chung: Refugee Trauma (Note 42).

[44] Kandiah: Refugee Mental Health (Note 8).

may be understood in terms of awareness, sensitivity, and empathy for the patient's values and beliefs.[45] One could argue that these skills are crucial to any form of mental health practice. Yet, in the context of treating patients from a different cultural background, this competence needs refinement, since practitioners are often confronted with a set of values or beliefs they are not familiar with. It is highly questionable whether practitioners are adequately prepared for this task. Appropriate training in cultural sensitivity seems to be the exception, not the norm in the different European healthcare systems.[46]. This is not only an issue of mental health, but healthcare in general. As a result, patients may not receive treatment in a manner that is acceptable to them. Furthermore, this puts a certain pressure on practitioners, since they are confronted with a situation where their skills are insufficient to reach their patients.

Another challenge for practitioners arises from the very intention of treating their patients in a culturally sensitive way. Cultural sensitivity and awareness are important skills for practitioners, but overemphasizing the transcultural aspect of treating refugees might be a moral hazard:[47] Attaching a cultural or religious label to the individual patient entails the risk of reducing said patient to a certain role. When patients are mainly seen as »cultural strangers«,[48] they are in danger of being de-individualized by ascribing to them specific attitudes towards mental health treatment, specific concepts of mental health and illness, etc. On the one hand, this de-individualization of patients can be a threat to their autonomy. On the other hand, there is a risk that well-meaning practitioners could anticipate certain cultural factors in patients that are not necessarily given. As a result of what could be called cultural over-framing, patients may not get the treatment they really need due to presumed cultural characteristics.

Recently, new approaches have been developed in order to provide culturally sensitive mental healthcare without culturally overframing the treatment. Most notably is the attempt to develop a con-

---

[45] Jinger G. Hoop, Tony DiPasquale, Juan M. Hernandez, Laura Weiss Roberts: Ethics and Culture in Mental Health Care. In: Ethics and Behavior 18 (2008), pp. 353–372.
[46] Janne Sorensen, Marie Norredam, Jeanine Suurmond, Olivia Carter-Pokras, Manuel Garcia-Ramirez, Allan Krasnik: Need for ensuring cultural competence in medical programmes of European universities. In: BMC Medical Education 19 (2019), p. 21.
[47] Kramer et al.: Sleepless nights (Note 12).
[48] Kramer et al.: Sleepless nights (Note 12), p. 483.

cept of global mental health for research as well as clinical practice.[49] The aim is a mental health practice that integrates social and biomedical sciences, thus being able to provide mental healthcare services to patients regardless of their ethnic or social background. Global mental health can be seen as the most recent step in a development that has been going since the early 20$^{th}$ century[50]. At the beginning of this development stood the transcultural approach, according to which cultural factors like cultural identity, language, or religion are crucial to understanding behavior or suffering of individuals. Although the transcultural approach recognizes the need for integrating anthropological and sociological knowledge into psychological concepts, it has mainly been a theoretical approach. In order to make use of this theoretical knowledge for clinical practice, especially given the effects of globalization, the cultural competence approach was developed.[51] This included training of psychiatric residents in the sociocultural, ethnic, gender, spiritual, and other factors that shape the psychological development of a person. Although patients generally benefit from a treatment provided by a culturally competent practitioner, serval pitfalls of this approach have been noted. The focus on cultural competences tends to regard culture as static and essentialist, thus leading to a situation where patients are seen primarily as belonging to a certain group with specific, clear-cut characteristics. Global mental health aims at overcoming this static concept of culture and instead advocates a dynamic view that is sensitive to the individual experience.[52] Global mental health programs encourage residents to work with underserved populations outside of high-income countries. This clinical endeavor is based on bidirectionality, meaning a partnership for the mutual benefit for both sides. In the light of refugee mental healthcare, the paradigm of global mental health may be an opportunity to provide a more fitting treatment and to overcome the risk of cultural over-framing.

---

[49] Diana M. Robinson, Joseph Otonichar, Souraya Torbey, Maria Moreno, Richard L. Merkel: From Transcultural Psychiatry to Global Mental Health: The Development of a Global Mental Health Program at the Department of Psychiatry and Neurobehavioral Sciences at the University of Virginia. In: Sam Okpaku (Ed.): Innovations in Global Mental Health. Cham 2019, pp. 1–21.

[50] Robinson et al.: From Transcultural Psychiatry (Note 49).

[51] Robinson et al.: From Transcultural Psychiatry (Note 49).

[52] Robinson et al.: From Transcultural Psychiatry (Note 49).

## 4. Access to mental health services

Since mental disorders are prevalent among refugees and there is a high need for treatment, access is a crucial topic. From the perspective of ethics, matters of access are connected to the principles of beneficence and equity. Therefore, it has to be asked which factors constitute access barriers in this context. When it comes to access to mental health services, two groups of access barriers have to be distinguished. The first group consists of legal regulations and structural factors. One could consider these as hard barriers since they are difficult to overcome from the perspective of practitioners. Political decisions and legal subtleties are involved that go beyond the reach of practitioners. The second group consists of psychosocial, cultural, and individual factors. These could be seen as soft barriers since options to overcome them are available and have in certain cases already been implemented.

### *4.1 Hard access barriers: Legal regulations and structural factors*

Since regulations for accessing mental health services vary between European countries and can be complex even within one single country, this is not the place to discuss these regulations in detail. The example of Germany will suffice. According to the Asylum Seekers Benefits Act (*Asylbewerberleistungsgesetz*, AsylbLG), refugees and asylum seekers are entitled to limited healthcare services in the first 15 months after arrival.[53] Healthcare is provided to people with acute illness or pain and pregnant women. People with special needs, i.e. children, victims of torture and physical, psychological, or sexual violence, and people with disabilities are entitled to a broader range of services and to be given particular consideration. This is in accordance with the EU-Directive 2013/33/, which prohibits the limitation of healthcare services for vulnerable groups within the populations of refugees and asylum seekers.[54] The practical implementation of these

---

[53] Asylbewerberleistungsgesetz in der Fassung der Bekanntmachung vom 5. August 1997 (BGBl. I S. 2022), das zuletzt durch Artikel 4 des Gesetzes vom 17. Juli 2017 (BGBl. I S. 2541; 2019 I 162) geändert worden ist. Here: Art. 2; 4; 6. https://www.gesetze-im-internet.de/asylblg/BJNR107410993.html (accessed 9/24/2019).

[54] Directive 2013/33/Eu of The European Parliament and of The Council of 26 June 2013 laying down standards for the reception of applicants for international protec-

legal regulations differs within Germany:[55] In some Federal States, refugees receive a treatment voucher (*Behandlungsschein*) from a government agency, e.g. the social services department (*Sozialamt*) in case of acute illness. In other Federal States, refugees receive an electronic health care card (*Gesundheitskarte*) with which they can consult a physician directly. However, treatment for chronological illnesses, dental prosthetics, and psychotherapy are seldom granted.[56] Since in many cases, long-term interventions are needed that may take longer than 15 months, the need for mental health treatment often remains unmet. From an ethical perspective, this is a severe violation of patient well-being and the beneficence principle. It might be argued that especially persons with an unclear legal status cannot be entitled to healthcare services in the same way as persons who finance the insurance system. This would raise questions of justice and economic reasonableness. However, as we have seen, post-migration stressors can have an aggravating effect on symptoms of mental illness, thus also affecting the acculturation and integration process. In the long run, providing mental healthcare to a greater extend might thus be not only beneficial for the patient, but also contribute to a successful integration, which is in the interest of society as a whole.

When it comes to structural factors, there are several aspects to consider. First, many refugees do not have local access to mental health service, which makes transport to specific facilities necessary.[57] Transportation costs are often seen as a crucial issue in this respect. Second, the lack of interpreters and language services may in many cases prevent patients from being able to seek treatment.[58] The language barrier also poses the risk of misdiagnosis and mistreatment, resulting in negative long-term outcomes for the patient.[59] Third,

---

tion (recast). https://eur-lex.europa.eu/legal-content/EN/TXT/PDF/?uri=CELEX:32013L0033&from=DE (accessed 9/24/2019).

55 Federal Ministry for Health: Health Guide for asylum seekers in Germany. https://www.bundesgesundheitsministerium.de/fileadmin/Dateien/5_Publikationen/Gesundheit/Broschueren/Ratgeber_Asylsuchende_EN_web.pdf (accessed 9/24/2019).

56 Sabine Klotz: The right to health for all? Debates surrounding access to healthcare for asylum seekers in Germany. In: Katja Kuehlmeyer, Corinna Klingler, Richard Huxtable (Eds.): Ethical, Legal and Social Aspects of Healthcare for Migrants: Perspectives from the UK and Germany. Oxford 2019, pp. 125–144.

57 Satinsky et al.: Mental health care utilization (Note 3).

58 Satinsky et al.: Mental health care utilization (Note 3).

59 Deutsche Gesellschaft für Psychiatrie und Psychotherapie, Psychosomatik und

refugees are often unaware of available services or unsure where to seek support.[60] This lack of knowledge sometimes also extends to healthcare professionals and other staff members in refugee camps and similar facilities. As a consequence, a better communication strategy addressing both refugees and staff members is needed in order to provide information on the availability of services.

### 4.2 *Soft access barriers: Psychosocial, cultural, and individual factors*

Apart from the hard access barriers associated with legal regulations and structural factors, soft access barriers can be identified. As with mental healthcare in general, there exists a gap between availability and utilization of services in refugees. Although mental health needs are high in refugees, a recent meta-review by Satinsky et al.[61] shows that mental healthcare services in many European countries are under-utilized. The reasons are fear of stigma, the wish to seek help within the community first, and other factors related to different cultural attitudes toward mental health treatment that have already been discussed in section 3.2. As discussed before, measures can be implemented to overcome these barriers. These measures include a family- and community-centered approach as well as refugees as cultural mediators.

## 5. Conclusion and recommendations for mental health practice

The ethical analysis shows that several issues arise regarding refugees in need of mental health interventions. Overemphasizing pre- and peri-migration stressors may lead to an inappropriate treatment, thus threatening patient well-being and violating the beneficence principle. The same holds for the lack of cultural competence on behalf of

---

Nervenheilkunde (DGPPPN): Positionspapier: Psychosoziale Versorgung von Flüchtlingen verbessern (3/22/2016). https://www.dgppn.de/_Resources/Persistent/c03a6dbf7dcdb0a77dbdf4ed3e50981431abe372/2016_03_22_DGPPN-Positionspapier_psychosoziale%20Versorgung%20Fl%C3%BCchtlinge.pdf (accessed 9/24/2019).

[60] Satinsky et al.: Mental health care utilization (Note 3).

[61] Satinsky et al.: Mental health care utilization (Note 3).

practitioners as well as for hard and soft access barriers. The autonomy of patients may be violated by a cultural insensitive treatment that is unaware of specific values, beliefs, attitudes, and concepts of mental illness as well as its treatment. At the same time, overemphasizing the cultural background of patients may lead to a de-individualization, which also violates their autonomy. Several recommendations for mental health practice can be deduced from these results: Awareness of cultural differences and characteristics should follow the paradigm of global mental health, combining cultural sensitivity with a person-centered approach. Since many practitioners have not or only insufficiently been trained in global mental health, these trainings should be provided. Another important aspect is the empowerment of agency on behalf of refugees. Practitioners should be encouraged to use community-based approaches that activate available resources and focus on agency instead of victimization. One example is the already mentioned SCCM, which aims at linking different service providers, empowers patient autonomy and participation, emphasizes patient information, and integrates peer-to-peer counsellors. The focus is on refugees' resources for participating in creating structures of mutual aid. As cultural mediators, refugees can engage in projects for helping each other, use their intrinsic cultural knowledge, their knowledge of specific concepts of illness, and their language skills as resources. Thus, agency and autonomy can be empowered by a therapeutic approach that focusses on social support. Finally, practitioners could actively take part in policy-making by informing the public on mental health issues in refugees and using their expert knowledge to help modify existing regulations and structures for the benefit of their patients.

*Vera Vogel*

# Healthcare for refugees suffering from psychiatric disorders: an overview of the current care provision in Germany

Abstract
Over the past decade, more than two million refugees have resettled in Germany. Approximately 40 % of them fulfill the criteria of post-traumatic stress disorder (PTSD). This article endeavors to analyze the current situation in Germany by providing an overview of existing services in the field of mental health care for refugees, as well as highlighting some of the main weaknesses challenging the health care system. Focusing on the need for psychosocial and medical support for refugees, the current mental health care system is described according to the following four criteria: accessibility, availability, affordability, and acceptability. Furthermore, attention is paid to the trauma-related mental disorders that most commonly affect refugees, pointing out some of the most significant difficulties in the process of diagnosis, therapy and prevalence rate estimation. The cultural-sensitive approach of modern transcultural psychiatry is shown to be essential for the effective treatment of refugees suffering from mental illness.

## 1. Introduction

Over the past decade more than two million refugees have resettled in Germany.[1] Generally speaking, refugees are individuals who have fled their home countries due to natural disasters, war, or for fear of persecution for political, religious, or personal beliefs.[2] Between 30 and 50 % of them report having undergone traumatic experiences like war, torture, physical or sexual abuse.[3] As a consequence, asylum-

[1] Bundesamt für Migration und Flüchtlinge: Aktuelle Zahlen zu Asyl. http://www.bamf.de/DE/Infothek/Statistiken/Asylzahlen/AktuelleZahlen/aktuelle-zahlen-asyl-node.html (accessed 9/24/2019).

[2] Kelly Polcher, Susan Calloway: Addressing the Need for Mental Health Screening of Newly Resettled Refugees: A Pilot Project. In: Journal of Primary Care & Community Health 7 (2016), pp. 199–203.

[3] Patricia J. Shannon, Gregory A. Vinson, Tonya L. Cook, Evelyn Lennon: Character-

seekers are at risk of developing a range of trauma-related psychiatric disorders such as posttraumatic stress disorder (PTSD), major depression, anxiety disorders and drug or alcohol addiction.[4]Although the estimated prevalence rates vary considerably between different studies and populations, approximately 40 % of the refugees resettled to Germany fulfill the criteria for PTSD.[5] This fact presents a serious challenge for the country's public health system. Although research suggests that improvement in medical health care for asylum-seekers is needed,[6] there are few superregional studies with high caseloads that could help to quantify these needs in order to develop focused strategies.[7]

This article endeavors to analyze the current situation in Germany by providing an overview of existing provision and services in the field of mental health care and support for refugees, as well as highlighting some of the main weaknesses challenging the health care system.

In order to do so, I will first focus on trauma-related mental disorders that commonly affect refugees, pointing out some of the most significant difficulties in the process of diagnosis, therapy and prevalence rate estimation. Furthermore, I consider it important to provide a brief overview of the field of transcultural psychiatry, since its cultural-sensitive approach is nowadays considered essential for the effective treatment of refugees suffering from mental illness. Finally, I will turn to the need for psychosocial and medical support for refugees and describe the current mental health care system using the following four criteria: accessibility, availability, affordability, and acceptability.[8]

---

istics of Successful and Unsuccessful Mental Health Referrals of Refugees. In: Administration and Policy in Mental Health and Mental Health Services Research 43 (2016), pp. 555–568.

[4] Shannon et al.: Characteristics of Successful (Note 3), p. 556.

[5] Ulrike Gäbel, Martina Ruf, Maggie Schauer, Michael Odenwald, Frank Neuner: Prävalenz der Posttraumatischen Belastungsstörung (PTSD) und Möglichkeiten der Ermittlung in der Asylverfahrenspraxis. In: Zeitschrift für Klinische Psychologie und Psychotherapie 35 (2005), pp. 12–20.

[6] Laura Frank, Rahsan Yesil-Jürgens, Oliver Razum, Kayvan Bozorgmehr, Liane Schenk, Andreas Gilsdorf, Alexander Rommel, Thomas Lampert: Gesundheit und gesundheitliche Versorgung von Asylsuchenden und Flüchtlingen in Deutschland. In: Journal of Health Monitoring 2 (2017), pp. 24–47.

[7] Frank et al.: Gesundheit und gesundheitliche Versorgung (Note 6), p. 35.

[8] Jean Edward, Vicki Hines-Martin: Exploring the Providers Perspective of Health

## 2. Trauma-related disorders: prevalence, symptoms and diagnostic criteria

The definition of the term »trauma« has presented a major challenge to modern psychiatry and has undergone considerable changes since its introduction to the psychiatric classification systems (DSM; American Psychiatric Association and ICD; World Health Organization) in 1980.[9] Whether trauma witnessed only through media exposure, for instance, or an indirect trauma experience can be considered a qualifying experience has been repeatedly discussed over the past 35 years and has led to significant changes in the definition of PTSD.[10] Moreover, the co-existence of two main classification systems, the Diagnostic and Statistical Manual of Mental Disorders (DSM) and the International Classification of Diseases (ICD), makes it difficult to compare prevalence rates and the trauma definition itself on an international scale.[11]

The modern definition of trauma distinguishes between type I and type II trauma. Type I trauma is defined as a unique, time-limited event such as an accident or a natural disaster. Type II trauma, on the contrary, refers to recurrent, prolonged and unpredictable traumatic experiences.[12] A further differentiation is made between so-called »man-made disasters«, such as experiencing violence, torture or sexual abuse, and natural catastrophes. Research indicates that man-made disasters (especially torture and cumulative exposure to trauma) are more likely to affect the human psyche thereby causing trauma-related disorders.[13]

For many years, trauma-related disorders were classified as a subgroup of anxiety disorders. Only in the latest version of the

---

and Social Service Availability for Immigrants and Refugees in a Southern Urban Community. In: Journal of Immigrant and Minority Health 17 (2015), pp. 1185–1191.

9 Carol S. North, Alina M. Surís, Rebecca P. Smith, Richard V. King: The evolution of PTSD criteria across editions of DSM. In: Annals of Clinical Psychiatry 28 (2016), pp. 197–208.

10 North et al.: The evolution of PTSD (Note 9), p. 205.

11 North et al.: The evolution of PTSD (Note 9), p. 205.

12 Esther Kleefeldt, Barbara Wolff, Lotta de Carlo: Flüchtlinge in unserer Praxis. Informationen für ÄrztInnen und PsychotherapeutInnen. Bundesweite Arbeitsgemeinschaft der Psychosozialen Zentren für Flüchtlinge und Folteropfer (BAfF e. V.). Berlin 2016.

13 Kleefeldt, Wolff, de Carlo: Flüchtlinge in unserer Praxis (Note 12), pp. 21–22; Shannon et al.: Characteristics of Successful (Note 3), p. 556.

DSM (DSM V, 2013) was an individual section named »Trauma- and Stressor-Related Disorders« introduced, followed by a profound revision of the PTSD criteria.[14] Here trauma is defined as an »event involving actual or threatened death, serious injury, or sexual violence«,[15] differentiating four main exposure types: direct exposure, witnessed exposure, indirect exposure through others (family members or close friends), and repeated or extreme exposure to aversive episodes of trauma, e.g. exposure through electronic media, television, movies, or pictures (only if work related).[16] In DSM V, besides criterion A (the »stressor criterion«, corresponding to the traumatic event itself), PTSD includes a total number of 20 symptoms, classified in four groups: criterion B (intrusion, e.g. re-experiencing the event in the form of nightmares), C (avoidance of distressing memories of the event), D (alterations in cognition and mood), E (alterations in arousal and reactivity, like aggression or self-destructive behavior, insomnia or hypervigilance).[17] According to the time-criterion F, the symptoms start within 3 months of the traumatic event and last more than a month. DSM V further added a dissociative specifier (depersonalization, derealisation) and antisocial features, e.g. reckless or self-destructive behavior, to group E symptoms.[18] Although the total number of symptoms increased from 12 (DSM III) to 20 (DSM V),[19] the definition of the traumatic event itself, being defined precisely as a physical threat or injury, has become stricter, compared to DSM IV.[20]

A revision of the ICD-classification is pending and the new version is expected to be introduced in January 2022.[21] While the ICD-10, which is currently used in Germany, takes a rather broad diagnostic approach, the ICD-11 proposes to remove unspecific symptoms in

---

14 DSM V, 2013, quoted from: North et al.: The evolution of PTSD (Note 9), p. 198.

15 DSM V, 2013, quoted from: North et al.: The evolution of PTSD (Note 9), p. 201.

16 DSM V, 2013, quoted from: North et al.: The evolution of PTSD (Note 9), p. 201.

17 Rikinkumar S. Patel, Geetha Manikkara, Priya Patel, Jupi Talukdar, Zeeshan Mansur: Importance of Behavioral Therapy in Patients Hospitalized for Post-Traumatic Stress Disorder (PTSD) with Opioid Use Disorder. In: Behavioral Sciences 8 (2018), doi:10.3390/bs8080073.

18 North et al.: The evolution of PTSD (Note 9), pp. 200–203.

19 North et al.: The evolution of PTSD (Note 9), p. 200.

20 North et al.: The evolution of PTSD (Note 9), p. 207.

21 Deutsches Institut für Medizinische Dokumentation und Information: ICD-11. Revision der ICD der WHO. https://www.dimdi.de/dynamic/de/klassifikationen/icd/icd-11/ (accessed 9/24/2019).

order to increase the specificity of the diagnosis.[22] In addition, the proposed ICD-11 template differentiates between a simple and a complex form of PTSD, the latter characterized by more complex and persistent symptomatology with disorders of affect regulation, changes in sexual behavior, dissociative symptoms and persistent changes in personality.[23] The criteria of the currently valid ICD-10 for PTSD are the exposure to an exceptionally threatening event of a catastrophic nature and the symptom triad »intrusive trauma-related imagery or nightmares«, »avoidance of situations that remind them of the trauma«, and either »partial amnesia of the trauma« or »prolonged hypervigilance that causes irritability or frequent outbursts of anger, concentration problems, sleeping problems and/or an exaggerated startle response« (F43.1, ICD-10).[24] The symptoms should begin within six months from the traumatic event and last more than four weeks.

Even if the same diagnostic system is used, estimated prevalence rates vary considerably according to different studies (6.7–76.7 %).[25] Several reasons can be mentioned to explain this phenomenon. On the one hand, case numbers and composition of the samples may be important influencing patterns. On the other, heterogeneity of cultures and countries of origin as well as inconsistency of testing methods also influence the level of PTSD diagnostic identification.[26]

Although PTSD is the most frequent psychiatric disorder among refugees (its prevalence being over ten times higher compared to the

---

[22] Anna C. Barbano, Willem F. van der Mei, Richard A. Bryant, Douglas L. Delahanty, Terri A. deRoon-Cassini, Yutaka J. Matsuoka, Miranda Olff, Wei Qi, Andrew Ratanatharathorn, Ulrich Schnyder, Soraya Seedat, Ronald C. Kessler, Karestan C. Koenen, Arieh Y. Shalev: Clinical implications of the proposed ICD-11 PTSD diagnostic criteria. In: Psychological Medicine 49 (2018), pp. 483–490.

[23] Anna C. Barbano, Willem F. van der Mei, Terri A. deRoon-Cassini, Ettie Grauer, Sarah Ryan Lowe, Yutaka J. Matsuoka, Meaghan O'Donnell, Miranda Olff, Wei Qi, Andrew Ratanatharathorn, Ulrich Schnyder, Soraya Seedat, Ronald C. Kessler, Karestan C. Koenen, Arieh Y. Shalev: Differentiating PTSD from anxiety and depression: Lessons from the ICD-11 PTSD diagnostic criteria. In: Depression and Anxiety 36 (2019), doi: 10.1002/da.22881.

[24] Bolette Daniels Beck, Steen T. Lund, Ulf Søgaard, Erik Simonsen, Thomas C. Tellier, Torben O. Cordtz, Gunnar H. Laier, Torben Moe: Music therapy versus treatment as usual for refugees diagnosed with posttraumatic stress disorder (PTSD): study protocol for a randomized controlled trial. In: Trials 19 (2018), doi: 10.1186/s13063–018–2662-z.

[25] Frank et al.: Gesundheit und gesundheitliche Versorgung (Note 6), p. 35.

[26] Frank et al.: Gesundheit und gesundheitliche Versorgung (Note 6), p. 35.

general population, which in Germany is 1.5–3.5 %),[27] there are other trauma-related disorders, which show high prevalence rates and a high co-occurrence with PTSD.[28] According to a German study, 87.5 % of the refugees affected by PTSD suffer from at least another psychiatric disease, 77.5 % from two or more.[29] Meta-analyses showed prevalence rates of 20–88 % for anxiety disorders and 2–80 % for major depression among refugees.[30] Several studies have also shown a strong relationship between PTSD and substance abuse, especially alcohol and opioids.[31] A possible explanation for opioid abuse might be relief from anxiety and the urge to escape re-experiencing a traumatic event.[32] Similar mechanisms may also explain the high rate of alcoholism among patients suffering from PTSD. According to a recent Swiss study, exposure to potentially traumatic events and chronic stressors are strongly linked to mental health disorders, such as PTSD and depression.[33] In fact, the proportional incidence of acute or mixed-alcohol intoxication among asylum seekers in Swiss emergency departments was 3.7 % compared to 1.6 % among the Swiss-national patients and was associated with a younger age and the male gender. Not surprisingly, the primary complaints among asylum-seeking patients with alcohol-related issues were trauma and psychiatric distress.[34] As Brown claims, »alcohol-related illness among displaced persons and asylum seekers is noticeably understudied by the healthcare community«, which, according to the author, »represents a major gap in our understanding of the health care needs of a highly vulnerable population«.[35]

---

[27] Andreas Maercker, Simon Forstmeier, Birgit Wagner, Heide Glaesmer, Elmar Brähler: Posttraumatische Belastungsstörung in Deutschland. In: Der Nervenarzt 79 (2008), pp. 577–586.

[28] Kleefeldt, Wolff, de Carlo: Flüchtlinge in unserer Praxis (Note 12), p. 25.

[29] Axel Perkonigg, Ronald C. Kessler, Stephanie Storz, Hans-Ulrich Wittchen: Traumatic events and post-traumatic stress disorder in the community: prevalence, risk factors and comorbidity. In: ActaPsychiatrica Scandinavica 101 (2000), pp. 46–59; quoted from Kleefeldt, Wolff, de Carlo: Flüchtlinge in unserer Praxis (Note 12), p. 31.

[30] Daniels Beck et al.: Music therapy versus treatment (Note 24), p. 301.

[31] Patel et al.: Importance of Behavioral (Note 17), p. 73.

[32] Patel et al.: Importance of Behavioral (Note 17), p. 73.

[33] Adam D. Brown, Martin Müller, Trevor Hirschi, Jonathan F. Henssler, Katharina Rönz, Aristomenis K. Exadaktylos, David Srivastava: Acute and mixed alcohol intoxications in asylum seekers presenting to an urban emergency department in Switzerland. In: BMC Public Health 19 (2019), doi: 10.1186/s13063–018–2662-z.

[34] Brown et al.: Acute and mixed (Note 33), p. 536.

[35] Brown et al.: Acute and mixed (Note 33), p. 536.

In addition, it has been suggested that PTSD increases the risk of physical illness, especially for cardiovascular diseases such as strokes or myocardial infarction.[36] A Danish study has proved that refugees have a significantly higher risk for the above-mentioned diseases, independently of other risk factors such as smoking or alcohol abuse.[37] Moreover, studies with American Indian and Alaskan Native (AIAN) populations showed a high co-occurrence of PTSD with psychiatric conditions such as anxiety and depression, as well as physical diseases such as diabetes, cardiovascular disease, and pain reactions.[38] Finally, co-occurrence has also been found between PTSD and immunological diseases, such as arthritis, asthma and eczemas, as well as chronic obstructive pulmonary disease (COPD) and rheumatoid diseases.[39] Also of considerable importance is the high association between trauma and suicide risk. Suicidal tendencies have been associated with traumatic events such as war, sexual abuse and natural disasters, among others.[40] Studies have reported suicide-risk rates as high as 10.2 % among refugees.[41]

In summary, besides the inconsistency of diagnostic systems, post-traumatic stress disorder describes a syndrome characterized by a temporal and conceptual link to a traumatic event as well as a large number of specific (e. g. flashbacks, nightmares, avoidance of triggering factors) and unspecific (e. g. hyperarousal, insomnia, difficulties in concentration) symptoms, which deeply affect the daily life of those suffering from it.[42] Furthermore, research has shown that traumatic experiences can be passed on to subsequent generations not only through religious and spiritual beliefs and practices but also biologically through changes to the DNA.[43] The science of epigenetics inves-

---

[36] Kleefeldt, Wolff, de Carlo: Flüchtlinge in unserer Praxis (Note 12), p. 31.

[37] Kleefeldt, Wolff, de Carlo: Flüchtlinge in unserer Praxis (Note 12), p. 31.

[38] Karina L. Walters, Jane M. Simoni: Reconceptualizing Native Women's Health: An »Indigenist« Stress-Coping Model. In: American Journal of Public Health 92 (2002), pp. 520–524.

[39] Kleefeldt, Wolff, de Carlo: Flüchtlinge in unserer Praxis (Note 12), p. 31.

[40] Jelena Jankovic, Stephen Bremner, Marija Bogic, Dusica Lecic-Tosevski, Dean Ajdukovic, Tanja Franciskovic, Gian Maria Galeazzi, Abdulah Kucukalic, Nexhmedin Morina, Mijailo Popovski, Matthias Schützwohl, Stefan Priebe: Trauma and suicidality in war affected communities. In: European Psychiatry 28 (2012), pp. 514–519, here p. 519.

[41] Jankovic et al.: Trauma and suicidality (Note 40), p. 516.

[42] North et al.: The evolution of PTSD (Note 9), pp. 201–202.

[43] Ann Pederson, Erin Nuetzman, Jennifer Gubbels, Leonard Hummel: Remembrance

tigates the heritability of trauma by examining the expression or suppression of genes based on environmental exposure. It has proved that epigenetic processes such as DNA-methylation, histone modifications or chromatin remodeling can affect physical and mental health and be transmitted to succeeding generations.[44]

## 3. Transcultural Psychiatry: a cultural-sensitive approach to psychiatric disorders

Establishing a culturally-responsive approach to the treatment of mental disorders is the declared aim of modern transcultural psychiatry. This sector of mental healthcare (also called intercultural or cross-cultural psychiatry) arose at the end of the nineteenth century as cooperation between psychiatry and ethnology[45], encompassing changing notions of culture, race and psychiatry over time.[46]

Some researchers consider Emil Kraepelin (1856–1926) to be the »founder« of transcultural psychiatry.[47] During his travels to northern Africa, North and Central America and above all to South Asia, he carried out comparative research on the symptomatology and epidemiology of psychiatric diseases in non-western populations; giving birth to a discipline he called »vergleichende Psychiatrie«.[48] Nevertheless, transcultural psychiatry was created as a distinct discipline only after World War II.[49] Dissociating explicitly from previous racist psychologies,[50] it addressed the question of whether psychiatric disorders can be considered universal conditions rather than cultural

---

and Resilience: How the Bodyself responds to Trauma. In: Zygon 53 (2018), pp. 1018–1035.

[44] Pederson et al.: How the Bodyself (Note 43), p. 1018.

[45] Emmanuel Delille, Ivan Crozier: Historicizing transcultural psychiatry: people, epistemic objects, networks, and practices. In: History of Psychiatry 29 (2018), pp. 257–262.

[46] Jatinder Bains: Race, culture and psychiatry: a history of transcultural psychiatry. In: History of Psychiatry 16 (2005), pp. 139–154.

[47] Holger Steinberg: Emil Kraepelin's ideas on transcultural psychiatry. In: Australasian Psychiatry 23 (2015), pp. 531–535.

[48] Delille, Crozier: Historicizing transcultural psychiatry (Note 45), p. 257; Steinberg: Emil Kraepelin's ideas (Note 47), pp. 531–532.

[49] Bains: Race, culture and psychiatry (Note 46), p. 139.

[50] Delille, Crozier: Historicizing transcultural psychiatry (Note 45), p. 258.

phenomena.[51] In the 1970s transcultural psychiatry moved from the US to Europe and Transcultural Psychiatry Societies were established in England, France and Italy.[52] Consequently its aims shifted from the earlier theoretic focus towards a multiracial, multidisciplinary and multicultural discipline, which promoted equality of mental health independently of gender, race or culture, especially in areas with high rates of ethnic minorities.[53] In Germany, the Confederation of Transcultural Psychiatry, Psychotherapy and Psychosomatics (Dachverband der transkulturellen Psychiatrie, Psychotherapie und Psychosomatik, DTPPP) was founded in 2008 to coordinate the activities of the transcultural health providers of the country. Considering the enormous influx of refugees and the high prevalence of psychiatric disorders among asylum-seekers, transcultural psychiatry has become a major field of investigation, as demonstrated by the numerous publications in physical and psychiatric medicine of the past few decades.

Turning to the actual treatment of trauma-related disorders, therapy is currently based on two approaches, psychotherapy and pharmacotherapy, the latter being considered efficient only if applied jointly with the former.[54] Psychotropic drugs are used mainly to treat insomnia and depression. Statistical evidence is available for selective serotonin reuptake inhibitors (SSRI) such as Paroxetine and Sertraline and the serotonin–norepinephrine reuptake inhibitor (SNRI) Venlafaxine.[55] Caution should be exercised when prescribing antidepressants as they may increase the risk of suicide or worsen previously existing sleep disturbance, inner unrest or limited impulse control.[56] In cases of strong restlessness and insomnia, Mirtazapine or tricyclic antidepressants such as Amitriptyline or Doxepine can be used. Strong states of anxiety may require the use of neuroleptics with a sedative effect like Promethazine, Risperidone or Quetiapine.[57] When working with refugees suffering from trauma-related disor-

---

[51] Bains: Race, culture and psychiatry (Note 46), p. 145.

[52] Bains: Race, culture and psychiatry (Note 46), p. 148.

[53] Bains: Race, culture and psychiatry (Note 46), p. 149.

[54] Kleefeldt, Wolff, de Carlo: Flüchtlinge in unserer Praxis (Note 12), p. 40.

[55] Guido Flatten, Ursula Gast, Arne Hofmann, Christine Knaevelsrud, Astrid Lampe, Peter Liebermann, Andreas Maercker, Luise Reddemann, Wolfgang Wöller: S3-Leitlinie Posttraumatische Belastungsstörung. ICD-10: F43.1. In: Trauma & Gewalt 3 (2011), pp. 202–210, here p. 206.

[56] Kleefeldt, Wolff, de Carlo: Flüchtlinge in unserer Praxis (Note 12), p. 41.

[57] Kleefeldt, Wolff, de Carlo: Flüchtlinge in unserer Praxis (Note 12), p. 42.

ders, experts recommend a multi-modal interpreter-mediated concept, which implies psychotherapy in combination with social and medical assistance,[58] as well as other therapeutic approaches such as occupational, music or art therapy.[59] Statistical evidence has proved the beneficial effects of several psychotherapeutic methods, especially cognitive behavioral therapy, narrative exposure therapy and testimony therapy.[60] The understanding of psychiatric conditions in other cultures may vary greatly from western ideals and this must be taken into consideration during treatment. Due to mental health stigma and lack of information, patients often do not see psychiatric conditions as a consequence of trauma and are therefore reluctant to disclose important aspects of their symptomatology.[61] Three main types of barriers should be taken into consideration: language barriers (due to different mother tongues as well as trauma-related symptoms such as avoidance), acculturation barriers, which include divergent cultural beliefs about psychiatric disorders and their treatment, and emotional barriers (feelings of guilt or shame, trauma-related relationship disorders, difficulties in establishing trust).[62] The aim of psychotherapy is not to erase the traumatic experience, but rather to allow a coherent and chronological integration of the events and the feelings connected with it. Patients should learn to control involuntary memories and trigger factors so that trauma can become an integrated part of their personal biography.[63] According to the S3 guideline for PTBS, trauma-therapy should therefore consist of three phases: examination of mental stability (and stabilization if needed), trauma processing, and psychosocial re-integration.[64]

---

[58] Kleefeldt, Wolff, de Carlo: Flüchtlinge in unserer Praxis (Note 12), p. 40.

[59] Flatten et al.: S3-Leitlinie (Note 55), p. 206.

[60] Colleen A. McFarlane, Ida Kaplan: Evidence-based psychological interventions for adult survivors of torture and trauma: a 30-year review. In: Transcultural psychiatry 49 (2012), pp. 539–567, here pp. 540, 552 and 556.

[61] Shannon et al.: Characteristics of Successful (Note 3), p. 556; Fabiana Kotovicz, Anne Getzin, Thy Vo: Challenges of Refugee Health Care: Perspectives of Medical Interpreters, Case Managers, and Pharmacists. In: Journal of Patient-Centered Research and Reviews 5 (2018), pp. 28–35.

[62] Kleefeldt, Wolff, de Carlo: Flüchtlinge in unserer Praxis (Note 12), p. 15.

[63] Kleefeldt, Wolff, de Carlo: Flüchtlinge in unserer Praxis (Note 12), p. 39.

[64] Kleefeldt, Wolff, de Carlo: Flüchtlinge in unserer Praxis (Note 12), p. 39.

## 4. Analysis of the current care provision in Germany

Over the past ten years 2.233.096 applications for asylum were submitted to the Federal Office for Migration and Refugees (Bundesamt für Migration und Flüchtlinge), 51.370 initial applications have been submitted in the current year 2019, with the largest groups fleeing from Syria, Iraq, and Nigeria.[65]

In what follows, we will explore the current situation of mental health care for refugees in Germany in more detail. In order to do so, we will analyze the system according to the 4 criteria of accessibility, affordability, availability and acceptability, as described by Edwards.[66] These criteria were first applied in primary health care but can easily be transferred to mental health providers. The two criteria accessibility and affordability will be used to describe the overall legal and environmental conditions of mental health care supply such as availability of services, reachability, and cost assumption, whereas availability and acceptability target the quality of the services provided regarding the special needs of refugees and the aspect of cultural sensitivity.

### *4.1 Accessibility and Affordability of health and social services for refugees*

The first question I will address concerns the extent to which refugees are able to access mental health services. Accessibility and affordability of mental health providers not only depend on the availability of services, but also on statutory conditions, transportation, language services, etc.[67] Concerning affordability, healthcare of asylum-seekers is covered by the Asylum Procedure Act (Asylverfahrensgesetz, AsylVfG), the Residence Act (Aufenthaltsgesetz, AufenthG), and the Benefits for Asylum Seekers Act (Asylbewerberleistungsgesetz, AsylbLG).[68] In accordance with paragraph 4.1 (AsylbLG), examination and treatment for asylum-seekers is guaranteed in cases of acute illness and pain, as well as during pregnancy.[69] Chronic diseases,

---

65 Bundesamt für Migration und Flüchtlinge: Aktuelle Zahlen (Note 1).
66 Edward, Hines-Martin: Exploring the Providers (Note 8), p. 1188.
67 Shannon et al.: Characteristics of Successful (Note 3), p. 565.
68 Kleefeldt, Wolff, de Carlo: Flüchtlinge in unserer Praxis (Note 12), p. 9.
69 Kleefeldt, Wolff, de Carlo: Flüchtlinge in unserer Praxis (Note 12), p. 9.

which, if left untreated, would turn into acute medical conditions, can also be treated according to AsylbLG. Within the first 15 months of stay, the costs are covered by the local Social Services Department (Sozialamt).[70]

With regard to psychiatric disorders, this regulation implies that acute conditions such as psychosis, psychological crisis, aggressive behavior or acute suicide risk, which require immediate in-patient admission to a psychiatric unit, can be treated, whereas follow-up treatment is not provided. Furthermore, asylum-seekers require a medical treatment voucher (*Behandlungsschein*) issued by the Social Services Department before accessing treatment. Children, pregnant women, people with disabilities and victims of torture and violence are considered particularly vulnerable; therefore, health care providers should give particular consideration to their needs.[71]

After the expiry of the fifteen-month deadline, the expenses for the health care of refugees are covered by statutory health insurance institutions (*gesetzliche Krankenkasse*) and asylum-seekers receive an electronic health care card (*elektronische Versicherungskarte*) which replaces the medical treatment voucher.[72] Access to the health care system is regulated in the respective federal states. In some states, asylum-seekers already obtain the electronic health care card within the first fifteen months of their stay in Germany. In Bremen, for instance, the card is issued around three months after the first registration, thereby avoiding the cumbersome application process for the medical treatment voucher at the social services department.[73] The fifteen-month deadline marks the threshold to access the services offered by the statutory health insurance.[74] According to the Benefits for Asylum Seekers Act (Asylbewerberleistungsgesetz), psychiatric treatment is considered acute care, whereas psychotherapy is usually not included within the services defined by statutory health insurance. To authorize the assumption of costs for psychotherapy paragraph 6 AsylbLG is considered, according to which at least short-time psychotherapy can be covered.[75]

---

70 Kleefeldt, Wolff, de Carlo: Flüchtlinge in unserer Praxis (Note 12), p. 55.

71 Bundesministerium für Gesundheit (Ed.): Health Guide for asylum seekers in Germany. Berlin 2016.

72 Kleefeldt, Wolff, de Carlo: Flüchtlinge in unserer Praxis (Note 12), p. 11.

73 Kleefeldt, Wolff, de Carlo: Flüchtlinge in unserer Praxis (Note 12), pp. 11–12.

74 Kleefeldt, Wolff, de Carlo: Flüchtlinge in unserer Praxis (Note 12), p. 11.

75 Frank et al.: Gesundheit und gesundheitliche Versorgung (Note 6), p. 39.

Another central issue of accessibility is the identification and referral of refugees needing mental health services.[76] Asylum-seekers suffering from mental disorders are frequently unaware of their illness or tend to hide them due to the significant stigma toward mental illness present among many refugee groups.[77] They rather complain about physical symptoms (pain, dizziness) and thus tend to utilize medical health care services rather than mental health services.[78] Therefore, experts advocate the introduction of routine mental health screening as part of the overall comprehensive health assessment for refugees.[79] In the US, mental health screening guidelines have recently been included in the recommendations for health screening for newly arrived refugees at the Centers for Disease Control and Prevention;[80] in Germany, on the contrary, there is no nationwide screening program. Questionnaires such as Refugee Health Screener-15 (RHS-15), Harvard Trauma Questionnaire and Posttraumatic Stress Diagnostic Scale were developed and validated especially for asylum-seekers and could be used by mental health care providers as well as in primary care.[81] The RHS-15, for instance, consists of fourteen questions scored on a Likert-type scale (from 0 to 4) and is currently available in fifteen languages. It screens for anxiety, depression, and PTSD and demonstrates high levels of sensitivity (0.81–0.95) and specificity (0.86–0.89).[82]

Finally, it should be noted that even if the possibility of adequate treatment is given, refugees have to face further logistical challenges. Shannon identified the lack of care coordination by providers as a major barrier to refugees accessing mental health services.[83] For newly arrived refugees, who are unfamiliar with the German system or those with limited language proficiency, using public transportation

[76] Shannon et al.: Characteristics of Successful (Note 3), p. 561.
[77] Kleefeldt, Wolff, de Carlo: Flüchtlinge in unserer Praxis (Note 12), p. 35.
[78] Priscilla M. Flynn, Jennifer L. Ridgeway, Mark L. Wieland, Mark D. Williams, Lindsey R. Haas, Walter K. Kremers, Carmen Radecki Breitkopf: Primary care utilization and mental health diagnoses among adult patients requiring interpreters: A retrospective cohort study. In: Journal of General Internal Medicine 28 (2013), pp. 386–391, here p. 390.
[79] Polcher, Calloway: Addressing the Need (Note 2), p. 199.
[80] Shannon et al.: Characteristics of Successful (Note 3), p. 555.
[81] Kleefeldt, Wolff, de Carlo: Flüchtlinge in unserer Praxis (Note 12), p. 28.
[82] Polcher, Calloway: Addressing the Need (Note 2), p. 200.
[83] Shannon et al.: Characteristics of Successful (Note 3), p. 563.

to reach therapeutic facilities can be a considerable challenge. In addition, due to the mental condition itself, many patients suffering from PTSD are not able to leave their accommodation independently and are therefore dependent on the assistance of volunteers, since institutional support (e.g. a taxi certificate) is usually not provided.

### *4.2 Availability and Acceptability of health and social services for refugees*

Despite having a formal right for mental health care, as delineated above, only a few mental health providers have specialized facilities for refugees. Under the keyword availability we will now point out some of the institutions that focus on providing mental health care for asylum-seekers.

Generally speaking, a distinction must be drawn between in-patient (*stationär*), semi-inpatient (*teilstationär*), and out-patient (ambulant) services. Refugees can potentially be referred to any psychiatric or psychosomatic department for in-patient treatment in Germany in cases of acute psychiatric conditions. Some hospitals have special transcultural in-patient and semi-impatient units for asylum-seekers, such as the Center for Transcultural Psychiatry and Psychotherapy (*Zentrum für Transkulturelle Psychiatrie und Psychotherapie, Klinikum Wahrendorff*) in Hannover. For out-patient care there is a wider range of specialized facilities, which can be independent services or subunits of the local health providers. Some examples are the Center for Intercultural Psychiatry (*Zentrum für interkulturelle Psychiatrie, Charité Berlin*), the Migation-Ambulance (*Migrationsambulanz, Universitätsklinikum München*), the Refugee-Ambulance (*Flüchtlingsambulanz, Universitätsklinikum Essen*), the Transcultural Psychiatric Ambulance (*transkulturelle psychiatrische Ambulanz, Universitätsklinikum Mainz*), the Transcultural Ambulance (*Transkulturelle Ambulanz, LVR-Klinikum Düsseldorf*), the Intercultural Ambulance (*interkulturelle Ambulanz, LVR-Klinikum Essen*), and the Psychiatric Ambulance (*Psychiatrische Institutsambulanz, Universitätsklinikum Tübingen*).

Furthermore, psychosocial centers (*psychosoziale Zentren*) play a major role in out-patient treatment of refugees suffering from mental illness. Currently there are 32 psychosocial centers in Germany, treating almost 20.000 patients (17.674 in 2016).[84] They provide culturally-responsive, multidisciplinary care which includes psychotherapy, assistance with paperwork and asylum procedures, consultation regarding accommodation, language classes and apprenticeships and establishing contacts with volunteers.[85]

All the institutions mentioned above share a cultural-sensitive approach and work with professional interpreters and culture mediators, who are essential for efficient treatment. The costs for interpreters are usually not covered by statutory health insurance.[86] Within the first fifteen months of stay, an application to the Social Services Department is possible but relatively complex and not always successful, since it is at the discretion of the single case-handler.[87] Once the fifteen-month deadline has expired, the expenses for medical treatment are covered by the statutory health insurance, so that the cost of interpreters can no longer be refunded according to AsylbLG. Nevertheless, in some cases the Social Services Department or the Job Center authorize cost assumption for interpreter services as an atypical need within the meaning of paragraph 73 of Social Security Code XI (atypischer Bedarf, Sozialgesetzbuch, SGB XI).[88]

Interpreters are essential not only for communication in a strict linguistic sense; they serve also as cultural brokers. This brings us to the aspect of acceptability: as already mentioned, refugees often struggle to accept the western concept of mental disorders. Interpreters therefore need special training in order to fulfill their role as culture mediators and avoid secondary traumatization for themselves. Agencies that provide specially trained interpreters in Germany are, for instance, SprInt (*Bundesweite Sprach- und Intergrationsmittlung*) and Bundesverband der Dolmetscher und Übersetzer e. V. (BDÜ).[89]

Finally, it should be pointed out that psychotherapeutic treatment takes a considerable amount of time, even more so in the case of refugees, where a consistent time slot is needed to establish a trustful patient-provider relationship and obtain acute mental stabilization.

---

[84] Bundesweite Arbeitsgemeinschaft der Psychosozialen Zentren für Flüchtlinge und Folteropfer (BAfF e. V.) (Ed.): Tätigkeitsbericht für das Jahr 2017. Berlin 2018, p. 60.

[85] BAfF e. V.: Tätigkeitsbericht (Note 84), p. 53.

[86] Kleefeldt, Wolff, de Carlo: Flüchtlinge in unserer Praxis (Note 12), p. 53.

[87] Kleefeldt, Wolff, de Carlo: Flüchtlinge in unserer Praxis (Note 12), p. 55.

[88] Kleefeldt, Wolff, de Carlo: Flüchtlinge in unserer Praxis (Note 12), p. 56.

[89] Kleefeldt, Wolff, de Carlo: Flüchtlinge in unserer Praxis (Note 12), p. 57.

Before the actual trauma-focused therapy begins, sufficient time should be dedicated to psychoeducation in order to provide information about the therapeutic setting and validate refugees' experiences.[90] Considering that long-term treatment is rarely covered by the insurance system, it is virtually impossible to accomplish adequate trauma-focused therapy. More often psychotherapy consists of crisis intervention, which is helpful in the acute situation of mental distress but not sufficient to prevent the long-term consequences of traumatization. The asylum process itself may hinder the progress of psychotherapy: impending deportation, uncertain residence status, notifications from the authorities are aspects which deeply influence the daily life of refugees and must often be prioritized in therapy since they may lead to acute stress response.[91]

## 5. Conclusion

In view of the above, mental health care for refugees presents a challenge for the national health system on various levels. Working with trauma-patients requires a systemic and holistic approach that addresses the multiple dimensions of trauma and reinforces strategies for maintaining resilience in the recovery process.[92] An accessible, culturally sensitive and coordinated mental health care system for refugees is required in order to guarantee adequate treatment of trauma-related disorders, as well as specialized centers with trained medical personnel. The providers currently available cover a mere fraction of the need for out-patient and in-patient health care for refugees.[93] In future, further training for medical staff working with asylum-seekers will be needed in order to promote awareness of the psychiatric disorders of refugees among physicians of all fields (especially general practitioners, psychiatrists and pediatricians) but also among nursing staff, occupational, music and art therapists.

[90] Kleefeldt, Wolff, de Carlo: Flüchtlinge in unserer Praxis (Note 12), pp. 35–36.

[91] Kleefeldt, Wolff, de Carlo: Flüchtlinge in unserer Praxis (Note 12), p. 40.

[92] Pederson et al.: How the Bodyself (Note 43), p. 1032.

[93] Deutsche Gesellschaft für Psychiatrie und Psychotherapie, Psychosomatik und Nervenheilkunde: Psychosoziale Versorgung von Flüchtlingen verbessern (3/22/16). https://www.dgppn.de/_Resources/Persistent/c03a6dbf7dcdb0a77dbdf4ed3e5098143 1abe372/2016_03_22_DGPPN-Positionspapier_psychosoziale%20Versorgung%20Fl %C3%BCchtlinge.pdf (accessed 9/24/2019).

This is all the more important considering the high prevalence rates of mental disorders among refugees and the fact that clinical symptoms, including suicidal behavior, might manifest years after the traumatic event itself, thus requiring even more attention in detecting cases of trauma-related disorders in the years to come.[94] Furthermore, the heritability of trauma, proved by the epigenetic studies, indicates the necessity for treatment in subsequent generations even in individuals without direct exposition to traumatic events. In this regard, standardized examinations in first accommodation facilities are essential to identify and refer asylum-seekers needing mental health services, as well as to improve nationwide data availability of the estimated need for physical and mental healthcare.[95]

The lack of mental health providers for refugees furthermore draws attention to a general deficit of licensed psychotherapists in private practice in Germany. Even if acute mental healthcare facilities are provided all over the country, there are long waiting lists for outpatient care and long-term therapy. This deficit is even more evident in the treatment of asylum-seekers since a special license is required to treat refugees and the complexity of the application process stands in the way of developing a nationwide therapists' network for refugee care.[96] In fact, only 5 % of the patients treated in psychosocial centers are currently referred to psychotherapists in private practice.[97]

Another serious deficiency is the lack of cost assumption for interpreters by the statutory health insurance funds, which are crucial for psychotherapy provision. Providers specialized in mental health care for refugees are therefore reliant on external funding (donations, sponsoring, project and private funds), state or municipal funds, or services covered by the statutory health insurance to cover the expenses for interpreter agencies.[98]

In order to guarantee sufficient accessibility to mental health providers, coordinated care which integrates on-site mental health care

---

[94] Jankovic et al.: Trauma and suicidality (Note 40), p. 514.

[95] Frank et al.: Gesundheit und gesundheitliche Versorgung (Note 6), p. 24.

[96] Bundesweite Arbeitsgemeinschaft der Psychosozialen Zentren für Flüchtlinge und Folteropfer (BAfF e. V.): Die Ermächtigung zur psychotherapeutischen Behandlung von Geflüchteten – ein wichtiges Instrument droht zu scheitern. http://www.baff-zentren.org/ermaechtigung/ (accessed 9/24/2019).

[97] BAfF e. V.: Tätigkeitsbericht für das Jahr (Note 84), p. 100.

[98] Kleefeldt, Wolff, de Carlo: Flüchtlinge in unserer Praxis (Note 12), p. 55.

for immediate consultation with primary care is needed.[99] In fact, according to Shannon, the main factor that contributes to successful referrals of asylum-seekers is culturally responsive care supported by active care coordination with proactive resolution of access barriers.[100] To this end, researchers advocate for a »patient-focused care that is comprehensive and delivered through inter-professional teams with strong communication«,[101] which at this point, despite many recent initiatives and growing networks of psychosocial centers in Germany, is still not sufficiently available.

---

[99] Meagan E. Williams, Sandra C. Thompson: The use of community-based interventions in reducing morbidity from the psychological impact of conflict-related trauma among refugee populations: A systematic review of the literature. In: Journal of Immigrant and Minority Health 13 (2011), pp. 780–794; Shannon et al.: Characteristics of Successful (Note 3), p. 561.

[100] Shannon et al.: Characteristics of Successful (Note 3), pp. 557–561.

[101] Shannon et al.: Characteristics of Successful (Note 3), p. 556; Josephine McMurray, Katherine Breward, Michael Breward, Rob Alder, Neil Arya: Integrated Primary Care Improves Access to Healthcare for Newly Arrived Refugees in Canada. In: Journal of Immigrant and Minority Health 16 (2014), pp. 576–585, here p. 577.

*Ivana Tucak*

# Cultural differences and informed consent

Abstract
Informed consent and the principle of autonomy have lately become the subjects of new academic controversies. Critics oppose the prevailing perception of autonomy as being atomistic or individualistic. It is particularly problematic regarding patients with a non-western background. In non-individualistic, community-oriented cultures, characterized by different family dynamics and different perception of the relationship between doctors and their patients, there are a number of ethical and legal challenges, which contemporary moral philosophers, bioethicists and jurists need to face in multicultural societies. The paper is divided in three parts. The first part aims to clarify the nature of informed consent. It offers a short overview of the most influential theoretical justifications of informed consent. The second part elaborates the cultural challenges that the doctrine of informed consent faces in today's culturally diverse societies. The third part explores the regulation of informed consent in the Republic of Croatia in order to determine whether the Croatian legal system can accommodate these cultural challenges.

## 1. Introduction

Informed consent and the principle of autonomy have lately become the subjects of new academic controversies. Critics oppose the prevailing perception of autonomy as being atomistic or individualistic. It is particularly problematic regarding patients with a non-western background. How can the informed consent process be carried out in non-individualistic, community-oriented cultures? In those cultures, characterized by different family dynamics and different perception of the relationship between doctors and their patients, there are a number of ethical and legal challenges, which contemporary moral philosophers, bioethicists and jurists need to face in multicultural societies.[1] The

[1] Roy Gilbar, José Miola: One Size Fits All? On Patient Autonomy, Medical Decision-

paper examines the justifiability of critiques of bioethics and allegations that it prefers western values. Those critiques stress that western values favoring the interests of individuals over the welfare of a society are incorporated into relevant international law. With respect to informed consent, the requests that an individual's social context needs to be taken into account are gaining popularity.[2] According to empirical research, the cultural affiliation of a patient influences his or her perception of health and illness, and consequently, his or her decision-making ability.[3] This raises the question which type of autonomy should deserve legal support.

In traditions in which an individual is primarily perceived as a family member, contemporary authors discuss the question whether to seek legal mechanisms, which could enable family members to participate in the informed consent process. Can disclosure of information and decision-making be transferred to the family or, depending on the principles of a respective society, to a particular family member? Such a concept of informed consent undoubtedly challenges its current fundamental components: voluntariness and freedom from other people's controlling influences. The paper agrees with the authors who highlight that regarding the application of the principle of informed consent in non-western cultures, all these open questions, their research and familiarization will contribute to better understanding of the concept of informed consent as well as of its nature and role in medical law and ethics.

The paper is divided in three parts. The first part aims to clarify the nature of informed consent. It offers a short overview of the most influential theoretical justification of informed consent, i.e. protection of a patient's individual autonomy. The second part elaborates the cultural challenges that the doctrine of informed consent faces in today's culturally diverse societies. The third part explores the regulation of informed consent in the Republic of Croatia. Is the current Croatian legal system up to these challenges?

---

Making, and the Impact of Culture. In: Medical Law Review 23 (2015), pp. 375–399; Mark Kuczewski, Patrick J. Mccruden: Informed Consent: Does It Take a Village? The Problem of Culture and Truth Telling. In: Cambridge Quarterly of Healthcare Ethics 10 (2001), pp. 34–46.

[2] Gilbar, Miola: One Size Fits All? (Note 1), p. 376.

[3] Linda Farber Post, Jeffrey Blustein, Elysa Gordon, Nancy Neveloff Dubler: Pain: Ethics, Culture, and Informed Consent to Relief. In: The Journal of Law, Medicine & Ethics 24 (1996), pp. 348–359.

## 2. Nature of Informed Consent

It is often said that informed consent neither contains »consistent central elements« nor has »a clear purpose«.[4] There are various notions of informed consent in law and ethics as well as various theoretical justifications of its existence. This part of the paper briefly touches upon the most influential theoretical justification of informed consent, i. e. the protection of a patient's individual autonomy. There is no doubt that individual autonomy is »deeply entrenched in Western cultures and law«.[5] Therein, the voluntary and consciously given consent of an individual represents one of the basic legal concepts. Its rule is equally important in law of contracts[6] and criminal law. In Schuck's opinion, such consent has priority in Western cultures, which is based on individualistic values promoting that »the individual should be the author of her own undertakings«.[7] This is perceived as a prerequisite of true respect for his or her dignity.[8] An individual may freely tailor the nature of his or her relationships with others and on such an occasion, the only limitation is the »coercive regulatory authority« of the state.[9]

One may say that this justification of informed consent is most discussed among bioethicists and legal scholars. A good example of such an attitude is Wendy Parmet's claim that patients', research subjects' and tissue donors' autonomy has been enhanced through informed consent since this concept provides them with information necessary to make a decision which reflects their values.[10]

Nowadays, informed consent appears as the cornerstone of bioethics and is incorporated into the most relevant international and European documents regulating the protection of patients' and research subjects' rights, such as UNESCO's Universal Declaration on Bioethics and Human Rights, adopted in 2005, and the Council of

---

[4] Wendy E. Parmet: Informed Consent and Public Health: Are They Compatible When It Comes to Vaccines? In: Journal of Health Care Law and Policy 8 (2005), pp. 71–110, here p. 83.

[5] Peter H. Schuck: Rethinking Informed Consent. In: Yale Law Journal 103 (1994), pp. 899–959, here p. 924.

[6] Schuck: Rethinking Informed Consent (Note 5), p. 900.

[7] Schuck: Rethinking Informed Consent (Note 5), pp. 900–901.

[8] Schuck: Rethinking Informed Consent (Note 5), pp. 900–901.

[9] Schuck: Rethinking Informed Consent (Note 5), pp. 900–901.

[10] Parmet: Informed Consent (Note 4), p. 101.

Europe Convention on Human Rights and Biomedicine (Oviedo Convention), which entered into force in 1999.[11] These documents protect the free choice of competent adult patients.[12] One may say that today the prevailing concept of informed consent involves the following elements: the mental capacity to make a medical decision, the right to information prior to the decision-making and the capacity to freely and independently decide on a medical intervention.[13] The autonomy is undoubtedly individual. For instance, Article 3 of the Declaration on Bioethics and Human Rights sets forth that the interests and welfare of an individual have priority over the interests of a society.

### 2.1 *Criticism of the Approach that Informed Consent is Important Due to the Protection of Patients' Autonomy*

Carl Wellman rejects Immanuel Kant's version of autonomy, according to which informed consent is needed to avoid treating a research subject as »a mere means« by the doctor and to facilitate taking patients' or research subjects' »practical rationality« into consideration.[14] The reason for the rejection is that informed consent does not turn the research subject into a researcher's »partner«. Even after giving informed consent, »the subject of medical research is typically acted on rather than an actor in the research«.[15]

In accordance with Onora O'Neil, the ethical importance of this concept cannot relate to the protection of individual autonomy since the concept is supposed to protect the choices of individuals who are »timid, conventional and lacking individual autonomy« as well as the choices of those who are featured by individual autonomy, i. e. those

---

[11] Universal Declaration on Bioethics and Human Rights adopted by UNESCO's General Conference on 19 October 2005. http://portal.unesco.org/en/ev.php-URL_ID=31058&URL_DO=DO_TOPIC&URL_SECTION=201.html (accessed 9/24/2019); Convention for the protection of Human Rights and Dignity of the Human Being with regard to the Application of Biology and Medicine: Convention on Human Rights and Biomedicine. https://www.coe.int/en/web/conventions/full-list/-/conventions/treaty/164 (accessed 9/24/2019).

[12] Roy Gilbar: Family Involvement, Independence, and Patient Autonomy in Practice. In: Medical Law Review 19 (2011), pp. 192–234, here p. 196.

[13] Gilbar: Family Involvement (Note 12), p. 196.

[14] Carl Wellman: An Approach to Rights: Studies in the Philosophy of Law and Morals. Dordrecht, London, Boston 1997, p. 88.

[15] Wellman: An Approach to Rights (Note 14), p. 88.

who are »self-assertive, self-knowing« and »critically reflective«.[16] Informed consent does not make all the medical procedures legitimate. The respect for autonomy can be subject to other moral considerations.[17] It is fully legitimate to restrain the autonomy of a patient if his or her choice may do harm to other people, e.g. jeopardize the health of a broader community.[18] Since healthcare represents an example of »a scarce good«, autonomy may be restrained on the occasion of its distribution.[19] Similarly, autonomy protection is not absolute with respect to the termination of a therapy in case of »medically futile treatment«, »dysthanasia«.[20]

O'Neill accentuates that informed consent bears certain ethical relevance, which is more elementary than autonomy: it prevents patients, research subjects and tissue donors from being deceived or coerced.[21] Patients and others must have »control« over the situation they are facing: over the amount of received information prior to a medical intervention or research. Along with the possibility to decline the intervention, they are entitled to »rescind« the given consent thereto at any time.[22]

The real meaning of informed consent refers, as claimed by Wellman, to the legitimation of researcher's action imposing a risk.[23] Consent is necessary, thinks Wellman, when someone's conduct threatens or breaches one or more rights of another person. Informed consent is required in medical research due to the need for protection of the following »fundamental« rights of research subjects: »the right to privacy«, »the right to personal security«, in extreme circumstances even »the patient's right to life«, »the right to the truth«, »the right to freedom from exploitation«, »the right to the best health care possible«.[24] By giving informed consent, an individual waives those

[16] Onora O'Neil: Some Limits of Informed Consent. In: Journal of Medical Ethics 29 (2003), pp. 4–7, here p. 5.
[17] Tom L. Beauchamp, James F. Childress: Principles of Biomedical Ethics. 5th Edition. Oxford, New York 2001, p. 65.
[18] Beauchamp, Childress: Principles of Biomedical Ethics (Note 17), p. 65.
[19] Beauchamp, Childress: Principles (Note 17), p. 65.
[20] Iva Sorta Bilajac: Informirani pristanak – konceptualni, empirijski i normativni problem. In: Medicina Fluminensis 47 (2011), pp. 37–47, here p. 41.
[21] O'Neill: Some Limits (Note 16), pp. 4–5.
[22] O'Neill: Some Limits of Informed Consent (Note 16), p. 6.
[23] Wellman: An Approach to Rights (Note 14), p. 90.
[24] Wellman: An Approach to Rights (Note 14), p. 89.

rights, which protect them from any act of the doctor or researcher.[25] In other words, an individual »does not only express agreement« but also authorizes the doctor to carry out a medical intervention or the researcher to conduct research.[26]

## 3. The Challenges of Multiculturalism

Regardless of the cultural circle a patient belongs to, his or her attitude towards health and diseases is always culturally dependent.[27] There are numerous definitions of culture. For the sake of this paper, Gibar and Miola's definition of culture is used. These authors define culture as:

> a set of shared attitudes, values, beliefs, language, rituals, and practices that distinguish a particular social group, or as a set of guidelines that people inherit as members of a particular community, that guide them how to view the world and how to behave in relation to other people.[28]

Moreover, culture is »a lens through which the world is perceived and understood«.[29] The experience of pain by a patient and the response of the caregivers depend, beside his or her gender, age and social class, on his or her cultural affiliation too.[30]

This implies that the caregivers in Europe are facing new challenges due to the new wave of migrations. In the light of healthcare delivery, »cultural pluralism« is more a rule than an exception, particularly in urban centers.[31] In scientific discussions on health protection and clinical research, scholars pay more and more attention to this phenomenon. The political philosophy of contemporary societies

---

25 Wellman: An Approach to Rights (Note 14), p. 91.

26 Beauchamp, Childress: Principles of Biomedical Ethics (Note 17), p. 78.

27 American Academy of Pediatrics Policy. Policy Statement. Organizational Principles to Guide and Define the Child Health Care System and/or Improve the Health of All Children. Committee on Pediatric Workforce: Ensuring Culturally Effective Pediatric Care: Implications for Education and Health Policy. In: Pediatrics 114 (2004), pp. 1677–1685, here p. 1679; Farber Post et al.: Pain: Ethics, Culture (Note 3).

28 Gilbar, Miola: One Size Fits All? (Note 1), p. 377.

29 Farber Post et al.: Pain: Ethics, Culture (Note 3), p. 355.

30 Farber Post et al.: Pain: Ethics, Culture (Note 3), p. 350 and 355.

31 Patricia A. Marshall, Barbara A. Koenig, Paul Grifhorst, Mirjam van Ewijk: Ethical Issues in Immigrant Health Care and Clinical Research. In: Sana Loue (Ed.): Handbook of Immigrant Health. Boston, MA, 1998, pp. 203–226, here p. 203.

characterized by cultural and religious diversity has shaped the idea of multiculturalism. In the descriptive sense, the term »multicultural« denotes »the fact of diversity in a society«.[32] It also entails a number of prescriptive meanings, all of which reject the idea of »a melting pot«.[33] Minority group members are not expected to assimilate, but they are encouraged to preserve their collective identity and habits. Multicultural policies provide better conditions for migrant integration.[34] This section of the paper sheds light on what this means for the healthcare sector.

### *3.1 Differences between the Western and non-Western cultures*

Empirical studies show that patients belonging to the Western cultural circle particularly appreciate »self-determination, rights and open communication with clinicians«.[35] In the West, a direct and open communication between clinicians and their patients, and a full access to relevant information occur to be »the golden rule« in their relationship.[36] What needs to be strived for is that patients become fully aware of their illness and available treatments, and that the clinicians provide answers to all of the patients' questions and encourage them to get involved in making decisions on their own health.[37]

On the other hand, patients from non-Western cultures are guided by other values, which raises the fundamental challenge in multicultural societies: how to adequately protect their beliefs.[38] Unlike Europe and North America, other regions in the world, from the Middle to the Far East and Africa, deem other values as more important than the protection of individual autonomy. This can be even said

---

[32] Sarah Song: »Multiculturalism«. In: Edward N. Zalta (Ed.): The Stanford Encyclopedia of Philosophy (Spring 2017 Edition). https://plato.stanford.edu/archives/spr2017/entries/multiculturalism/ (accessed 9/24/2019).

[33] Song: »Multiculturalism« (Note 32).

[34] Song: »Multiculturalism« (Note 32).

[35] Gilbar, Miola: One Size Fits All? (Note 1), p. 377; Mahati Chittem, Phyllis Butow: Responding to Family Requests for Nondisclosure: The Impact of Oncologists' Cultural Background. In: Journal of Cancer Research and Therapeutics 11 (2015), pp. 174–180, here p. 174.

[36] Gilbar, Miola: One Size Fits All? (Note 1), p. 397.

[37] Chittem, Butow: Responding to family requests for nondisclosure (Note 35), p. 174.

[38] Gilbar, Miola: One Size Fits All? (Note 1), p. 377.

for some minority groups who have resided in the West for a long time.[39] In those non-Western cultures, it is not so unusual to fully deprive patients of the right to information and to consult their families when making medical decisions relating to their health.[40] Members of non-Western cultures put the emphasis on »family-determination, moral responsibility to others and limited disclosure.«[41]

For example, in the United States, there was a request to exclude members of the Navajo nation from the enforcement of the Patient Self-Determination Act (PSDA).[42] The request was based on the fact that members of the Navajo nation believe in the causal power of discussing negative information.[43] Similar challenges are faced by Western oncologists who are requested by immigrant families not to disclose the cancer diagnosis to the affected family member.[44] Western physicians are placed in ethical and moral dilemmas by requests for »non-direct communication« and non-disclosure of relevant medical information.[45] However, they can violate »the cultural integrity« and »personal dignity« of patients coming from minority groups if they are not aware of those cultural differences and thus insist on getting informed consent in the inherited »patient-centered manner«.[46]

There are growing requests to broaden the concept of autonomy and grant patients the power to waive the right to informed consent and assign the power to make relevant medical decisions to their families.[47] It should be stressed that physicians also have their own clinical culture and health-related values: to provide treatment and

---

39 Fabrizio Turoldo: Relational Autonomy and Multiculturalism. In: Cambridge Quarterly of Healthcare Ethics 19 (2010), pp. 542–549, here p. 545.

40 Gilbar, Miola: One Size Fits All? (Note 1), pp. 377–378.

41 Gilbar, Miola: One Size Fits All? (Note 1), p. 377.

42 Kuczewski, Mccruden: Informed Consent (Note 1), pp. 41–42.

43 Joseph A. Carrese, Lorna A. Rhodes: Western Bioethics on the Navajo Reservation. In: JAMA 274 (1995), pp. 826–829, here p. 826; Kuczewski, Mccruden: Informed Consent (Note 1), p. 41.

44 Chittem, Butow: Responding to family requests for nondisclosure (Note 35), pp. 174–180.

45 Chittem, Butow: Responding to family requests for nondisclosure (Note 35), p. 174; Insoo Hyun: Waiver of Informed Consent, Cultural Sensitivity, and the Problem of Unjust Families and Traditions. In: The Hastings Center Report 32 (2002), pp. 14–22, here p. 14.

46 Hyun: Waiver of Informed Consent (Note 45), p. 14.

47 Hyun: Waiver of Informed Consent (Note 45), p. 15.

extend human lives.[48] Highly educated healthcare professionals may easily assume that all the others share their values, which can put the entire development of the protection of patients' rights in jeopardy since the doctrine of informed consent first appeared in the West and its purpose was to protect the autonomous choice of a patient from his or her doctor.[49] As a result of the historical development of informed consent, western bioethicists are suspicious of all forms of social influence on an individual when making medical decisions.[50] Hence, can the wishes of members of minority groups to include their families in the medical decision-making process be fulfilled at all?[51]

When working with their patients, doctors and other caregivers can personally witness that even Western patients are not »self-sufficient entities« despite the ideal type propagated by bioethics and law. Respect for a patient's autonomy usually implies ›a process of collaborative decision-making‹, involving, beside the patient and his or her physician, the patient's relatives or family members.[52] This opens up the possibility to recognize the legitimate role of the family in the medical decision-making process.[53]

### 3.2 *Relational autonomy*

The prevailing viewpoint on informed consent has lately been challenged theoretically in several ways. This paper concentrates on the critiques describing informed consent as a Western concept and as such, it is regarded as an inappropriate mechanism for treating individuals who belong to other cultures. Yet, criticism of individual autonomy as the foundation of informed consent can be heard in the West too.[54] The authors who question informed consent from the aspect of the so-called Western imperialism rely their critiques on some originally Western theories, particularly on feminist ethics of

---

48 Kuczewski, Mccruden: Informed Consent (Note 1), p. 40.
49 Kuczewski, Mccruden: Informed Consent (Note 1), p. 40.
50 Gilbar, Miola: One Size Fits All? (Note 1), p. 383.
51 Gilbar, Miola: One Size Fits All? (Note 1), p. 379.
52 Kuczewski, Mccruden: Informed Consent (Note 1), p. 34.
53 Kuczewski, Mccruden: Informed Consent (Note 1), p. 34.
54 Peter I. Osuji: Relational autonomy in informed consent (RAIC) as an ethics of care approach to the concept of informed consent. In: Medicine Health Care and Philosophy 21 (2017), pp. 101–111, here p. 101.

care.[55] As highlighted by Osuri, ethics of care does not consider people as isolated individuals but regards all human beings as »ontologically relational«, which is why this ethics prefers relational over individual autonomy.[56]

The roots of relational autonomy can be found in feminist theory[57] which deems the main Western concept of autonomy as »inherently masculinist or fundamentally individualistic and rationalistic«.[58] Feminist scholars tackle individual(istic) autonomy for its neglect of »mutual responsibility, cooperation and care towards others«.[59] Advocates of relational autonomy point out that people are rarely completely independent and that their identity, needs and interests, and autonomy itself are always tailored by their relationships with other people, individuals, and groups.[60]

Since social relationships come as part of every person's identity, this social relationship needs to be acknowledged when making medical decisions as well.[61] It is necessary to legally regulate a mechanism, which could enable inclusion of the family in the respective process.[62] As an integral part of the prevailing informed consent doctrine, independence gets endangered in the event of inclusion of a patient's close relatives in making relevant medical decisions on his or her health.[63] Instead of independence, relational autonomy sheds light on »interdependence«.[64] A person is perceived »as a caring interdependent being« and not as »a rationalistic« and »abstract individuality«, stripped of all emotions and friendly and family ties.[65] Individuals are no longer self-sufficient but dependent beings.[66] As emphasized by Dove et al.:

---

[55] Osuji: Relational autonomy (Note 54), p. 101.
[56] Osuji: Relational autonomy (Note 54), p. 108.
[57] Gilbar, Miola: One Size Fits All? (Note 1), p. 379.
[58] Turoldo: Relational Autonomy (Note 39), pp. 544–545.
[59] Edward S. Dove, Susan E. Kelly, Federica Lucivero, Mavis Machirori, Sandi Dheensa, Barbara Prainsack: Beyond individualism: Is there a place for relational autonomy in clinical practice and research? In: Clinical Ethics 12 (2017), pp. 150–165, here p. 153.
[60] Dove et al.: Beyond individualism (Note 59), p. 151.
[61] Gilbar, Miola: One Size Fits All? (Note 1), p. 379.
[62] Gilbar, Miola: One Size Fits All? (Note 1).
[63] Gilbar: Family Involvement (Note 12), p. 196.
[64] Dove et al.: Beyond individualism (Note 59), p. 153.
[65] Osuji: Relational autonomy (Note 54), p. 107.
[66] Osuji: Relational autonomy (Note 54), p. 108.

Relational autonomy can be viewed as a conception of autonomy that places the individual in a socially embedded network of others. Relationships (with family, community and society), responsibility, care and interdependence are key attributes of relational autonomy: people develop their sense of self and form capacities and life plans through the relationships they forge on a daily and long-term basis. Relational autonomy asserts, therefore, that social surroundings and relationships are crucial for developing autonomy, and encourages us to act in ways guided by an ethic of trust and care.[67]

Relational autonomy is, accordingly, a »reciprocal« and »collaborative« process because it attempts to achieve a balance between individuals who are part of each other's lives and the recognition of their interdependence when trying to accomplish their goals.[68]

Osuri has formulated a concept of »relational autonomy in informed consent (RAIC)«:

Care creates relationships and interdependence, and the concept of relational autonomy implies that we as relational beings become autonomous in relation to family, friends, relations, and others. Therefore, decisions are made not just in relation to others but with them, that is, involving them: family members, friends, relations, and others. Little wonder then that as we saw above, ethics of care emphasizes a process approach to decision making wherein the input of relevant others to one's decision making is vital.[69]

According to Osuri, the relationship between healthcare providers and patients should be based on »human interrelatedness and interdependence.«[70] This corresponds to human universal experience not only in the private but also in the public sphere, both national and international. Informed consent based on relational autonomy appears as a dynamic process as well.[71]

### 3.3 *Some Difficulties Related to the Concept of Relational Autonomy*

Some bioethicists see relational autonomy as a dubious concept.[72] There is no consensus about the value of relationality. As believed

---

[67] Dove et al.: Beyond individualism (Note 59), p. 153.
[68] Gilbar: Family Involvement (Note 12), p. 198.
[69] Osuji: Relational autonomy (Note 54), p. 109.
[70] Osuji: Relational autonomy (Note 54), p. 110.
[71] Osuji: Relational autonomy (Note 54), p. 110.
[72] Gilbar: Family Involvement (Note 12), p. 198.

by Dove et al., we all can agree that social relations are of key importance for human progress and this cannot be contested even by the keenest advocates of individualistic autonomy. However, what is controversial is the question whether an utterance of the importance of social relations for human beings should be regarded as a »description of a social fact or whether it should have deeper analytical and also normative implications.«[73] The approach of ethics of care to this problem, hold the above authors, reflects in the standpoint that »relationality« implies »normative implications« for the fashion in which we treat other people.[74]

Turoldo speaks about limitations in multiculturalism.[75] In his opinion, only individuals, not cultures, can possess rights. Individuals are entitled, thinks Turoldo, to subject individual autonomy to other values which they consider important, such as trust in a good clinician or family. Turoldo classifies such a perspective as »liberal multiculturalism« and believes that it is the only multicultural perspective that does not challenge individual human rights and therefore, he depicts it as the best interpretation of relational autonomy.

In the bioethical context, there is a disagreement on the role and scope of family inclusion in the medical decision-making process.[76] According to Roy Gilbar and José Miola, the main issues affecting medical practice refer to passive patients who delegate the medical decision-making process to dominant male relatives.[77] Is full respect for the autonomy and cultural values of patients contrary to the foundations of Western democratic societies, such as gender equality? These authors propagate integration of the concept of relational autonomy into contemporary law and bioethics, yet their starting point is the existence of a particular »level of individual autonomy«, and justice and equality within the family.[78]

The proposed changes encompass, among other things, legal abandonment of »the reasonable patient test for disclosure of information to patients«,[79] according to which reasonable patients are those with Western values. Instead, a new test should be developed

---

[73] Dove et al.: Beyond individualism (Note 59), p. 153.
[74] Dove et al.: Beyond individualism (Note 59), p. 153.
[75] Turoldo: Relational Autonomy (Note 39), p. 548.
[76] Gilbar: Family Involvement (Note 12), p. 198.
[77] Gilbar, Miola: One Size Fits All? (Note 1), p. 397.
[78] Gilbar, Miola: One Size Fits All? (Note 1), p. 397.
[79] Gilbar, Miola: One Size Fits All? (Note 1), p. 397.

and the scope of disclosure therein needs to be adapted to the information-seeking needs of particular patients (»the particular patient test«).[80] Such a test would be useful to all patients, irrespective of their cultural affiliation since physicians would be expected to devote more time to knowing their cultural and personal values.[81]

Insoo Hyun indicates the need for protection of only the »authentic values« of a person and not those resulting from a certain manipulation.[82] All the autonomy theories which do not fulfil »the authenticity condition« are not satisfactory since they cannot differentiate between people acting autonomously and in accordance with their own values, and those acting following other people's values.[83] Hyun suggests and Gibar and Miola support that suggestion that a person may waive his or her right to informed consent if the following four requirements have been met:[84] 1) In a private conversation, the healthcare provider has pointed to the patient's right to informed consent and to the possibility that this right does not have to exclude his or her family if that is what he or she wishes; 2) the patient clearly communicates his or her decision to fully waive his or her right to informed consent, without being forced to do so by his or her family or someone else; 3) the patient's wish to empower his or her family to make medical decisions on his or her behalf fulfils the authenticity condition; 4) the patient's family is willing to take full responsibility for the decision-making. On such an occasion, the patient's welfare or general well-being has been recognized as a legitimate goal.

## 4. Informed consent in the Republic of Croatia

When it comes to the protection of the right to informed consent in the Republic of Croatia, it is important to stress the role of the Supreme Court of the Republic of Croatia therein. In two of its frequently quoted decisions, one dated in 1967 and the other one in 1975, the Supreme Court protected the patient's autonomy prior to

---

80 Gilbar, Miola: One Size Fits All? (Note 1), p. 398.

81 Gilbar, Miola: One Size Fits All? (Note 1), p. 397–398; Farber Post et al.: Pain: Ethics, Culture (Note 3), pp. 351–352.

82 Hyun: Waiver of Informed Consent (Note 45), pp. 14–22.

83 Hyun: Waiver of Informed Consent (Note 45), p. 16.

84 Hyun: Waiver of Informed Consent (Note 45), p. 19; Gilbar, Miola: One Size Fits All? (Note 1), p. 399.

the adoption of any legal document referring to informed consent.[85] In 1967, the Supreme Court drew the following conclusion:

Interference with the bodily integrity of a particular person by a third-party professional for the sake of medical treatment shall lose its illegal character only if accompanied with the informed consent of the sick person and in case of its lack, only if the patient is incapacitated to provide informed consent and his/her condition could be life-threatening if an urgent medical intervention is not performed.[86]

The 1975 decision of the Supreme Court contains the following formulation:

It is inadmissible and against the principle of inviolability of the physical integrity to perform a surgical intervention on a person against his/her will, even in case when this would be of benefit for this person, except if the reasons are not special and justify such procedure, like endangered life and condition of the sick person, making it impossible for this person to give consent.[87]

The 1990 Croatian Constitution contains several clauses which bear relevance for the protection of a patient's autonomy.[88] Article 23 (1) clearly envisages the need for informed consent when conducting »medical or scientific experiments«, Article 35 relates to »the protection of each person's private and family life, dignity, and reputation«

[85] Saša Nikšić: Načelo autonomije pacijenta u hrvatskom zakonodavstvu. In: Ksenija Turković, Sunčana Roksandić Vidlička, Aleksandar Maršavelski (Eds.): Hrestomatija hrvatskoga medicinskog prava. Zagreb 2016, pp. 585–591, here pp. 590–591.

[86] Zlatan Stipković: Protupravnost kao pretpostavka odgovornosti za štetu. Zagreb 1991, p. 81; Nikšić: Načelo autonomije (Note 85), p. 591; Ksenija Turković: Pravo na odbijanje medicinskog tretmana u Republici Hrvatskoj. In: Medicina Fluminensis 44 (2008), pp. 158–170, here p. 163.

[87] Decision of the Supreme Court of Croatia in 1975, (1554/74, ZSO, book 1., band 4. page 204). Translated by Maja Proso: Some Legal Issues on Informed Consent in Croatian Legislation and Practice, p. 1341, footnote 7. http://nugo.dife.de/bioethics/16th_World_Congress_on_Medical_Law/ARTICLES/pdf/334.pdf (accessed 9/24/2019); Petar Klarić: Odštetno pravo. Zagreb 2003, p. 403; Nikšić: Načelo autonomije (Note 85), pp. 590–591.

[88] Maja Proso: Neka pravna pitanja informiranog pristanka u Hrvatskoj legislativi i praksi. In: Zbornik radova Pravnog fakulteta u Splitu 43 (2006), pp. 103–114, here p. 104, footnote 1; Ksenija Turković, Sunčana Roksandić Vidlička, Juraj Brozović: Informirani pristanak djece u hrvatskom zakonodavstvu. In: Turković, Roksandić Vidlička, Maršavelski (Eds.): Hrestomatija hrvatskoga medicinskog prava (Note 85), pp. 572–584, here p. 572, footnote 3.

and Article 40 protects »freedom of conscience and religion«.[89] The first explicit provisions on informed consent were incorporated into Article 29 of the 1991 Healthcare and Health Insurance Act.[90] Then came the 1998 Criminal Code which, inspired by Austrian criminal legislation, regulated unauthorized medical treatment in its Article 241.[91] Two articles from the current Criminal Code bears particular relevance for elaboration of this issue – Medical Malpractice (Article 181), Illicit Removal and Transplantation of Human Body Parts (Article 182).[92]

### *4.1. Act on the Protection of Patients' Rights*

The Act on the Protection of Patients' Rights[93] was adopted to align the national legislation with the 1997 Council of Europe Convention for the Protection of Human Rights and Dignity of the Human Being with regard to the Application of Biology and Medicine (Oviedo Convention).[94] It does not explicitly mention the term informed consent but it regulates the patient's right to information and participation in the decision-making with respect to the intervention he or she is about to undergo. The Croatian legislator has thus embraced the so-called shared decision-making model instead of a pure informed consent model. According to Article 6 of the above Act, »[t]he patient's right to shared decision-making comprises the patient's right to in-

---

[89] The consolidated text of the Constitution of the Republic of Croatia as of 15 January 2014. Edited and translated by the Constitutional Court of the Republic of Croatia. https://www.usud.hr/sites/default/files/dokumenti/The_consolidated_text_of_the_Constitution_of_the_Republic_of_Croatia_as_of_15_January_2014.pdf (accessed 9/24/2019).

[90] Turković: Pravo na odbijanje medicinskog tretmana (Note 86), p. 158.

[91] Sunčana Roksandić Vidlička: Aktualna pitanja pojedinih kaznenih djela protiv zdravlja ljudi u svjetlu donošenja nacrta izmjena hrvatskog Kaznenog zakona. In: Godišnjak Akademije pravnih znanosti Hrvatske 1 (2010), pp. 93–145, here p. 120; Turković: Pravo na odbijanje medicinskog tretmana (Note 86), p. 163.

[92] Criminal Code: The Official Gazette of the Republic of Croatia no. 125/11, 144/12, 56/15, 61/15, 101/17, 118/18.

[93] The Act on the Protection of Patients' Rights: The Official Gazette of the Republic of Croatia no. 169/04, 37/08.

[94] Sanja Babić Bosanac, Ana Borovečki, Kristina Fišter: Patients' Rights in the Republic of Croatia – between the Law and Reality. In: Medicinski glasnik 5 (2008), pp. 37–43, here pp. 39–40.

formation and acceptance or refusal of a diagnosis or therapy.«[95] Some authors claim that the fact that the law has not accepted a pure informed consent model indicates a patient's autonomy restriction.[96] Other Croatian authors, e.g. Vučemilo et al., rightly notice that that is not case here. In fact, this is the third existing model of regulation of the relationship between doctors and their patients. The other two are the paternalistic and the pure informed consent model. In terms of the shared decision-making model, scientific literature qualifies it as advantageous with respect to the pure informed consent one. Vučemilo et al. assert that this model requires equal participation of doctors and their patients in the decision-making process, facilitates information exchange and encourage patients to take the responsibility for their treatment.[97]

Pursuant to Article 8 of the Act on the Protection of Patients' Right, a patient is entitled to obtain comprehensive information on his or her health, recommended examination, potential advantages or risks of their performance, and possible alternatives. Following a verbal request, relevant information is provided in a manner that is understandable to the patient and adapted to his or her age, qualifications and mental ability. In compliance with his or her written and signed statement, a patient with legal capacity has the right to waive his or her right to receive information on his or her health, the expected outcome of his or her treatment and proposed measures (Article 14). Article 15 (1) foresees the only exception in regard to waiving the right to information and it refers to the situation in which »a patient with legal capacity shall be aware of the nature of his or her illness, so as to avoid jeopardizing other people's health.«

The Croatian law protects a patient's autonomy concerning his or her wish to provide someone else, including his or her family members, with the right to obtain notice on his or her health status. According to Article 15 (2), a patient »shall have the right to appoint another person to receive information on his or her condition«.

---

95 When translating provision of this Act, I used the existing translation of the specific provisions from the following article: Babić-Bosanac, Borovečki, Fišter: Patients' Rights in the Republic of Croatia – between the Law and Reality (Note 94), pp. 37–43.
96 Proso: Some Legal Issues on Informed Consent (Note 87), p. 1346.
97 Luka Vučemilo, Sanja Babić-Bosanac, Silvio Altarac, Ana Borovečki: Pristanak obaviještenog pacijenta s posebnim osvrtom na Hrvatsku. In: Liječnički vjesnik 136 (2014), pp. 104–109, here p. 105.

From the aspect of the protection of patients' rights, Article 16 (1) seems to be the most controversial one. In accordance therewith, a patient shall have:

> the right to accept or refuse individual diagnostic or therapeutic procedures, except in the event of a need for an urgent medical intervention when his or her life and health would be endangered or when it could come to his or her permanent impairment or health deterioration if the intervention was not preformed.

This means that a patient shall not decline a medical intervention if the rejection could endanger his or her life or cause permanent health problems. The same Article leads some prominent Croatian authors to conclude that a patient's autonomy is not appropriately protected in the Republic of Croatia. According to Saša Nikšić,[98] this Act differs from other legal regulations in the Croatian legal system, which deals with the protection of patients' rights, particularly from the Criminal Code and Oviedo Convention. Article 16 (1) is a clear evidence thereof and the author believes that the Act on the Protection of Patient's Rights is based on the principle of paternalism. According to another Croatian author, Ksenija Turković, the Act on the Protection of Patient's Rights has imposed both broader and narrower restrictions of the right to patient self-determination than the Oviedo Convention.[99] The restrictions in this Act are narrower than in Oviedo Convention since the latter offers more reasons for restriction of patients' rights, such as public safety, prevention of criminal offences, the protection of public health and the rights and freedoms of other people that are not comprised by the scope of the Croatian Act on the Protection of Patient's Rights.[100] The only explicit restriction of the patient's right to making own decisions in the Act on the Protection of Patient's Rights refers to an individual's health status (Article 7). On the other hand, the Croatian Act on the Protection of Patient's Rights contains broader restriction of patients' rights than the Oviedo Convention does.[101] This particularly relates to the legal provision stipulating that

---

[98] Nikšić: Načelo autonomije (Note 85), pp. 585–591.

[99] Turković: Pravo na odbijanje medicinskog tretmana (Note 86), p. 164.

[100] Convention for the Protection of Human Rights and Dignity of the Human Being with regard to the Application of Biology and Medicine, Article 26 (1). https://www.coe.int/en/web/conventions/full-list/-/conventions/rms/090000168007cf98 (accessed 9/24/2019).

[101] Turković: Pravo na odbijanje medicinskog tretmana (Note 86), p. 164.

a patient shall not decline a medical intervention if such a rejection can lead to permanent health deterioration or death. In the part which deprives patients of the right to refuse treatment that could prevent jeopardizing or permanently deteriorating his or her health, Turković regards Article 16 (1) of the Act on the Protection of Patient's Rights as invalid since it is contrary to the Oviedo Convention which is in the Croatian legal system as a ratified international treaty superior to the former Act and other laws shall be harmonized therewith.[102]

Turković stresses that a doctor's failure to take into consideration patient's refusal of proposed treatment represents unauthorized medical treatment, which is a criminal offence (Article 181 of the applicable Croatian Criminal Code) defined as medical malpractice.[103] Beside the doctor's criminal liability, acting contrary to the patient's also implies civil liability in such cases.[104] Cases in which a patient refuses a medical intervention and can thus put his or her life in danger should be, holds Turković, perceived differently. Neither the European Convention on Human Rights nor the Oviedo Convention fully prefers the principle of individual autonomy, so from the doctors' perspective, Article 16 (1) of the Act on Protection of Patients' Right had better be adhered to.[105]

With respect to the protection of patients' rights in the Republic of Croatia, one should definitely mention the Code of Medical Ethics and Deontology adopted by the Croatian Medical Chamber.[106] Considering the issue of inclusion of the patient's family in making medical decisions relating to his or her health status, two clauses of the above Code bears the greatest relevance. They provide the family with a more important role than the Act on the Protection of Patients' Rights does.

According to Article 2 (4) of the Code, physicians shall respect the rights of mentally competent and conscious patients to freely accept or refuse a certain physician or recommended medical treatment. In case of patients who are not capable of making medical decisions, the referring decision shall be made by their legal representative. Ac-

---

102 Turković: Pravo na odbijanje medicinskog tretmana (Note 86), p. 164.
103 Turković: Pravo na odbijanje medicinskog tretmana (Note 86), p. 164.
104 Turković: Pravo na odbijanje medicinskog tretmana (Note 86), p. 164.
105 Turković: Pravo na odbijanje medicinskog tretmana (Note 86), p. 169.
106 Kodeks medicinske etike i deontologije, pročišćeni tekst. 2016. Hrvatska liječnička komora. https://www.hlk.hr/EasyEdit/UserFiles/3-kodeks-medicinske-etike-i-deonto logije-procisceni-tekst.pdf (accessed 9/24/2019).

cording to Article 2 (5) of the Code, medical aid shall be provided to children and minors, if that has been approved of by their parents or guardians or »elderly family members with legal capacity«. In this light, the Code broadens the circle of potential decision makers with respect to the referring Act. The Act governs that children may be represented only by their legal representatives or guardians (Article 17) whereas the Code envisages the possibility of their representation by competent adult family members.[107]

Article 5 (1), generally dealing with tissue and organ transplantation, sets out that in the event of the brain death of a patient, the physician shall inform the patient's nuclear family about the intention to remove for transplantation purposes his organs and that the removal of organs without the consent of the patient's family is not ethical. This implies that the will of the family is sometimes superior to the autonomy of the patient itself. In compliance with Article 17 (1) of the Croatian Act on the Transplantation of Human Organs for Medical Treatment Purposes,[108] organs from a brain-dead patient may be removed for transplantation purposes unless the individual objected thereto in writing during his or her life. Croatia has accepted the so-called opt-out system, according to which all members of a society can be regarded as potential donors (implied consent model).[109] This puts physicians in an unfavorable position when their patients did not object organ transplantation during their life, but their families do not agree therewith.

## 5. Conclusion

Migration is today depicted as »a defining issue of our time«.[110] It is clear why is that so when the fact that there are one billion migrants in the world today is taken account of, out of which 258 million of

---

107 Pravo pacijenta na suodlučivanje. http://klinika.pravo.unizg.hr/content/pravo-pacijenta-na-suodlucivanje (accessed 9/24/2019).

108 The Official Gazette of the Republic of Croatia no. 144/12.

109 Tomislav Nedić: Pristanak obitelji za uzimanjem organa ili tkiva od preminule osobe radi presađivanja u Republici Hrvatskoj. In: Pravni vjesnik: časopis za pravne i društvene znanosti Pravnog fakulteta Sveučilišta J. J. Strossmayera u Osijeku 33 (2017), pp. 31–50; Murat Civaner, Zümrüt Alpinar, Yaman Örs: Zašto bi opt-out sustav za pribavljanje organa bio pravedniji? In: Synthesis philosophica 25 (2010), pp. 367–376.

110 Lawrence O. Gostin, Ibrahim Abubakar, Ranieri Guerra, Sabina F Rashid, Eric A

migrants have crossed state borders.[111] Modern European and North American countries are faced with rising cultural pluralism, which imposes new challenges on caregivers and healthcare providers since the cultural affiliation of an individual affects people's conduct within a healthcare system.[112] This paper has investigated growing body of literature, which highlights the need to abandon the West-centered concept of informed consent based on individual autonomy and adequately recognize the significant role that family has in the life of individuals with a non-Western background. This literature, as asserted by Insoo Hyun, requires re-conceptualization of autonomy in a way that could enable individuals to act in line with their own values.[113] The idea of relational autonomy pervades in non-Western cultures, such as African and Asian countries with community-oriented individuals, which cannot be said for Western culture where the emphasis is put on notions like »rights, non-interference, self-direction and rational control«.[114]

Yet, there is a major question whether this aspiration for »less individualistic, more process-oriented notion of informed consent« should be welcomed or not.[115] The protection of individual autonomy represents, beyond any doubt, a positive shift from the paternalistic relationship between doctors and their patients, which had been the dominant medical practice until the second half of the 20$^{th}$ century.[116] Does the concept of relational autonomy enrich the current model of informed consent[117] or does it threaten progress in respecting the autonomy of an individual, which has been achieved in the West relatively recently?

All the efforts towards improvement of the self-determination of patients who are members of different non-Western cultures should be greeted.[118] A patient's autonomy, think Kuczewski and Mccruden, can be achieved if the decision on medical treatment is made in the

---

Friedman, Zsuzsanna Jakab: WHO takes action to promote the health of refugees and migrants. In: The Lancet 393 (2019), pp. 2016–2018, here p. 2016.

111 Gostin et al.: WHO takes action (Note 110), p. 2016.

112 Gilbar, Miola: One Size Fits All? (Note 1), p. 377.

113 Hyun: Waiver of Informed Consent (Note 45), p. 15.

114 Osuji: Relational autonomy (Note 54), p. 109.

115 Kuczewski, Mccruden: Informed Consent (Note 1), p. 35.

116 Dove et al.: Beyond individualism (Note 59), p. 151.

117 Osuji: Relational autonomy (Note 54), p. 110.

118 Gilbar, Miola, One Size Fits All? (Note 1), p. 398–399.

same way as other patient's life decisions.[119] Taking account of values in other cultures is supposed to enrich the existing bioethical principles.[120] On that occasion, one should remember that cultures are not »stable, unchanging and harmonious« but »adaptive, open-textured and permeated with opposing interests«.[121] Therefore, one should foster the perception that »(…) beyond the usual cultural norms of the patient's ethnic community and focus more locally on the dynamics of that patient's family and the circumstances surrounding that patient's desire to relinquish his or her decision-making authority.«[122]

The paper supports Turoldo's thesis that in this context, it is individuals and not cultures who are holders of human rights. A good example thereof is Article 25 of the Declaration of Helsinki, proclaimed by the World Medical Association, which confirms that the interests of people and groups are connected with other individuals and groups, but the final decision on the participation in a research study is up to the individual concerned.[123] The Declaration acknowledges that when performing medical research, it may be appropriate to ask for an opinion of family members or of community leaders of research subjects, but such an opinion can never replace patients' freedom of choice.

As far as the Republic of Croatia is concerned, it can be asserted that in this light, it keeps track with European trends, but with a certain delay. Croatia had not legally regulated informed consent until the beginning of the 1990s. For the sake of its European aspirations, Croatia has mostly harmonized its legislation with European standards. Nevertheless, the real nature of the most relevant law governing this issue – the Act on the Protection of Patients' Rights has remained controversial. This Act has not completely embraced the principle of a patient's autonomy and in its Article 16 (1), it favors the paternalistic principle and hence in a certain way, individuals are protected from themselves since they, from the legal viewpoint, cannot reject a medical intervention, which could seriously put their health or life in danger.

---

119 Kuczewski, Mccruden: Informed Consent (Note 1), pp. 34–46.
120 Osuji: Relational autonomy (Note 54), p. 101.
121 Hyun: Waiver of Informed Consent (Note 45), p. 15.
122 Hyun: Waiver of Informed Consent (Note 45), p. 15.
123 Dove et al.: Beyond individualism (Note 59), p. 153.

How legal regulations are implemented in the Republic of Croatia is a completely different issue. Recent research indicates that all the previous legal efforts have not been much of a success and that for cultural and social reasons, the legislation has not managed to improve the real status of a patient in the Croatian legal system.[124] Vučemilo's research has revealed that as much as 54 % of Croatian patients did not gave their consent in writing before a certain medical intervention. A large number of examinees (39 %) disclosed that the doctors made the decision on their treatment totally independently whereas half of them revealed that despite a conversion with their doctors, they did not feel as equal participants in the medical decision-making process.[125]

With respect to the recognition of the role of the family in making medical decisions in Croatia, the Code of Medical Ethics plays an important role, which, in the context of organ transplantation, provides the family with a right that is not even incorporated in referring legal regulations.

---

[124] Babić-Bosanac, Borovečki, Fišter: Patients' Rights in the Republic of Croatia (Note 94), pp. 37–43.

[125] This passage is quoted according to: Marija Selak, Informed Consent Between Bioethical Theory and Medical Practice: A Call for Active Vulnerability. In: Facta Universitatis Series: Law and Politics 15 (2017), pp. 171–179, here p. 174; Luka Vučemilo: Uvažavanje prava bolesnika na obaviještenost o medicinskom postupku tijekom bolničkoga liječenja u Hrvatskoj, PhD dissertation, Medical School, University of Zagreb. Zagreb 2015.

*Pranab Rudra*

# Physician-patient relationship models in Bangladesh and Germany

Abstract
Differences in healthcare services between Bangladesh and Germany are evident. Germany introduced its first health insurance system in 1883, but even after 48 years of independence, Bangladesh is yet to introduce any such system in the country. Conditions in the health sector in Bangladesh remain unsatisfactory, and many reforms are needed. Here I explore the different patient-doctor relationship models in Bangladesh and Germany to improve culturally sensitive understanding of health, thereby contributing to the disease and illness among migrants and emerging public health issues in a globalized world.

## 1. Introduction

The size of Germany is twice as big as Bangladesh but the population number of Bangladesh is significantly higher with respect to Germany. Bangladesh is booming with 158.9 million people.[1] Germany has a total population of 82 million people.[2] Population growth rate in Bangladesh (1.07 %)[3] has decreased over time but is still higher than Germany (0.37 %)[4]. Life expectancy in Bangladesh is 7 years less

---

[1] Bangladesh Statistics: Bangladesh Bureau of Statistics (BBS) Statistics and Informatics Division (SID) Ministry of Planning (2017). http://bbs.portal.gov.bd/sites/default/files/files/bbs.portal.gov.bd/page/a1d32f13_8553_44f1_92e6_8ff80a4ff82e/Bangladesh%20%20Statistics-2017.pdf (accessed 9/24/2019).

[2] Destatis: Statistisches Bundesamt (2017). https://www.destatis.de/DE/Themen/Gesellschaft-Umwelt/Bevoelkerung/Bevoelkerungsstand/Tabellen/liste-zensus-geschlecht-staatsangehoerigkeit.html (accessed 9/24/2019).

[3] The World Bank (2017). https://data.worldbank.org/indicator/SP.POP.GROW?locations=BD (accessed 9/24/2019).

[4] The World Bank (2017). https://data.worldbank.org/indicator/SP.POP.GROW?locations=DE (accessed 9/24/2019).

than in Germany[5] and 12.9 % are living under extreme poverty[6]. 15.2 % of the whole population is undernourished.[7] Compared to Bangladesh, the economy of Germany is at a better state (1 euro equivalents to 95 taka).

When healthcare system between the two countries comes into play, Bangladesh still lacks a functioning health insurance system while Germany introduced its first health insurance system in 1883.[8] Having no health insurance system in Bangladesh, sickness often has fatal consequences, especially for the poor. Unfortunately, patients still need to buy all the medicines from outside the hospitals with no financial support. Moreover, healthcare workers are poorly qualified, low paid and therefore insufficiently motivated and often absent, especially in remote regions of Bangladesh. These add further burden to the physician-patient relationship that is central in medical ethics and is integral to the delivery of high-quality health care in the diagnosis and treatment of ailments.

There are some points to consider when we take the German healthcare system into account. First, it is mandatory to be insured when living, studying, or working in Germany – exception may include some working groups or a particular population.[9] Second, there is a dual system for Germans containing compulsory insurance and a private insurance. Each of these two insurances has their pros and cons. The compulsory insurance, in particular, is based on a concept of a welfare state, meaning that all Germans pay money into the system. Those becoming sick or having an accident receive money from the system for their treatment. However, not every person gets all of the money back he or she has paid in. Until or unless the person is sick, that person cannot receive money from the insurance. However, the system is made as such that everybody pays for those in

---

[5] Central Intelligence Agency: The World Factbook (2017). https://www.cia.gov/library/publications/the-world-factbook/rankorder/2102rank.html (accessed 9/24/2019).

[6] The World Bank (2016). https://www.worldbank.org/en/news/feature/2017/10/24/bangladesh-continues-to-reduce-poverty-but-at-slower-pace (accessed 9/24/2019).

[7] The World Bank (2016). https://data.worldbank.org/indicator/SN.ITK.DEFC.ZS?locations=BD (accessed 9/24/2019).

[8] Reinhard Busse, Miriam Blümel, Franz Knieps, Till Bärnighausen: Statutory health insurance in Germany: a health system shaped by 135 years of solidarity, self-governance, and competition. In: The Lancet 390 (2017), pp. 882–897.

[9] German Healthcare System – Germany Health Insurance System. http://www.germanyhis.com/ (accessed 9/24/2019).

need of help. The majority of people living in Germany have compulsory insurance. The financial income of the person determines how much he or she needs to pay for the insurance. Those who earn less or no money are given the chance to be insured for small amounts. In contrast, with private insurance one needs to pay an amount depending on age and health. The older the person gets, the higher the insurance payment gets in addition to whether he or she have been sick before. The topic of health insurance is very important in Germany not due to its obligation but also the safety concern of the citizens.

When it comes to registered physicians, Germany has almost 4.5 times more physicians than Bangladesh.[10] 68 % of the German physicians are at least 50 years old.[11] The rural areas of Bangladesh have only 1.1 doctors per 10,000 population and 18.2 doctors per 10,000 in urban areas.[12] The patient-physician ratio is quite high in Bangladesh as many doctors are absent or dissatisfied with their current position. Under-five year mortality rate per 1000 live birth is high in Bangladesh (32.4) because the neonatal care is not that developed as in Germany (3.7).[13] Leading cause of death in Bangladesh is cancer (13 %) as there are many cancer-causing pollutants in Bangladesh.[14] In Germany, on the other hand, heart disease (14 %) predominates, mainly due to adiposity.[15]

When we consider the patient-physician relationship, we understand a relationship between physician and patient that is considered as an important determinant of quality healthcare. It has been and remains a keystone of care: the medium in which data are gathered, diagnoses and plans are made, compliance is accomplished, and heal-

---

[10] Bangladesh Statistics (Note 1); Bundesärztekammer. Statistik (2018). https://www.bundesaerztekammer.de/fileadmin/user_upload/downloads/pdf-Ordner/Statistik2018/Stat18AbbTab.pdf (accessed 9/24/2019).

[11] Destatis: Statistisches Bundesamt. https://www.destatis.de/EN/Themes/Society-Environment/Health/Health-Personnel/health-personnel.html (accessed 9/24/2019).

[12] Syed M. Ahmed, Timothy G. Evans, Hilary Standing, Simeen Mahmud: Harnessing pluralism for better health in Bangladesh. In: The Lancet 382 (2013), pp. 1746–1755.

[13] The World Bank: Mortality rate, under-5. https://data.worldbank.org/indicator/SH.DYN.MORT?locations=BD-DE (accessed 9/24/2019).

[14] Centers for Disease Control and Prevention: Global Health – Bangladesh. https://www.cdc.gov/globalhealth/countries/bangladesh/default.htm (accessed 9/24/2019).

[15] State of Health in the EU: Country Health Profile 2017 – Germany https://ec.europa.eu/health/sites/health/files/state/docs/chp_de_english.pdf (accessed 9/24/2019).

ing, patient activation, and support are provided.[16] A trusting and responsive relationship between physician and patient is important for better communication, guiding patients by listening to concerns, better decision making, and negotiating a plan to improve well-being, even when therapeutic interventions fail and alternative therapies should be proposed.

Here I discuss some major factors influencing patient-physician relationship. Physician consultation time plays a major role in physician-patient relationship. Then I explain different physician-patient relationship models. Finally, I explore what could possibly be a relationship model for a German physician and a Bangladeshi patient.

## 2. Factors influencing physician-patient relationship

Overpopulation and poverty significantly affect the decision-making process in the clinical setting. This is currently the situation in Bangladesh. The physicians are underpaid and therefore to live up to their standards they look for scope in private practice, consultation in private hospitals, and so on. Many physicians are generous to look after patients in government hospitals free of charge. However, at the end of the day, they have little or no time left to do so. In a metropolitan city like Dhaka, physicians are even busier and involved in multiple jobs, such as private practice or consultation in private hospitals and have hardly any time available for government hospitals. On the other hand, the patient spends a huge amount of money doing expensive diagnosis either by selling household goods or by taking loans. In many cases, the outcome results in poor or no long-term health improvements. This creates a situation where people are vulnerable economically, physically, and emotionally, that would instead require care with sympathy, active and proper treatment while guiding patients by listening carefully to their concerns, communication and sufficient health information. When patients are burdened with poor economic, physical and emotional state, they are vulnerable and hence undecided to make their own decision for their wellbeing. Their vulnerable state is misused by the physicians since the physicians takes over power to decide what is better for the patient and not let

[16] Mark Lipkin, Sanuel M. Putnam, Aaron Lazare (Eds.): The Medical Interview: Clinical Care, Education, and Research. Berlin 1995.

the patient decide for her/himself. Such burden results in a physician-patient relationship to be very paternalistic.

Since there is only one doctor per 10,000 populations, each physician has to deal with a large number of patients every day. Due to poverty or lack of proper insurance system, many people do not visit physicians until they are really sick. When people from rural areas get sick, they are socially used to taking medicine from the nearby pharmacy or village doctor without any prescription or consulting a registered physician. The drug seller or village doctor has very little training in medicine and provides medicine based on their common sense and experience. The two major reasons that inspire the patients' actions to take service from the village doctor are free consultation and an intimate social relationship towards the villagers. In case the patient sees no improvement, or the illness rapidly gets worse, they then visit the local government hospital.

Transparency International Bangladesh, a Berlin-based global organization against corruption, mentions three main types of corruption in the healthcare system: harassment and bribery, private business by government physicians, and expensive pathological tests.[17] Around 77 % of the physicians are dissatisfied with the present status and aims to do post-graduation for financial solvency and better social status.[18] Little or no emphasis is given on humanities or medical ethics subjects in the medical curriculum, which may also be another reason for poor moral values of the physician.[19] Lack of sufficient nurses and other medical assistants, lack of sufficient medical equipment, and a small number of facilities for training have been reported.[20]

Another important focus in physician-patient relationship is the consultation time between physicians and patient. A systematic review of 67 countries has been performed to find an average primary

[17] Transparency International Bangladesh (2008): National Household Survey 2007 on Corruption in Bangladesh. https://www.ti-bangladesh.org/research/HHSurvey07full180608.pdf pp. 28–30 (accessed 9/24/2019).

[18] Mohidur Rahman, Shibley Rahman, Noreen Begum, A. K. M. Asduzzaman, Md. Shahjahan, Ahmad Firoz, Morshida Sikder Metul: Client Expectation From Doctors: Expectation-Reality Gap. In: Kathmandu University Medical Journal 5 (2007), pp. 566–573.

[19] Munir Talukder: On Patient-Physician Relationships: A Bangladesh Perspective. In: Asian Bioethics Review 3 (2011), pp. 65–84.

[20] Rahman et al.: Client Expectation (Note 18), p. 570.

care physician consultation time.[21] In the review, it is stated that in Germany, the average consultation time is 7.6 minutes, whereas in Bangladesh consultation time averages to merely 2 minutes. However, since these data have been given as average, the range in Bangladesh has been found to be around 48 seconds. Surprisingly, a large proportion of the global population receives only a few minutes of consultation time from their physicians. More specifically, the authors found 18 countries that represent about 50 % of the global population spends around 5 minutes or even less with their physicians. The authors concluded that such an alarmingly short consultation timeframe would hugely influence not only the patient healthcare but also the physician workload.

Another study in Charité Hospital Berlin conducted on 501 patients showed that physicians interrupt patient's conversation after an average time of 19 seconds.[22] When physicians were asked how long the patient would talk unhindered, they expected an average time of around three and a half minutes. Differences in language and culture seem to have an influence on the average length of the patients' monologue. The study suggested physician to listen to a patient for at least a minute without fear of being overwhelmed by their patients' complaints. Therewith the physician gains perspectives that expand the physician's options for treating the patient.

## 3. Different physician-patient relationship models

Emanuel and Emanuel suggested four models based on physician-patient relationship, which are widely used in Western societies.[23] They are described below in detail.

---

[21] Greg Irving, Ana L. Neves, Hajira D. Miller, Ai Oishi, Hiroko Tagashira, Anistasiya Verho, John Holden: International variations in primary care physician consultation time: a systematic review of 67 countries. In: BMJ Open 7 (2017), doi:10.1136/bmjopen-2017-017902.

[22] Teresa Bär: Die spontane Gesprächszeit von Patienten zu Beginn des Arztgesprächs in der hausärztlichen Praxis (9/18/2009). https://refubium.fu-berlin.de/handle/fub188/5268?show=full (accessed 9/24/2019).

[23] Ezekiel Emanuel, Linda Emanuel: Four Models of the Physician-Patient Relationship. In: The Journal of the American Medical Association 267 (1992), pp. 2221–2226.

### *3.1 Paternalistic model*

A traditional and influential model for the physician-patient relationship is paternalism. This model has been widely used in almost all medical codes such as Hippocratic Oath and American Medical Association codes until the mid-20th century.[24] According to Emanuel and Emanuel, paternalistic model consists of physician-patient interaction where physicians are morally obliged to act for the benefit of patient. This means that physicians are obliged to diagnose, identify the etiology, and reduce patient's sufferings by all means. In this model, the physician generally takes the role of the patient's guardian to take rightful initiative for the well-being of the patient. This model has similarity to Veatch's proposed »priestly model« where physicians have the full authority to make their own moral judgments that would benefit the patient.[25] Veatch suggests the physician to act on the »Benefit and do no harm to the patient«.[26]

According to Talukder[27], there are two main criticisms against paternalism: First, Paternalism compromises the patient's autonomy and respect. Buchanan mentions:

> There are two main types of arguments against paternalism. First are the arguments that rely upon a theory of moral rights rooted in a conception of personal autonomy (…). Second are the arguments that meet the paternalist on his own ground and then attempt to cut it from beneath him by showing that his arguments are defective.[28]

Second, paternalism is difficult to practice since it is difficult to be sure, what is best for the patient.[29] When things go wrong in treatment, many paternalists do agree to stake the responsibility to live with the risks involved. However, it all comes down to patients that ultimately have to live the mistakes of the physicians.[30] As an example, Childress and Siegler mention regarding the meaning of health

---

[24] Talukder: On Patient-Physician Relationships (Note 19).
[25] Talukder: On Patient-Physician Relationships (Note 19).
[26] Robert M. Veatch: Models for Ethical Medicine in a Revolutionary Age. In: The Hastings Center Report 2 (1972), pp. 5–7.
[27] Talukder: On Patient-Physician Relationships (Note 19).
[28] Allen Buchanan: Medical Paternalism. In: Philosophy and Public Affairs 7 (1978), pp. 370–390.
[29] Buchanan: Medical Paternalism (Note 28).
[30] Brian McKinstry: Paternalism and the doctor-patient relationship in general practice. In: British Journal of General Practice 42 (1992), pp. 340–342.

and disease that »when the physician insists that cigarette smoking is a disease, but the patient claims that it is merely a nasty habit«.[31] The degree of autonomy has been criticized by Matthews who argues that physicians giving degrees of autonomy to patients only take into account their patients' wishes when they concur with their own.[32] O'Neill adds that consent for each and every aspect of treatment is not necessary; however, consent must be obtained for fundamental aspects of actions or proposals.[33]

### 3.2 *Informative model*

This model focusses primarily on patients since the physician aims to provide patients with all relevant information, including risks, benefits, and alternatives, and then asks them to select their individual medical intervention. Therefore, the patient can choose the best treatment to be given while the physician will offer correct, up-to-date, truthful, and relevant information based on his or her skills. The physician informs the patient of his or her disease condition, the nature of diagnosis that he or she needs to undertake, and the therapeutic inventions. This model is all about facts and patient's values with a very limited role for physician's values. The physician is obliged to act for the patient's will even if he or she believes otherwise. The physician here promotes his or her technical expertise by providing important and truthful information, while consulting others when their knowledge is insufficient. Unlike any other model, the patient's autonomy is given the highest priority.

According to Talukder, this model does not qualify it as an ideal patient-physician model due to minor physician's influence.[34] The author adds that physicians are morally responsible to advise patients in a neutral way regarding the best treatment. The physician should not only inform patients but also suggest the best available treatment option to be able to recover from the disease.

---

[31] Ames F. Childress, Mark Siegler: Metaphors and models of doctor-patient relationships: Their implications for autonomy. In: Theoretical Medicine 5 (1984), pp. 17–30.
[32] Eric Matthews: Can paternalism be modernised? In: Journal of Medical Ethics 12 (1986), pp. 133–135.
[33] Onora O'Neill: Paternalism and partial autonomy. In: Journal of Medical Ethics 10 (1984), pp. 173–178.
[34] Talukder: On Patient-Physician Relationships (Note 19).

Verweij and Lelie reject the informative model since »it obliges the physician to provide the patient with value-free information«.[35] Another criticism by Verweij and Lelie to reject the model is that it »simplifies and impoverishes the physician-patient relationship«.[36] The authors provide four reasons for that. The first reason is that the informative approach lacks empathy of doctors towards their patients. The neutral perspective of facts and information has only a limited place for an empathetic attitude. The second reason would be to not justify or discuss anything regarding patient's preference, since the view of patients is not the concern of the physician. Third, this model does not allow discussing the physician's moral beliefs and experiences with patients. Refraining from such discussion compromises the patient in developing preferences on treatment. Fourth, there is a distinct lack of physician's role to listen, talk and adjust preferential treatment to patients during the course of illness.[37]

### *3.3 Interpretive model*

Patients want their physician not only to provide them with facts or freedom to make their own decisions. They eagerly look upon a counselor or advisor who understands the values to guide them through their illness. Therefore, in this model the physician determines the patient's values and what he or she actually wants. This aids the patient to select the medical intervention that realizes these values. Here the physician takes the role of a counselor or advisor to provide the patient with all the information that is true, correct, and relevant to help the patient in the decision-making process. The physician not only provides mere information but also explains the information with a suggestive approach. According to Veatch, such a model can resemble as a »collegial model« where physician and patient are seen equal like colleagues with a common goal to fight the disease.[38] The relationship between the physician and the patient is based on trust

---

[35] Annique Lelie, Marcel Verweij: Futility without a dichotomy: Towards an ideal physician-patient relationship. In: Bioethics 17 (2003), pp. 21–31.
[36] Lelie, Verweij: Futility without (Note 35), p. 25.
[37] Lelie, Verweij: Futility without (Note 35), pp. 25–26.
[38] Veatch: Models for Ethical Medicine (Note 26).

and compassion without superiority of either side. Rather, respect, mutual understanding, autonomy, and values are taken into account.

According to Talukder, the interpretive model has some limitations.[39] First, there might be differences in the values of the physician and the patient. Since a physician deals with different types of patients and their values, it may sometimes be difficult for a physician to advise their patient according to the value appropriate for that particular patient. Moreover, limited consultation time might also come as a disadvantage. As a result, the physician's values may come as an imposition towards the patient having his or her own value, ultimately going back to a paternalistic model. To this Emanuel and Emanuel say, »[s]uch circumstances may push the interpretive model towards the paternalistic model in actual practice.«[40]

### *3.4 Deliberative model*

Like the informative and interpretive model, this final model focuses on the moral deliberation of patient's values. This means that the physician-patient interaction will encourage the patient to determine and choose the most suitable health-related values (i.e. conscious health behaviors and increased motivation for health-enhancing pursuits) among many different treatment interventions. The physician here is obliged to portray precisely the patient's clinical situation and help clarify certain values that would be preferable to the patient. Both the physician and the patient deliberatively decide what kind of health-related value would be the best to pursue. The deliberation needs to be, in its strict sense, moral and not coerced. Immersing in moral deliberation would help both the physician and patient to judge the importance of alternative values through dialogue and learn to implement the worthy value for clinical treatment. This means that the physician is willing to realize the origin of his values, which may come from her or his family or teachers in medical school, and be more willing to explore other options and negotiate rather than demand patients to comply in clinical settings where values are in conflict. Here, the physician takes the role of a teacher or friend, being more empathetic towards the patient.

---

39 Talukder: On Patient-Physician Relationships (Note 19), p. 74.

40 Emanuel, Emanuel: Four Models (Note 23).

Emanuel and Emanuel mention three fundamental objections related to this model.[41] Some physician may emphasize values more than others, which can conflict with other physicians or patients. Second, recommendations and care should not defer based on an individual physician's value and judgment on patient's value. Third, patients should refrain from revising their values or engage in moral deliberation. This can then easily lead to paternalistic physician-patient interaction.

Talukder criticizes Emanuel and Emanuel's deliberative model mentioning that the physician's role as »teacher« and »friend« are two separate types of relationship. A friend shares an intimate relationship whereas a teacher helps students grow wiser, thus putting them into two distinct dimensions. Furthermore, the author adds that moral deliberation is a lengthy process of discussing values and the significance of a particular treatment, which can, however, be time-consuming.

Despite such drawbacks Emanuel and Emanuel claim that the deliberate model is to be the preferred model and provide six points to justify the preference.[42] First, the ideal version of autonomy is maintained, i. e. patients critically assess, reflect and justify their own actions, values, and preferences whether it is desirable or not. Second, an ideal physician instills the information from literature, art, and culture and reflects the values while making a recommendation to the patient that would best suit and promote his or her well-being. Third, the ideal physician »persuades« the patient and does not »impose« values that might lead to a paternalistic relationship. Fourth, it is important for the patient to understand the health-related values of the physician. A patient can choose a physician based on the matching health-related values of the physician. This means that the patient can switch physicians based on a particular physician's approach, attitude, or values. Fifth, physicians should not only limit themselves to therapy interventions but also promote broader health-related values for the well-being of the patient. Finally, changes in medical care and education should be implemented to address physician's deficiencies in training. Moreover, the physician should not just »spend more

---

41 Emanuel, Emanuel: Four Models (Note 23), p. 2225.

42 Emanuel, Emanuel: Four Models (Note 23), pp. 2225–2226.

time in physician-patient communication but to elucidate and articulate the values underlying their medical care decisions«.[43]

Reach considers patient autonomy as a link between the previous three models and suggests patient education as an ethical pathway.[44] According to the author,

> patient education is the empowering process that in chronic care not only provides information to the patients but also leads them to an interpretation of their own preferences and a deliberation between their, and the HCP's, preferences.[45]

Here the HCP or health care provider primarily focuses on prevention of long-term complications of disease to the patient. Between informative model and interpretative model, there is empathy which transfers down to patient education. According to the author, »empathy consists of imagining what is good from the point of view of the person«.[46] Between interpretative and deliberative model there should be sympathy involved which according to the author is »is imagining what is good for that person«.[47] The physician should not only ask for patient's preference (empathy) but also provide their own preference (sympathy) towards a given therapy. The author adds, instead of speaking to a »patient«, the physician should speak to an autonomous person who according to Frankfurt and Dworkin[48] has the ability to deliberately change their mind while going from informative model (physician first gives the fact) to interpretative model (physician helps patient to elucidate own preference) and finally to deliberative model (the patient gets to choose between different treatment interventions). When such a condition prevails, care has no relation to paternalism or manipulation. Since the deliberative model is reached at the end of the pathway, it is therefore different from the paternalistic model. According to the author, there is no antinomy between autonomy and care as well as between autonomy and patient

---

[43] Emanuel, Emanuel: Four Models (Note 23), p. 2226.

[44] Gérard Reach: Patient autonomy in chronic care: solving a paradox. In: Patient Preference and Adherence 8 (2014), pp. 15–24.

[45] Reach: Patient autonomy (Note 44), p. 20.

[46] Reach: Patient autonomy (Note 44), pp. 15–24.

[47] Reach: Patient autonomy (Note 44), pp. 15–24.

[48] Gerald Dworkin: The Theory and Practice of Autonomy. In: Ethics 102 (1991), pp. 129–139; Harry G. Frankfurt: Freedom of the will and the concept of a person. In: Journal of Philosophy 68 (1971), pp. 5–20.

education, provided that the patient is regarded as an »autonomous person« and not as a »patient«.

## 4. The appropriate model to the Bangladeshi Perspective

Paternalism that undermines a patient's autonomy is a ubiquitous model in Bangladesh. This model is deeply rooted in society and culture. Malpractice and misconduct by physicians while exercising their dominant power are common problems of the public in Bangladesh. Many patients die, or become disabled for life, due to malpractice of the physician.[49] Recently, the trend is that the paternalistic norm is changing and the concept is being questioned.[50]

According to Talukdar, the informative model is too formal for Bangladesh, as this model would be challenging owing to insufficient physicians and patients who are under poverty level. The model may work if both the physician and patient obey moral rules with free legal system.[51] In particular, the private health sector of Bangladesh largely uses this model. Moreover, this model may not be suitable for Bangladesh since many people in rural areas are illiterate or since physicians may exaggerate information in order to attract more patients.

In terms of interpretive model, Talukder believes that health counseling is a necessity for Bangladeshi patients.[52] However, the author adds that the model is inappropriate for Bangladesh since there is a chance that physician's or patient's interpretation may turn biased and the physician can impose his or her values. Unfortunately, there is nobody to verify a particular interpretation as correct or true or take the responsibility if a patient is misguided by physician. Since the moral law (i.e. rules of behavior of people that determine what is »right« or »wrong« but not necessary part of legal and formal law) is still not held firm, Bangladesh would need physicians as counselor with firm moral values to guide patients for overall well-being.

---

49 Talukder: On Patient-Physician Relationships (Note 19).
50 Country Report: Bangladesh. Health ethics in six SEAR countries, World Health Organization (WHO) publication 1991. https://www.who.int/ethics/regions/en/searo_ethics.pdf (accessed 9/24/2019).
51 Talukder: On Patient-Physician Relationships (Note 19).
52 Talukder: On Patient-Physician Relationships (Note 19).

According to Talukder, the last model, the deliberative model that is considered by Emanuel and Emanuel to be the best model, may, unfortunately, be inappropriate for Bangladesh due to the consultation time the physicians have to spend on patients. Unfortunately, patients in Bangladesh cannot afford long consultation time due to poor financial conditions.[53] Moreover, the author believes that since many patients are illiterate, it might not be possible to follow correctly the physician's moral deliberation.

Bangladesh is slowly recovering from corruption. Until or unless corruption is eradicated or controlled, following any of the model mentioned above would be to consider corruption alongside cultural problems, illiteracy and poverty. Nevertheless, patients nowadays expect care, advice, and sympathy from the physician rather than an overly formal relationship.[54] For Bangladesh, an appropriate model can be foreseen where both patient's autonomy and a physician's influence are in balance.[55] Such an alternative model would comprise major components of quality healthcare: reliability, responsiveness, assurance, tangibles (i.e. physical evidence like hospital appearance, equipment, personnel etc.), communication, empathy, and process features (i.e. orderly management of the physician in maintaining proper visiting schedule, structured visiting hours etc.).[56] According to Talukder, in this model physicians' »attitude and practices towards patients« should be changed and physicians would treat their patients as a »care seeker« rather than »client« or »customer« while the patients would perceive their physicians as »caregivers«.[57]

## 5. Physician-patient relationship model in Germany

According to Bertelsmann Stiftung, 80 % of the population in Germany agrees to have a shared-decision making model where both the doctor's and patient's values are respected.[58] The treatment informa-

[53] Talukder: On Patient-Physician Relationships (Note 19); Emanuel, Emanuel: Four Models (Note 23), p. 2226.

[54] Talukder: On Patient-Physician Relationships (Note 19), p. 78.

[55] Talukder: On Patient-Physician Relationships (Note 19), p. 79.

[56] Syed S. Andaleeb, Nazlee Siddiqui, Shahjahan Khandakar: Patient satisfaction with health services in Bangladesh. In: Health Policy and Planning 22 (2007), pp. 263–273.

[57] Talukder: On Patient-Physician Relationships (Note 19), p. 80.

[58] Bertelsmann Stiftung (2018): Gemeinsam entscheiden Junge Ärzte bemängeln

tion is both medical as well as personal. »Shared decision making« (SDM) means that the doctor as well as the patient have the same say and decide together on the further course of treatment. During SDM, the physicians support deliberation on behalf of patients throughout the process.[59] The doctor is the expert in choosing the therapy interventions and judging their effects, whereas the patient contributes his or her personal experiences, needs, and preferences to the decision-making process. Key elements in this model are the exchange of information and – after clarification of all treatment options and coming to a decision – the active involvement of the patient in medical decisions.

SDM is based on »team talk«, »option talk«, and »decision talk«, that depicts a process of collaboration and deliberation.[60] In team talk, support is provided to the patients by making them aware of choices, and guide them through a decision-making process towards a goal. Option talk emphasizes the task to compare alternatives via risk communication principles. This means that the physician compares all the possible options to select one that is best suitable for the patient. Decision talk includes task of arriving at decisions that reflect on the patient's informed preferences, while the patient is guided by the physician's experience and expertise.[61]

In a study conducted in Germany, Thielscher and Schulte-Sutrum analyzed whether the physician-patient relationship has deteriorated during the last years from the perspective of the chambers and the statutory health insurance physician associations. In case the deterioration has occurred, the authors would then look upon the reasons behind the change and provide suggestions in what ways the relationship can be improved.[62] For that, the chairmen or presidents of cham-

---

schlechte Rahmenbedingungen für Patientenbeteiligung im Klinikalltag. https://www.bertelsmann-stiftung.de/fileadmin/files/BSt/Publikationen/GrauePublikationen/VV_SpotGes_Gemeinsam_entscheiden_final.pdf (accessed 9/24/2019).

[59] Glyn Elwyn: Shared Decision Making: A Model for Clinical Practice. In: Journal of General Internal Medicine 27 (2012), pp. 1361–1367.

[60] Glyn Elwyn, Marie A. Durand, Julia Song, Johanna Aarts, Paul J. Barr, Zackary Berger, Nan Cochran, Dominick Frosch, Dariusz Galasiński, Pål Gulbrandsen, Paul K. Han, Martin Härter, Paul Kinnersley, Amy Lloyd, Manish Mishra, Lilisbeth Perestelo-Perez, Isabelle Scholl, Kounosuke Tomori, Lyndal Trevena, Holly O. Witteman, Trudy V. Weijden: A three-talk model for shared decision making: multistage consultation process. In: British Medical Journal 359 (2017), pp. 1–7.

[61] Elwyn et al.: A three-talk (Note 60).

[62] Christian Thielscher, B. Schulte-Sutrum: Development of the Physician-patient

bers of medicine and associations of statutory health insurance physicians were comprehensively interviewed and 5 out of 10 chairmen stated a change from the paternalistic to the shared decision-making model. 5 respondents stated that patients' confidence in the entire medical profession has declined in the sense of a loss of image for the entire occupational group. On the other hand, none of the respondents said that trust in the individual physician-patient relationship is deteriorating. 8 out of 10 respondents stated that patients learn more about their illness, especially via the Internet. 4 out of 10 respondents agreed that patients have a higher expectation in the sense of a claim to heal. 4 out of 10 chairmen agreed that physicians are underpaid. Therefore, physicians communicate too little with the patients.[63]

## 6. A German physician – Bangladeshi patient relationship model

According to the Federal Statistical Office, there are around 14,150 Bangladeshi migrants in Germany from a total population of 10.9 million foreigners (2018).[64] Previously, we have seen that Bangladeshi individuals are accustomed to a more paternalistic model of relationship. Although it does take time to adapt to the freedom of speech in Germany, encouraging patient autonomy of Bangladeshi migrants may have a positive effect on therapeutic inventions. Cultural background also plays a major role within the physician-patient relationship. For instance, a Bangladeshi may have different expectations from the physician or they are used to involve family members to decide for them what would be a suitable therapeutic option. Moreover, culture-based norms relating to sex and gender can affect the relationship between physician and patient, e.g. rejection of gynecological treatment from a German male physician. Religious beliefs may also affect physician-patient communication and the patients' willingness to agree to particular treatments. To cope up with such differences, development of a good relationship with the patient with

Relationship in Germany during the Last Years from the Perspective of the Heads of Chambers and KVs. In: Gesundheitswesen 78 (2016), pp. 8–13.

63 Thielscher, Schulte-Sutrum: Development of the Physician-Patient (Note 62).

64 Destatis: Statistisches Bundesamt. https://www-genesis.destatis.de (accessed 7/07/2019).

a different background is necessary. Furthermore, experience in treating many foreigners may help understand their background and their mindset. Although a smooth communication is an important factor in such a relationship model, it is however not easy for physician and patient to understand each other. A lack of understanding may often result in difficulties in the relationship. Many physicians cannot feel or perceive what the patient actually thinks and reach a common ground.[65] As a result, physicians feel frustrated to encounter reserved behavior from the patient. Patients may insist on getting prescriptions and often, physicians that prescribe more medicaments, are seen as good ones by patients. Expression of pain varies from culture to culture and many times when married couples from Bangladesh are living in Germany, the husbands speak on behalf of their wives. Due to the language barrier, the Bangladeshi migrants do not feel that the physicians take their pain seriously or that the physician's response is insufficient. Moreover, many migrants may encounter discrimination based on their origin, nationality, or language.[66]

Betancourt and Cervantes propose a model for cross-cultural care where any patients irrespective of race, ethnicity, culture, class, or language receive the tools and skills for quality care.[67] This model is built on four aspects. First is the assessment of core cross-cultural issues. Here physicians may be unaware of »hot-button« issues that may result in patients losing trust in the physician. To avoid cross-cultural misunderstandings, the authors mention five issues which should be taken into account: »styles of communication; mistrust and prejudice; decision-making and family dynamics; traditions, customs and spirituality; and sexual and gender issues«.[68] Second is exploring the meaning of illness from the perspective of the patient. The patient's explanation can be exotic or mundane, but understanding their perspective would come very useful for the physician. Third is determining the social context, which is further divided into migra-

[65] Kristina Würth, Wolf Langewitz, Stella Reiter-Theil, Sylvie Schuster: Their view: difficulties and challenges of patients and physicians in cross-cultural encounters and a medical ethics perspective. In: BMC Medical Ethics 19 (2018), pp. 1–10.
[66] Würth et al.: Their view (Note 65).
[67] Joseph R. Betancourt, Marina C. Cervantes: Cross-cultural medical education in the United States: Key Principles and Experiences. In: The Kaohsiung Journal of Medical Sciences 25 (2009), pp. 471–478.
[68] Betancourt, Cervantes: Cross-cultural (Note 67), p. 473.

tion, literacy and language, life control, social stressor and supports.[69] Finally, both physician and patient should engage in negotiation. Diverse sociocultural backgrounds add complexity to the situation and therefore the physician should skillfully try to convey messages to patients that they can easily comprehend while valuing their belief system.

## 7. Conclusion

Understandably, there seems to be no ideal model that encompasses all cultures and all societies. As we have seen, each model has some pros and cons and draws attention to improve it further. Overall, the consultation time, physician-patient ratio, balance of patient autonomy and physician's influence, healthcare framework, and socio-economic conditions can all be improved to instill an efficient physician-patient relationship model. As with time, the patient-physician relationship has gone through significant evolution and is still evolving. Further research is warranted to sort out more determinants or to predict any further change in the model of patient heterogeneity that will be needed to cope with the future.

[69] Betancourt, Cervantes: Cross-cultural (Note 67), p. 474.

*Sylvia Agbih*

# Understanding vulnerability and deliberations on justice – the case of health care for refugees and asylum seekers in Germany

Abstract
The main concern of this contribution is to further develop an understanding of human vulnerability and what it means for us from an ethical perspective both in general as well as in the particular situation of health care for refugees and asylum seekers. After an introduction to this situation, the next and major part explores the meaning of the term vulnerability as well as the current debate on concepts of vulnerability. Both the term as well as the use of concepts of vulnerability seem inherently ambiguous. Coming from this more abstract and general level of deliberation into concrete questions of health care for refugees and asylum seekers is taken on by testing the taxonomy of vulnerability developed by Mackenzie, Rogers and Dodds. This test confirms that navigating the positive and negative effects of using vulnerability as a guideline for the practical necessity of distributing resources remains a challenging task. Yet, the conclusion is not to forfeit those concepts. The use and usefulness of the taxonomy as a method needs to be tested, reflected, and discussed in more detail but the focus of the last brief part of this paper turns to basic questions of how our understanding of vulnerability is linked to matters of justice.

## 1. Introduction: The Situation of Refugees and Asylum Seekers concerning Health Care in Germany

The terms »refugee«, »asylum seeker« and »asylum entitlement« are legally strictly defined according to the Geneva Refugee Convention and the German asylum law. Entitlement and access to health care depend on approval according to these legal frameworks. Since the need for health care does not depend on legal status, ethical considerations apply to a wider group here, even if they are not legally approved. So, the terms »refugee« and »asylum seeker« in this text include all people who come seeking protection from war, persecution, natural catastrophe, hunger, poverty, or other for them unbearable situations.

The German Health Care System is a public-private-partnership system based on compulsory membership in mostly statutory but also private health insurances with joint state and expert control over reimbursement of medical services. The sickness funds provide immediate treatment without or with very low out-of-pocket expenses. This means that generally everybody who is part of the system has access to health care provisions. Since membership is compulsory, the cost of the insurance is carried jointly by the employer and the employee. Self-employed persons are obliged to join a private insurance. In case of unemployment the cost of health care is taken on by the social aid according to the Social Code Book XII. So, over all, most people living in Germany are insured.

Yet there are persons or groups of persons who are not absorbed by this system for different reasons e.g. homeless people who do not register anywhere, persons without papers, migrants from European countries or elsewhere whose health insurance is no longer valid and others[1]. Even though emergency care could be provided de jure, de facto there is no public facility taking care of the health needs of persons without papers that does not pose the threat of informing authorities about their undocumented status. This leads to the situation that health care is not accessible for them.

NGOs like Doctors of the World offer very good support but the capacity of voluntary organizations is limited.[2] They cannot fully take on a responsibility of the state. This situation raises serious ethical concerns regarding (public) health care.

Healthcare for refugees and all asylum seekers who are legally registered is not part of the insurance system but regulated by a federal law, the Asylum Seekers' Benefits Act[3] (AsylbLG) and funded by

---

[1] Maren Mylius, Andreas Frewer: Zugang zu medizinischer Versorgung von MigrantInnen ohne legalen Aufenthaltsstatus. Zwischen Notfallversorgung, Infektionsschutz und humanitärer Hilfe. In: Zeitschrift für Menschenrechte 9 (2015), pp. 102–120; Maren Mylius: Die medizinische Versorgung von Menschen ohne Papiere in Deutschland. Studien zur Praxis in Gesundheitsämtern und Krankenhäusern. Bielefeld 2016; Zentrale Ethikkommission der Bundesärztekammer: Versorgung von nicht regulär krankenversicherten Patienten mit Migrationshintergrund. Stellungnahme. In: Deutsches Ärzteblatt 110 (2013), pp. A 899–A 903.

[2] Dagna Frydryszak, Anne-Laure Macherey: Legal Report On Access To Healthcare In 17 Countries. MdM International Network 2016. https://mdmeuroblog.files.wordpress.com/2016/11/mdm-2016-legal-report-on-access-to … (accessed 9/24/2019).

[3] Deutscher Bundestag: Asylbewerberleistungsgesetz. AsylbLG 1993; Georg Classen: Stellungnahme zur öffentlichen Anhörung des Gesundheitsausschusses.https://www.

the municipality asylum seekers are attached to, not by the statutory health insurance. So, refugees and asylum seekers are excluded from the common solidarity system of the sickness funds.

This applies for the first 18 months as long as they are in the application process. During this period, according to §4 of the AsylbLG, access to Health Care is restricted to the treatment of acute diseases and pain; maternity care and vaccinations are provided, chronic conditions and assistive appliances e. g. for disabled persons are not covered. According to §6 of the AsylbLG some exceptions could be made so that e. g. victims of violence and torture or children might be granted treatment on a case-by-case level.

Moreover, under the AsylbLG access to healthcare in many communities requires a more complicated administrative procedure.[4] These procedures vary in the different German states and communes since the details of the implementation of the AsylbLG underlie the authority of the states. The initial system requires a so called Behandlungsschein (treatment voucher) granted by the communal administration as well as an approval of the particular treatment. This means that the final decision about a medical intervention is taken by administrative staff with no medical training. In recent years, some states have opted for the so-called Bremer Modell providing asylum applicants with an E-Health-Card (EHIC) which does not change the restrictions nor the difference in financing of the AsylbLG but lowers the administrative work load both for medical practitioners as well as for the patients.

After these 18 months or once the applicant gains a status as refugee according to the Geneva Refugee Convention or asylum according to the German Constitution or subsidiary protection, health care and social aid are regulated according to the Social Code Books (II, V, XII) analog to German citizens. However, according to legal amendments of the AsylbLG[5] (last made 2016, 2017 and 2019) social benefits including health care can be downgraded under specific circumstances, basically as a form of sanction if asylum applicants are

---

bundestag.de/resource/blob/426800/f496b296a808fe481c3a4285cd22a7f1/ESV-Georg-Classen-data.pdf (accessed 9/24/2019).

[4] Wolfgang Günther, Renate Reiter, Phillip Florian Schmidt: Migration, Integration und Gesundheit. In: Oliver Decker, Steffen Kailitz, Gert Pickel, Antje Röder, Julia Schulze Wessel (Eds.): Handbuch Integration. Wiesbaden 2019, pp. 1–14.

[5] Deutscher Bundestag: Asylbewerberleistungsgesetz (Note 3), §1a.

judged not to be compliant especially regarding proves of their identity.[6] So, restricted entitlement to health care can be extended beyond 18 months.

Apart from the restrictions in entitlement it is important to note that even once full access to healthcare is granted by law, asylum seekers face many obstacles receiving adequate medical care and treatment due to language problems in the absence of trained and paid interpreters in the system, lack of procedural knowledge concerning the German health care system and (perceived) cultural barriers.

In summary it can be stated that health care for asylum applicants is restricted and impeded on all levels of entitlement to, access to and quality of care.[7]

This seems odd when at the same time refugees and asylum seekers are often described as a vulnerable group. Does this not imply they may need more (health) care rather than less? Indeed, the seemingly neutral description of people as vulnerable is mostly used to make a normative claim and legitimize special interventions and supportive measures for a particular group or population. More or less explicitly and intuitively these normative claims refer somehow to principles of justice. What constitutes the normative basis? What exactly do we mean with vulnerable? What other effects does it have to describe a whole heterogeneous group of people as vulnerable? And how exactly are refugees vulnerable?

---

[6] Deutscher Bundestag: Sachstand. Sanktionen im Leistungsrecht für Asylbewerber und Flüchtlinge Asylbewerberleistungsgesetz, Zweites und Zwölftes Buch Sozialgesetzbuch. Wissenschaftliche Dienste WD 6 – 3000 – 053/16. Berlin 2016; Ulrike Davy: Refugee Crisis in Germany and the Right to a Subsistence Minimum: Differences that ought not to be. In: Georgia Journal of International and Comparative Law 7 (2019) pp. 367–450.

[7] Günther, Reiter, Schmidt: Migration, Integration und Gesundheit (Note 4), pp. 1–14; Sylvia Agbih: Gesundheitsversorgung für Flüchtlinge aus ethischer Perspektive: Wo fangen die Fragen an? In: Andreas Frewer, Lutz Bergemann, Caroline Hack, Hans G. Ulrich (Eds.): Die kosmopolitische Klinik. Globalisierung und kultursensible Medizin. Jahrbuch Ethik in der Klinik, Band 10. Würzburg 2017, pp. 41–75; Judith Wenner, Oliver Razum: Die gesundheitliche Versorgung Geflüchteter – von Gleichheit und Ungleichheit. In: Andreas Frewer, Lutz Bergemann, Caroline Hack, Hans G. Ulrich (Eds.): Die kosmopolitische Klinik. Globalisierung und kultursensible Medizin. Jahrbuch Ethik in der Klinik, Band 10. Würzburg 2017, pp. 75–93.

## 2. Reflecting on Vulnerability

### *2.1 The term vulnerability – approaching meaning*

#### 2.1.1 Vulnerability – term and meaning in every-day language

A first step to understand what we mean with vulnerability and which repercussion, side-effects or implicit consequences it may have to call someone vulnerable, is a reflection of the meaning we generally connect more or less implicitly to the word. Following I do not offer a complete analysis of the term but some initial explorations.

The term vulnerability stemming from the Latin word vulnus meaning wound, expresses that somebody (or something) could be wounded by somebody or something. It expresses a possibility or potential to be harmed and is often defined as susceptibility to harm or as being at higher risk of harm. Yet, vulnerability and risk are not the same. Vulnerability seems to describe a particular relation of risk to resources or something we might want to call resilience (without going into the discussion on the different concepts of resilience, what is meant here is a capacity to cope with adverse events to maintain health and well-being). So, vulnerability as exposure to harm while there is – for different reasons – a lack of resources, protective factors or coping capacity to deal with this exposure. The risk of harm as such is not necessarily special since all human beings and in fact all life is in constant danger of being harmed. The reasons why someone cannot defend or protect herself or himself are manifold and the particular vulnerability seems to be due to these reasons. Vulnerability is not just a higher risk but seems a higher risk or exposure to harm in connection with the lack of means to protect oneself or develop resilience.

#### 2.1.2 Synonyms

The general use of the term vulnerability includes both being susceptible to physical injury as well as to emotional or psychological harm. What exactly harm is would be worth thinking about but is not further explored here due to the scope of this paper. Different situations entail the risk for particular kinds of harm and in what way a person is especially vulnerable depends on the individual circumstances – which is exactly what needs to be figured out when we think of due measures of protection.

Looking at synonymous expressions and exploring the meaning of being vulnerable we find descriptions like being fragile, frail, exposed, naked, defenseless, helpless, weak, unsound, powerless, needy, dependent and therefore at someone's mercy. Literally thinking about vulnerability to the end confronts us with our dependency, our limits and finitude. Therefore, being vulnerable is generally regarded as not desirable and carries a touch of the unwanted and dangerous. Needs and neediness, dependency and vulnerability seem to undermine our autonomy and somehow seem to be a source of shame and maybe even feelings of guilt since we perceive ourselves as indebted to those helping us. We rather like to conceive of ourselves as independent, skillful, competent, and autonomous. Therefore, we might repress feelings of vulnerability although we know how vulnerable we are even as healthy grown-ups. Moreover, as Scully[8] analyses sharply scrutinizing how people with disability are regarded as vulnerable: there are vulnerabilities and dependencies tagged as permitted and normal in contrast to those defined as not normal and not acceptable. According to Scully

> permitted dependencies are naturalized and normalized. They are met and supported without question, and in doing so the vocabulary of vulnerability is never used. Other people, and groups, will have needs that fall outside the normative limit. These are nonpermitted dependencies. They are figured as abnormal and classed as rendering those people as especially vulnerable.[9]

The crucial question is: who defines this? Scully describes the social construction of vulnerability from a feminist perspective as follows:

> Normative dependencies are, tautologically, the dependencies of the normative citizen, and for reasons exhaustively articulated by feminist theorists the normative citizen of moral and political philosophy is likely to be male, white, and heterosexual. He will probably be nondisabled as well[.][10]

And certainly, the normative citizen is not a refugee.

---

[8] Jackie L. Scully: Vulnerability and Dependence: On Bodies, Disability and Power. In: Catriona Mackenzie, Wendy Rogers, Susan Dodds (Eds.): Vulnerability. Oxford 2014, pp. 204–222.

[9] Scully: Vulnerability and Dependence (Note 8), pp. 204–222, here p. 217.

[10] Scully: Vulnerability and Dependence (Note 8), pp. 204–222, here p. 217.

### 2.1.3 Contrasting meaning

Looking at the contrast of vulnerability we find what we attribute to our super heroes and goddesses: being (almost) invulnerable, invincible, powerful, strong, robust, healthy, resilient, well-fortified, independent, unlimited, even endless or everlasting. Interestingly though, the heroes we admire most do struggle with some kind of weak point and vulnerability. Otherwise, it seems there would be no story to tell. As much as we adore strength, invulnerability seems inhuman and we like those heroes who have some human sides, some vulnerable sides, so we can identify with them. In close social relationships like in friendship and partnership one essential feature is trust, so that we can show and share our weaknesses and vulnerability and still feel safe. It seems a relief to have spaces where we can let go of the masks of invulnerability.

So, our evaluation of vulnerability and invulnerability is somewhat ambiguous. We place very high value on independence and since vulnerability is closely related to neediness, dependence and being at someone's mercy, we associate it more with negative experiences, we rather do not have vulnerability. Yet, since we cannot achieve being invulnerable, we build strategies of permitted, normal vulnerabilities and special, abnormal ones. Do we categorize in order to cope with our neediness and not to feel too vulnerable? And at the same time, we somehow value vulnerability as human. Vulnerability might enable us to develop empathy. Zagorac suggests that vulnerability could be a positive force motivating richer personal development as well as richer social contacts – if we accept our vulnerabilities.[11] A similar line is followed by Brené Brown.[12]

The ambiguity remains. Even though there are positive aspects – and for both our theoretical understanding of vulnerability as well as for our self-conception as human beings it seems crucial to look at them more closely – the negativity is not washed away. It is important to recognize this since labelling other people as vulnerable has more than one effect. My thesis here is that vulnerability is not merely descriptive even though it is often attempted to use it as a

---

[11] Ivana Zagorac in her contribution and discussion during the BMBF Symposium Ulm (3/14/2019); Ivana Zagorac: What Vulnerability? Whose Vulnerability? Conflicts of Understanding in the Debate on Vulnerability. In: Facta Universitatis, Law and Politics 15 (2017), pp. 157–169.

[12] Brené Brown: Verletzlichkeit macht stark. München 2013.

description of e. g. a population or group in social and health sciences. Typically, this goes along with a claim for special protection and interventions for this vulnerable group. But since the term vulnerability in itself carries a normative level more or less explicitly (and I would say a more negative one) it has side-effects. This seems to be at the core of the growing critical discourse on concepts of vulnerability, which we now turn to.

## *2.2 Concepts of Vulnerability*

### 2.2.1 Critical points

Concepts of vulnerability seem to have appeared first in research ethics. The use of the term vulnerable group became popular since the 1980ies through the Belmont Report[13] published in 1979. Since then concepts of vulnerability are being widely used in research ethics as well as in public health practice, health policy documents, and health research.[14] The term and concepts of vulnerability can also be found in other fields like philosophy, theology, social and political science or environmental studies and ecology[15]. Brown, Ecclestone and Emmel call it a buzzword of our time and state that

> the concept of vulnerability has come to play a prominent role in academic, governmental and everyday accounts of the human condition. Policy makers and practitioners are now concerned with addressing vulnerability through an expansive range of interventions.[16]

---

[13] The National Commission for the Protection of Human Subjects of Biomedical and Behavioral Research: The Belmont Report. Ethical Principles and Guidelines for the Protection of Human Subjects of Research. 1979. https://www.hhs.gov/ohrp/regulations-and-policy/belmont-report/read-the-belmont-report/index.html (accessed 9/24/2019).

[14] Verina Wild: Vulnerabilität. In: Christian Lenk, Gunnar Duttge, Heiner Fangerau (Eds.): Handbuch Ethik und Recht der Forschung am Menschen. Heidelberg, Berlin 2014, pp. 297–298; Florencia Luna: Elucidating the Concept of Vulnerability. Layers not Labels. In: International Journal of Feminist Approaches to Bioethics 2 (2009), pp. 120–138.

[15] Daniel Burghardt, Markus Dederich, Nadine Dziabel, Thomas Höhne, Diana Lohwasser, Robert Stöhr, Jörg Zirfas (Eds.): Vulnerabilität. Pädagogische Herausforderungen. Stuttgart 2017.

[16] Kate Brown, Kathryn Ecclestone, Nick Emmel: The Many Faces of Vulnerability. In: Social Policy & Society 16 (2017), pp. 497–510, here p. 497.

The dominant traditional accounts of vulnerability describe certain populations and subpopulations like the elderly, women, children, refugees and others as vulnerable. The proclaimed purpose of this classification is to identify who needs protection and support. At a first glance this may seem laudable. But this labelling of a whole diverse group as generally vulnerable has led to substantial criticism,[17] namely: Labelling populations and subgroups is too simplistic overlooking real complexities. It is in fact stereotyping and has a stigmatizing effect since, as explored earlier on, there are generally mostly negative connotations to vulnerability. Depicting a whole actually diverse group of people as vulnerable leads to overlooking their capacities, their agency, resources and potentials and fosters a common picture of e.g. »the« refugee as a powerless object of our charity. In this way, using vulnerability could give rise to paternalistic practices.

Moreover, labelling some people as vulnerable assumes that there are others who are not vulnerable, who are – normal? There is an implicit assumption of a kind of average baseline of strength or health or resilience and those below are defined as vulnerable.[18] This supports Scully's analysis of permitted and non-permitted vulnerabilities.

Apart from identifying those in need, concepts of vulnerability are used for prioritization: who needs support most and first? These are uncomfortable questions we may be forced to ask in situations when we face limited resources. The search for criteria to make such decisions is a deeply challenging one. The danger here is to deem vulnerability as neutral not reflecting assumptions and pre-conditions of our evaluation. The judgement on who is vulnerable is tied very closely to evaluations of who is worthy and deserving. This again is entangled with unspoken concepts of normal and permitted needs and vulnerabilities.

---

[17] Carol Levine, Ruth Faden, Christine Grady, Dale Hammerschmidt, Lisa Eckenwiler, Jeremy Sugarman: The limitations of »vulnerability« as a protection for human research participants. In: The American Journal of Bioethics AJOB 4 (2004), pp. 44–49; Luna: Elucidating the Concept (Note 10), pp. 120–138; Anthony Wrigley, Angus Dawson: Vulnerability and Marginalised Populations. In: Drue H. Barrett, Gail Bolan, Angus Dawson, Leonard Ortmann, Andreas Reis, Carla Saenz (Eds.): Public Health Ethics: Cases Spanning the Globe. Public Health Ethics Analysis. Cham 2016, pp. 203–240; Brown, Ecclestone, Emmel: The many faces (Note 16), pp. 497–510; Florencia Luna: Identifying and evaluating layers of vulnerability – a way forward. In: Developing World Bioethics 19 (2018), pp. 86–95.

[18] Luna: Elucidating the Concept (Note 14), pp. 120–138.

Brown, Ecclestone and Emmel analyze this critically on a socio-political level by looking at what implications the use of vulnerability concepts might have on our understanding of citizenship and the relations between state and citizen.[19] One of their main concerns is an expansion of state-sponsored social control, going along with a diminished view of the human subject, and a paradoxical effect of labelling people as vulnerable since »individuals regulate their own behavior in ways that conform to particular norms about ›correct‹ or ›appropriate‹ behaviors.«[20] This means that people tend to behave more helpless since this is expected of them as vulnerable persons. Finally, this cycle leads to patronizing disempowerment and in fact increased lived vulnerability.

According to the authors challenges and tasks for further research are: a clearer definition of the term, thereby also clarifying differing operationalizations; being aware of implicit normativity bearing the danger of social control as well as psychologisation and individualization of social problems; overcoming imbalance in research since there are more theoretical debates and not enough empirical research into experiences of different stakeholders.

### 2.2.2 Encompassing two basic conceptions of vulnerability

In the discussion on vulnerability, two main concepts of understanding vulnerability can be discerned: a broad view of vulnerability as universal feature or condition of human life and a more narrow understanding of vulnerability as being tied to concrete circumstances, groups, certain phases in life or other specific attributes.[21] Both views encompass important aspects and both views face some criticism at the same time.

The broad view is said to be simply too broad since according to this understanding all human beings and in fact all life in general is vulnerable. Luna argues: »Whilst it is true that everyone is exposed to suffering, deterioration, and death, this is not the relevant point. (…) It is not the universal human condition that public policies target but

[19] Brown, Ecclestone, Emmel: The many faces (Note 16), pp. 497–510.

[20] Brown, Ecclestone, Emmel: The many faces (Note 16), pp. 497–510, here p. 500.

[21] Wrigley, Dawson: Vulnerability and Marginalised (Note 17), pp. 203–240; Luna: Elucidating the Concept (Note 15), pp. 120–138.

specific persons or groups in need of safeguards, protection or empowerment.«[22]

According to Luna's understanding there could not be specific vulnerabilities if everyone is vulnerable which would make it impossible to use the concept to protect or empower those in need. At the same time though, some form of specific vulnerability could be found for almost every group of human beings so that even in a narrow view we face the problem of an inflationary use of the term vulnerability. This threatens to make the concept useless. Moreover, when the narrow view assumes that some people are vulnerable and others are not, this is what easily leads to the aforementioned processes of stereotyping and stigmatization.

So, is the concept useless? What does it help if no one even knows what it is? Should we forfeit such a concept?

It seems to me that there are good reasons to at least try and rescue vulnerability before discarding it completely. Mainly – to put it very briefly – because we experience and see situations in human life that we can hardly describe and understand otherwise. Moreover, in practical contexts, vulnerability is already established as concept and every concept has and will always have flaws, there is no perfect one. This lies in the nature of conceptualization. Whilst this ought not to be a cheap excuse, the task remains to keep observing and reflecting the effects of the use of such a concept critically. Then, how should we understand and frame vulnerability?

I want to argue that we need both conceptions and need to understand vulnerability as both broad and narrow. Looking at the meaning of the term reflected on before, we can already see elements of both understandings. An encompassing understanding discerns two levels or dimensions of vulnerability rather than two different, separate concepts. To my mind it seems very true or adequate to describe vulnerability as part of our human condition. This human condition the way I understand it is not to be taken as a list of attributes we possess and it is far from trying to define what or who we human beings are as such. It is rather an insight into the conditions we find ourselves living in. An insight we gain through experience.[23] It is in the reflec-

---

[22] Florencia Luna: ›Vulnerability‹, an Interesting Concept for Public Health: The Case of Older Persons. In: Public Health Ethics 7 (2014), pp. 180–194, here p. 185.
[23] Wilhelm Kamlah: Philosophische Anthropologie. Sprachkritische Grundlegung und Ethik. Mannheim, Wien, Zürich 1972.

tion on our life that we find ourselves fundamentally vulnerable. Which does not mean that we feel vulnerable all the time in our everyday lives (though our life is in fact vulnerable every second). Rather, this fundamental vulnerability manifests itself in certain situations, phases and under specific circumstances. These situations are not the same for every individual and are not uniform across similar situations at different times. I might feel very weak and vulnerable when sick and in pain today, tomorrow the same situation may evoke my resistance, resilience or even anger, which in turn might make me feel and be very strong in the way I cope with the situation. Despite differences, we all know what it means to feel and be vulnerable – this insight into our shared human condition could be a safeguard against stigmatization of those who are in a vulnerable situation.

We are very likely to find many similarities and commonalities looking at when people are vulnerable and how vulnerability manifests. But at the same time these manifestations differ in each individual person and situation. So, (in my view, differing from Luna's analysis) universal vulnerability does not mean that we are all vulnerable in the same way all the time. Therefore, on the basis of an understanding of vulnerability as feature of our human condition, it is not only possible but even called for to develop a pragmatic concept of vulnerability that is more specific and context-bound in order to help us to discern situations that entail a higher risk of exposing people to harm they cannot protect themselves from. In this respect Luna's conception of layers of vulnerability could be very fruitful because it enables us to reflect the complexities of concrete living conditions, the multiple structural determinants and their interfaces and interplay that render people indeed vulnerable.

Acknowledging different sources of vulnerability, namely inherent, dispositional and pathogenic, the taxonomy of vulnerability developed by Mackenzie, Rogers and Dodds[24] takes both universal and specific vulnerability into account. Adding two different states of vulnerability – dispositional and occurrent – discerns more acute risks from dormant ones and therefore offers hints which exacerbations or cascade effects could still be prevented.

---

[24] Catriona Mackenzie, Wendy Rogers, Susan Dodds: Introduction: What Is Vulnerability and Why Does It Matter for Moral Theory? In: Catriona Mackenzie, Wendy Rogers, Susan Dodds (Eds.): Vulnerability. Oxford 2014, pp. 1–33.

While agreeing with Luna's criticism of taxonomies and categorization[25] because they always bear the danger and disadvantage of illusionary clarity, undue simplification and rigidity, this might at the same time be a necessary risk to run. Without some sort of framework or guideline to disentangle different intersections and layers of vulnerable situations we remain with the vulnerable-group-generalization. The challenge seems to be to keep up the awareness that this taxonomy, like any other categorical system, is not concrete reality but an analytical instrument with its limitations and that we are responsible for the kind of categories we build as well as for the way we use them. With this critical notion in mind a taxonomy could be used as one of the steps or means to gain understanding and necessary differentiation.

## 2.3 *How are refugees in Germany vulnerable concerning their health?*

### 2.3.1 Using the taxonomy by Mackenzie et al.

This section shows a first attempt to use the taxonomy of vulnerability by Mackenzie, Rogers and Dodds for assessing health vulnerability of refugees. Considered are health conditions and access to health care for adult refugees/asylum seekers in Germany. Admittedly, this is still a very generalized group and the category refugee/asylum seeker includes very heterogeneous people with very different stories. At the same time the fact of flight itself constitutes specific situational features that affect health and shape the possibilities of access to the German health care system. This does not imply that the whole group is vulnerable the same way. Rather, the purpose is to map out different kinds of situational vulnerabilities. Therefore, it seems useful to start with this categorization and then subsequently analyze more differentiated and finer grained after this first assessment e.g. for accompanied versus unaccompanied minors, people from specific religious, political or sociocultural backgrounds etc. Building up further exploration from there, it would be interesting to see whether and how intersectionality is reflected in the taxonomy.

The taxonomy of vulnerability according to Mackenzie, Rogers and Dodds discerns two states of vulnerability which helps to differ-

---

[25] Luna: Identifying and evaluating (Note 17), pp. 86–95, here p. 90.

entiate dispositions that are basically there but dormant in the sense of not acute (dispositional state) from those that occur acutely in a specific situation (occurrent state). Both states could stem from different sources: while inherent vulnerabilities are those we find tied to universal conditions of human life (like corporeality, basic physical and psychological needs, aging, and others), the situational sources refer to the context specific features both long- and short term. The pathogenic source aims to capture specific situational factors that exacerbate already existing vulnerabilities by way of paradoxical effects of interventions or structures that are meant to support; or by abuse and dysfunctional personal relationships, social, or political systems.

For the following taxonomy of vulnerability regarding health and health care for refugees and asylum seekers in Germany, influencing factors are grouped into dispositional and occurrent states according to a time-line. The cut-off mark is the entry into Germany. Factors people bring along are taken as acquired dispositions (therefore in the field of dispositional in the table) while influencing factors that occur due to the specific situation in the German health care system are taken as occurrent (therefore titled as »after flight/as asylum seeker«).

| **States**<br>**Sources** | **Dispositional** | **Occurrent** |
|---|---|---|
| **inherent** | Like all human beings:<br>risk of illness, injury, trauma, disability; inherited or acquired | Longstanding, adverse conditions pre-flight that affect health in a long-term like malnourishment, lack of health care, lack of education, etc.<br>>> multiple risks at the same time less chances to develop resources/ resilience; |
| **situational** | High exposure to acute risks of infections, accidents, trauma, abuse<br>pre-flight due to acute adverse conditions (war, famine, dysfunctional system etc.)<br>during flight due to unsafe travelling conditions, lack of food, sanitary facilities, health care, protection, privacy | After flight/ as asylum seeker<br>Low social status, lack of social support, social exclusion, adverse living conditions through inadequate housing for a longer period, long waiting times concerning decisions about asylum application, trauma and psychological problems not recognized and/or not treated, language/ cultural barriers exacerbated; lack of interpreters/ mediators |

| States<br>Sources | Dispositional | Occurrent |
|---|---|---|
| | after flight/ as asylum seeker<br>strain of acculturation/ new socialization, loss of family and friends, insecurity of perspective, language and cultural barriers, lack of system-knowledge<br><br>Undocumented migrants/ refugees:<br>>> no legal access to state support structures, difficulties accessing health care | Undocumented migrants/ refugees:<br>>> no access to legal support structures<br>>> alternative support (NGOs, church groups etc.) not always available |
| **pathogenic** | Exposure to violence and human rights violations, asymmetric power-relations and multiple dependencies, lack of protection and of possibilities to claim (human) rights<br><br>Pre-flight: experience of war, violence, persecution, torture, abuse, dysfunctional systems<br><br>During flight: exploitation and abuse by smugglers, authorities, care-takers, human trafficking; unsafe vessels and refusal of aid/ rescue; denial of right to asylum<br><br>exacerbated in case of undocumented migrants/ refugees | After flight: AsylbLG >> restriction of entitlement to health care (for 18 months, in case of sanctions maybe longer), abuse/ denial of rights and entitlements, dependency, hindrance to earn own income, lack of participation in society and decision-making processes, othering, racism, disempowering structures, highly contradictory political and legal frame in Germany and Europe due to ambiguous measures of deterrence<br><br>Undocumented migrants/ refugees:<br>*De jure* limited access to health care possible (AsylbLG) but *de facto* not given/ not accessible<br>– Care provider obliged to notify immigration authority according to immigration law (§87 Abs. 2 Nr. 1 AufenthaltG)<br>– request for refunding of cost from municipalities not possible without notification |

Tab. 1: First attempt to use the taxonomy of vulnerability by Mackenzie et al. regarding health care for refugees and asylum seekers in Germany

Starting with inherent dispositional vulnerability as the first part of the matrix we obviously find that concerning their health all human beings are inherently vulnerable (universal human condition). This disposition turns into an occurrent state in case of adverse conditions which expose people to diverse health risks or even endanger survival. These kinds of situations (lack of means to secure livelihood, war, persecution, natural disasters etc.) are typical causes of migration and flight. Dealing with the situation in Germany these pre-flight conditions are taken into consideration as inherent and occurrent vulnerabilities in the sense that refugees arrive with the (mid- and long term) effects on their health they have already suffered. Moreover, poor health conditions in places already characterized by insufficiencies like weak infrastructure, could turn more adverse due to acute, added problems (renewed outbreak of civil war, breakdown of structures, new waves of persecution, floods). This is taken as situational source of (increased) vulnerability existing pre-flight. During their flight refugees face multiple serious risks to health and life. Maybe it could be assumed that in general there is an acquired dispositional vulnerability through flight? Again, this turns into an occurrent state if the specific circumstances after flight in the receiving country Germany are posing further burdens and stressors like long waiting times, unconducive housing etc.

To my understanding there are multiple sources of (health) vulnerabilities for refugees that have to be placed under pathogenic in the matrix, both due to paradoxical effects as well as due to sociopolitical structures: European and German laws, immigration regulations, restricted health care provision, general lack of adequate protection of Human Rights and of opportunities to participate in society. Refugees without legal papers are specially mentioned since they face particular problems accessing health care (and other support) in Germany.

### 2.3.2 Brief evaluation

The following remarks are some first, still theoretical reflections on using the taxonomy as a method:[26]

[26] Thanks for the discussion to the participants Anne Kasper, Lea Marie Mohwinkel and Corinna Stoexen of the working group on vulnerability at the FlüGe interdisciplinary graduate school, Bielefeld University.

The use of the taxonomy certainly needs more careful thought and not all critical doubts can be simply thrown overboard. But it proves at this stage its potential to map out and differentiate a situation that is often regarded as vulnerable. This differentiation leads a step away from a generalized view of vulnerability to more specific features of the context and particularly reveals structural determinants of social determinants of health[27] like access to health care systems or other facilities, opportunities for social, cultural, and political participation, strategic housing etc.

Though it is not always salient how to discern dispositional and occurrent states of vulnerability (which the authors acknowledge[28]), this is not necessarily only a flaw since it resonates the real intricacies and complexities. Moreover, the taxonomy is thereby open and flexible enough to take e.g. social determinants of health into account since it offers the possibility to capture developments over time by e.g. taking long-term (situational) threats to health in the past (like malnutrition) as dispositions that can turn into an acute or occurrent state in the presence.

As a taxonomy of vulnerability, the focus does somewhat remain on the deficits. It seems to require a conscious effort to spell out strengths and resources. The taxonomy could be further elaborated and may need additional methodical tools when used for practical purposes to identify necessary interventions in individual cases in such a way that individual resources are taken into account.

Combining it with Luna's approach of layers of vulnerability, with Hurst's[29] definition of vulnerability and the respective questions as guideline (like Durocher does[30]) or with other approaches, is likely to advance the use and development of the taxonomy especially if

---

[27] Philippe Bourgois, Seth M. Holmes, Kim Sue, James Quesada: Structural Vulnerability: Operationalizing the Concept to Address Health Disparities in Clinical Care. In: Academic medicine journal of the Association of American Medical Colleges 92 (2017), pp. 299–307.

[28] Mackenzie, Rogers, Dodds: Introduction: What Is Vulnerability (Note 24), pp. 1–33, here p. 8.

[29] Samia A. Hurst: Vulnerability in research and health care; describing the elephant in the room? In: Bioethics 22 (2008), pp. 191–202.

[30] Evelyne Durocher, Ryoa Chung, Christiane Rochon, Matthew Hunt: Understanding and Addressing Vulnerability Following the 2010 Haiti Earthquake: Applying a Feminist Lens to Examine Perspectives of Haitian and Expatriate Health Care Providers and Decision-Makers. In: Journal of human rights practice 8 (2016), pp. 219–238.

adjusted to the setting (clinical trial, clinical care, public health care etc.).

## 3. Understanding Vulnerability and Justice in Health Care – Questions arising

This first attempt to use the taxonomy of vulnerability as analytical instrument regarding health and health care for refugees in Germany helps to outline different sources and states of vulnerability at different phases in refugee migration. Assessing the current situation in Germany as receiving country shows many pathogenic sources of vulnerability. It makes visible the multiple risk-exposures regarding a wide range of threads and harm to physical, psychological and social health and at the same time diminished opportunities to keep or build up resources and coping capacities. Across the phases pre-, during and after flight vulnerability seems highly increased mostly due to adverse situational conditions, political, legal, and social structures. The restrictions and derogations of health care in Germany for refugees in entitlement, access and quality of care increase vulnerability to an extent that health and well-being are at stake. This is exacerbated dramatically in case of undocumented persons.

More often than not refugees arrive not only with an increased vulnerability but already emotionally wounded or even traumatized. In order to avoid increase of vulnerability or even further harm it seems noteworthy to point out that the taxonomy shows where preventive measures could and ought to be taken[31]: The transformation of some of the dispositional vulnerabilities to the occurrent states could be prevented e.g. by full entitlement and uncomplicated, culturally sensitive access to health care supported by trained interpreters in case of trauma, psychological stress or chronic conditions.

But why does understanding how vulnerable the situation is, lead us to what we ought to do? Or, as phrased by Mackenzie et al: »Why does vulnerability give rise to moral obligations and duties of jus-

[31] Mackenzie, Rogers, Dodds: Introduction: What Is Vulnerability (Note 24), pp. 1–33.

tice?«[32] Moreover, we could ask whether – if vulnerability gives rise to moral obligations – it also constitutes (human) rights.[33]

Realizing how vulnerable other people are in certain situations intuitively appeals to us as a reason to assist. It seems like seeing a person in need – we generally agree that we ought to help to fulfil a need if the person is not able to do so himself or herself, if it is an existential need and if we have the means to do so without considerable danger for our own life. But the number of »ifs« already indicates that things are not as easy as it might seem at first glance. Likewise, we have to ask whether every kind of vulnerability creates a reason to assist or intervene, what kind of vulnerabilities do so, why and to whom exactly they pose a responsibility. Another fundamental question is whether it is vulnerability itself that constitutes a moral obligation or whether it rather points to other sources of such an obligation – like needs.[34] But what are we doing exactly when we try to analyze, categorize and determine different types, forms, levels or layers of vulnerability? Are we not actually trying to determine need? Does being vulnerable not mean being (almost?) in need of support and protection? Certainly, as we saw when analyzing the term in the first section of this paper, there is a strong connection of vulnerability to helplessness, weakness, fragility and so on. Being vulnerable and in need means being dependent and constitutes an asymmetric social power relation. Therefore, vulnerability is often seen as opposite to autonomy. Here, questions arise how we can understand autonomy acknowledging our universal vulnerability at the same time. How vulnerability, dependency, social power hierarchies and autonomy are dynamically related seems to me at the heart of the matter. To disentangle these interconnected phenomena in our lives needs much further thought and to outline the already existing discussion is beyond the scope of this paper. It may be emphasized at least that the role of vulnerability and needs for deliberations on justice touches crucial questions that are still undertheorized and gain

---

[32] Mackenzie, Rogers, Dodds: Introduction: What Is Vulnerability (Note 24), pp. 1–33, here p. 8.

[33] Lutz Bergemann, Andreas Frewer (Eds.): Autonomie und Vulnerabilität in der Medizin. Menschenrechte – Ethik – Empowerment. Menschenrechte in der Medizin. Volume 6. Bielefeld 2019.

[34] Mackenzie, Rogers, Dodds: Introduction: What Is Vulnerability (Note 24), pp. 1–33, here p. 10.

even more importance in connection with questions of global justice and global health.[35]

## 4. Further questions and outlook concerning refugee health in Germany

Regarding matters of justice in health care it seems worthwhile to at least point out a few of the central, unsolved questions concerning refugee health. This outlines some of the major tasks we need to urgently face in empirical research, philosophical reflection as well as in practical terms.

Distribution of services in the German health care system claims to consider justice by distributing according to health needs assessed on the basis of medical knowledge and expert judgement. In case of restricting health care for refugees there are no medical reasons rather the common argument in public and political discussion points into a different direction: newcomers should have less entitlement in general including health care services in particular because they have not contributed to the common solidarity system. There is a shift of the principle of justice from need to merit. Why? Moreover, as far as I can see, this shift is not made explicit and (therefore) not debated. At least it has to be questioned whether and how different principles of justice ought to be considered. And what exactly does solidarity entail in the context of health? Health care for refugees is intertwined with wider matters of social justice. If we take the impact of social inclusion and social determinants of health serious then we need to consider participatory justice and we may have to reconsider the protective function of justice. Refugees do not have any other place to turn to than the state, society and health care system of their host country, where they mostly live at the very end of the social hierarchy with little or no means to help themselves in case of illness. Restricting health care (and other forms of social participation) for them seems to equal leaving someone in a helpless situation alone despite the fact that one could assist.

---

[35] Gillian Brock, David Miller: Needs in Moral and Political Philosophy. Stanford Encyclopaedia of Philosophy. Summer 2019. https://plato.stanford.edu/archives/sum 2019/entries/needs/ (accessed 9/24/2019).

Regarding health it is generally accepted that not all health disparities are necessarily unjust but as Norman Daniels argues »health inequalities among different social groups can be considered unjust when they result from unjust distribution in factors that are socially controllable that affect population health.«[36] Since refugees' health vulnerability is less person-bound but rather due to circumstances, political, legal structures, rules, and pathogenic sources, they are principally changeable. So, I would claim, understanding vulnerability informs us about matters of justice.

Under the basic moral and ethical guideline to prevent harm, there is enough evidence already to take up the issue of refugee health seriously. To detect avoidable harm is what working with concepts of vulnerability can help us do. In using them, we need to be aware of and carefully navigate paradoxical effects of our support efforts to keep the direction of empowerment, fostering agency and respecting autonomy.

---

[36] Norman Daniels: International Health Inequalities and Global Justice: Towards a Middle Ground. In: Solomon R. Benatar, Gillian Brock (Eds.): Global health and global health ethics. Cambridge 2011, pp. 97–107, here p. 101.

*Ivana Zagorac*

# The power of empathy in the treatment of vulnerable subjects

Abstract
The main task of this paper is to examine the challenges of employing empathy as an aid in improving attitudes toward the vulnerable. One of the challenges is the lack of a clear and widely accepted definition of empathy. In the first part of the paper, I shall present the development of the concept of empathy and current debates related to its definition. Then I shall briefly analyze forms of empathy. Finally, following findings that emotional strategy based on empathy can be more successful in improving attitudes toward the vulnerable than cognitive or behavior strategies, I shall examine the potential of forms of empathy for attitude change. I conclude that the careful implementation of perspective taking exercises in anti-prejudice and anti-stigmatization programs has a great potential for inducing a positive change in attitudes toward the vulnerable. However, there is no guarantee that increased empathizing will motivate helping behavior.

## 1. Introduction

In 2016, Gallup research and polling organization conducted a Word Poll on the acceptance of migrants.[1] According to the resulting *Migrant Acceptance Index,* Croatia was in the group of ten countries with the lowest inclination toward the acceptance of migrants among 138 countries. Out of possible 9 points and with global average of 5.29, Croatia scored 2.39 points. Survey included about 1000 participants from each country. Some of the other countries at the bottom of the Gallup's list were together with Croatia part of the so-called Balkan route formed during the 2015 migrant crisis.

When designing the study, Gallup's researchers assumed that the

[1] Neli Esipova, John Fleming, Julije Ray: New index shows least-, most-accepting countries for migrants. https://news.gallup.com/poll/216377/new-index-shows-least-accepting-countries-migrants.aspx (accessed: 9/24/2019).

acceptable degree of personal proximity with migrants reflects one's level of the acceptance of migrants.[2] In the first part of the study, participants were asked whether the following situations are good or bad things: 1) migrants living in their country, 2) becoming their neighbors, and 3) marrying into their families. Second part of this Gallup's survey included a question on whether the survey respondents personally knew a migrant living in their country (this question was not asked in Croatia). In 94 % of the countries, results indicated a positive correlation between personal contact and the acceptance of migrants.[3]

Findings were interpreted as a confirmation of the »contact theory«[4] which states that intergroup contact typically reduces intergroup prejudice.[5] One important finding of the contact theory is that the positive (i. e. prejudice reducing) effects of the contact »typically generalize beyond participants in the immediate contact situation«, thus enhancing »the potential of intergroup contact to be a practical, applied means of improving intergroup relations«.[6] This is a significant finding in the context of the present paper. Earlier studies have already demonstrated that empathy was one of the key mediators of the contact-prejudice effect.[7] Other observed mediators were knowledge (contact enables knowledge about the outgroup members and this knowledge reduces prejudice) and anxiety (contact reduces intergroup anxiety and threat). Mediating role of anxiety reduction and empathy induction proved to be stronger than the role of increased knowledge.[8] Significant effect of personal contact and empathy on

---

2 Neli Esipova, Anita Pugliese, Julie Ray: Acceptance of migrants increases with social interaction. https://news.gallup.com/poll/217250/acceptance-migrants-increases-social-interaction.aspx (accessed: 9/24/2019).

3 John H. Fleming, Neli Esipova, Anita Pugliese, Julie Ray, Rajesh Srinivasan: Migrant Acceptance Index: A global examination of the relationship between interpersonal contact and attitudes toward migrants. In: Border Crossing 8 (2018), pp. 103–132.

4 Gordon W. Allport: The nature of prejudice. Cambridge 1954; Thomas F. Pettigrew, Linda R. Tropp: A meta-analytic test of intergroup contact theory. In: Journal of Personality and Social Psychology 90 (2006), pp. 751–783.

5 Pettigrew, Tropp: A meta-analytic test (Note 4), pp. 751–783.

6 Pettigrew, Tropp: A meta-analytic test (Note 4), p. 766.

7 Thomas F. Pettigrew, Linda R. Tropp: How does intergroup contact reduce prejudice? Meta-analytic tests of three mediators. In: European Journal of Social Psychology 38 (2008), pp. 922–934.

8 Pettigrew, Tropp: How does intergroup contact reduce prejudice? (Note 7), pp. 922–934.

decreasing prejudice about the migrants was recorded in adolescents as well.[9] These findings are in line with the results of other studies that suggest an important role of empathy in the formation of positive attitudes toward outgroup members, reduction of stereotyping and prejudice, improvement of intergroup relations in general, and even in inducing helping behavior.[10]

The motivating question behind the present paper is whether empathy can be manipulated in order to improve attitudes toward migrants, which would further result in the increased level of the acceptance of migrants. I am interested in challenges of employing empathy as an aid in improving attitudes toward the vulnerable. More generally, I am interested in the power of empathy in the treatment of vulnerable subject. The strategy of this paper is to focus on the concept of empathy. It is noticeable that in describing the positive outcomes of empathy authors differently describe empathy itself. The confusion surrounding the very definition of empathy will be briefly described in the first part of the paper. Next, I shall examine the forms of empathy. I am especially interested in the connection between a particular form of empathy and the attitude change of the empathizer. My thesis is that not every form of empathy is equally suitable mediator for attitude change. The connection between forms of empathy, attitudes toward those in need, and helping behavior will be examined in the last section of the paper. I believe that the clarifi-

[9] Marta Miklikowska: Development of anti-immigrant attitudes in adolescence: The role of parents, peers, intergroup friendships, and empathy. In: British Journal of Psychology 108 (2017), pp. 626–648.

[10] Nicole Tausch, Miles Hewstone: Intergroup contact. In: John F. Dovidio, Miles Hewstone, Peter Glick, Victoria M. Esses (Eds.): The SAGE Handbook of Prejudice, Stereotyping, and Discrimination. London 2010, pp. 544–560; Walter G. Stephan, Krystina Finlay: The role of empathy in improving intergroup relations. In: Journal of Social Issues 55 (1999), pp. 729–743; Krystina A. Finlay, Walter G. Stephan: Improving intergroup relations: The effects of empathy on racial attitudes. In: Journal of Applied Social Psychology 30 (2006), pp. 1720–1737; John F. Dovidio, Samuel L. Gaertner, Kerry Kawakami: Intergroup contact: The past, present, and the future. In: Group Processes & Intergroup Relations 6 (2003), pp. 5–21; Andreas Beelmann, Kim Sarah Heinemann: Preventing prejudice and improving intergroup attitudes: A meta-analysis of child and adolescent training programs. In: Journal of Applied Developmental Psychology 35 (2014), pp. 10–24; John F. Dovidio, James D. Johnson, Samuel L. Gaertner, Adam R. Pearson, Tamar Saguy, Leslie Ashburn-Nardo: Empathy and intergroup relations. In: Mario Mikulincer, Phillip R. Shaver (Eds.): Prosocial motives, emotions, and behavior: The better angels of our nature. American Psychological Association, Washington 2010, pp. 393–408.

cations of this kind necessarily precede a systematic use of any of empathy variations in intervention programs[11] aimed to reduce prejudice or promote positive intergroup attitudes.

## 2. The development of the concept of empathy

The term empathy entered the scientific literature in 1909 in Edward J. Titchener's *Lectures on the Experimental Psychology of Thought Process*. Titchener introduced empathy as a translation for the German word »Einfühlung«.[12] In the 18th century, Johann Gottfried Herder (1744–1803) used the term *Einfühlung* to describe the unification between the subject and the object, Man and Nature.[13] In the 19th century the term *Einfühlung* was present in the aesthetic work of Friedrich Theodor Vischer (1807–1888), Karl Köstlin (1819–1894) and Rudolf Hermann Lotze (1817–1881), as well as in the work of Robert Vischer (1847–1933), especially in his *Über das Optische Formgefühl: Ein Beitrag zur Aesthetik* (1873).[14] With Theodor Lipps (1851–1915), the aesthetical dimension of the term *Einfühlung* was even more strongly associated with its psychological dimension.[15] Lipps transformed *Einfühlung* from a concept related to philosophical aesthetics into a crucial concept for philosophy in general; namely, he suggested that *Einfühlung* was an answer to the puzzling question of how we understand the mental states of others. It was this understanding of the term *Einfühlung* that Titchener had in mind when he translated it as *empathy*. At the beginning of the 20th century, German phenomenology was especially interested in the concept of *Einfühlung*. Edmund Husserl (1859–1938) and Edith Stein (1891–1942) both criticized Lipps' account of *Einfühlung*, while Max Scheler (1874–1928) developed a view that shared some characteristics with the long-present philosophical concept of sympathy. The concept of *sympathy* had an important place in the philosophy of David Hume

[11] Beelmann, Heinemann: Preventing prejudice (Note 10), pp. 10–24.
[12] Edward J. Titchener: Lectures on the Experimental Psychology of Thought Process. New York 1909, p. 21.
[13] Magdalena Nowak: The complicated history of Einfühlung. In: Argument 1 (2011), pp. 301–326, here p. 303.
[14] Robert Vischer: Über das Optische Formgefühl: Ein Beitrag zur Aesthetik. Leipzig 1873; Ivana Zagorac: Bioetički senzibilitet. Pergamena. Zagreb 2018, pp. 30–31.
[15] Nowak: The complicated history of Einfühlung (Note 15), pp. 305–307.

(1711–1776) and Adam Smith (1723–1790). Moreover, some modern scholars consider *sympathy* to be a historical antecedent of the modern concept of empathy.[16] Important further promotion of empathy in psychology and psychotherapy was done by Carl Rogers (1902–1987) and Heinz Kohut (1903–1981).

The last decades of the 20th century brought new research interest in empathy, which resulted in contributions from many scientific fields. Such a diverse interest is not surprising given that many of the empathy-researchers state that multidimensionality is one of the key characteristics of empathy.[17] Multidimensionality is reflected not only in the number of studies coming from many scientific fields and contributing to the empathy research, but also in various definitions of their main subject.[18] A somehow disappointing result of the increased interest in the concept and manifestations of empathy is that the vast literature produced confusion about empathy, instead of an improvement in its understanding. In his overview of the current empathy research, Batson listed eight different psychological states that have been named empathy.[19] This confusion seems to have worsened with time. In their quantitative review and conceptual analysis of empathy definitions, Hall and Schwartz also found great differences between definitions of empathy explicitly or implicitly stated in the analyzed studies.[20] The discrepancy mostly arose from an unclear relation between empathy and similar concepts (e.g. perspective taking, empathic concern, emotional contagion/emotional sharing, etc.). Additionally, the authors of the analyzed empathy studies were

---

[16] Derek Matravers: Empathy in the aesthetic tradition. In: Heidi L. Maibom (Ed.): The Routledge Handbook of Philosophy of Empathy. London, New York 2017, pp. 77–85; Amy Coplan, Peter Goldie: Introduction. In: Amy Coplan, Peter Goldie (Eds.): Empathy: Philosophical and Psychological Approaches. Oxford University Press, New York 2011, pp. ix–xi.

[17] Judith A. Hall, Rachel Schwartz: Empathy present and future. In: Journal of Social Psychology 159 (2019), pp. 225–243.

[18] Hall, Schwartz: Empathy present and future (Note 17), pp. 225–243; Benjamin M. P. Cuff, Sarah J. Brown, Laura Taylor, Douglas J. Howat: Empathy: A review of the concept. In: Emotion Review 8 (2016), pp. 144–153; Amy Coplan: Understanding empathy: Its features and effects. In: Amy Coplan, Peter Goldie (Eds.): Empathy: Philosophical and Psychological Approaches. Oxford University Press, New York 2011, pp. 3–18.

[19] Charles Daniel Batson: Altruism in humans. Oxford University Press, Oxford 2011, pp. 11–20.

[20] Hall, Schwartz: Empathy present and future (Note 17).

far from being unanimous in their understanding of crucial characteristics of empathy, for example whether it was a process, a trait, a capacity or competency, a response to observing another's experience, or an interpersonal behavior.[21] Similar are the findings of the study of Cuff et al.: 43 definitions of empathy that were included in the analysis between themselves did not reach a consensus on any of the eight themes that Cuff et al. listed as crucial to our understanding of empathy.[22]

Although the results of both Hall and Schwartz and Cuff et al. study point to the same conclusion – that the concept of empathy lacks clear definition – their final suggestions differ. Hall and Schwartz advocate for the complete avoidance of the terms empathy and empathic. Instead, they suggest using terminology which corresponds to the actual subject of the study, whether it is a research on perspective taking, sympathetic feelings, physiological arousal to others, etc.[23] Such strategy would surely enable further research with the benefit of avoiding the mismatching of terms and concepts that are related to but not identical with empathy. On the other side, Cuff et al. attempted at finding the dominant tendencies in eight selected themes related to the empathy research with the final aim of producing a unifying definition of empathy. Not surprisingly, that was not an easy task. Despite their detailed analysis, the authors provide an unclear answer to the very first issue they put forward: What is the relation of empathy to similar concepts? Following the trend in empathy research, the authors confirmed that empathy, sympathy, compassion, and tenderness are all different concepts. However, it remained unclear whether or not they believe that empathy represents an »overarching category, containing all associated concepts«?[24] Indeed, is empathy an umbrella term for all related concepts, as some authors think,[25] or is it a self-standing emotional event, only loosely connected to the similar ones?

---

[21] Hall, Schwartz: Empathy present and future (Note 17), p. 234.

[22] Cuff et al.: Empathy (Note 18).

[23] Hall, Schwartz: Empathy present and future (Note 17), pp. 236–237; Jean Decety, Jason M. Cowell: Friends or foes: Is empathy necessary for moral behavior? In: Perspectives on Psychological Science 9 (2014), pp. 525–537.

[24] Cuff et al.: Empathy (Note 18), p. 5.

[25] Hall, Schwartz: Empathy present and future (Note 17).

## 3. Overview of the forms of empathy

It seems that the controversy over the definition and forms of empathy starts with the distinction between cognitive and affective aspects of empathy. The issue of cognitive vs. affective components of empathy is one of the most debated in the empathy research. The first line of research defines empathy primarily as a cognitive phenomenon. Main focus in this area of study is on one's ability to perceive and differentiate between various mental states of others. Additional questions here are related to the accuracy of that process and the possibilities of measuring its effects. The second line of research views empathy as an affective phenomenon, i.e. a phenomenon that is primarily constituted of emotions and feelings. Even though some authors advocate for the exclusivity of either cognitive or affective understanding of empathy,[26] Cuff et al. review study confirmed that the prevailing view is that empathy consists of both the cognitive and affective dimension. Cognitive and affective empathic reactions are most probably two different processes, but they rarely occur independently from one another.[27] Obviously, we can understand the emotions of others without experiencing these emotions ourselves. However, common view is that empathy is an emotional event, thus the complete absence of an affective reaction would be considered as non-emphatic.

How do the cognitive and affective aspects of empathy translate into numerous forms of empathy? Most commonly debated variations include perspective taking, empathic concern (sympathy), personal distress, affective empathy, and emotional contagion. Roughly following the division between cognitive and affective empathy, some authors consider perspective taking (»imagine how the other feels«; »imagine how you would feel«) to be a representative of cognitive empathy,[28] or even use the general term empathy for perspective taking. The latter is often the case in studies that ground their research on the Interpersonal Reactivity Index (IRI). IRI seems to be the most often used instrument for measuring empathy.[29] Some authors alter-

[26] Hall, Schwartz: Empathy present and future (Note 17), pp. 230–231.
[27] Cuff et al.: Empathy (Note 18), pp. 7–8.
[28] Cuff et al.: Empathy (Note 18), p. 8; Pettigrew, Tropp: How does intergroup contact reduce prejudice? (Note 7); Tausch, Hewstone: Intergroup contact (Note 10); Stephan, Finlay: The role of empathy (Note 10), p. 730.
[29] Hall, Schwartz: Empathy present and future (Note 17), p. 228.

natively describe perspective taking as only a precursor to empathy.[30] For example, studies of Batson et al.[31] and Batson[32] demonstrated that people reacted to the perceived need of the other in two distinctive ways: either with personal distress, or with a genuine concern for the other. Interpretation of the experiment results suggests that in the first case one's actions are motivated by egoism, while in the second the motivation is altruistic. For Batson, altruism is a »motivational state with the ultimate goal of increasing another's welfare«, while egoism is »a motivational state with the ultimate goal of increasing one's own welfare«.[33] Batson famously concluded that empathic concern is the likely source of altruistic motivation.[34] That is the ground claim of his empathy-altruism hypothesis. Alternative reaction to perspective taking is personal distress. Personal distress might as well motivate helping behavior, however in that case the motivation for helping comes from the wish to reduce one's own stress, i. e. such behavior lacks the altruistic motivation. More often than not, personal distress results in escaping the stressful situation.[35] The conclusion of numerous experiments by Batson is that perspective taking is only a precursor to empathy, not a form of empathy.

In the last decades, Batson's experiments popularized the view that the only genuine form of empathy is empathic concern. Empathic concern is characterized as other-oriented emotion, often described as very similar or even identical to sympathy or compassion.[36]

---

[30] C. Daniel Batson, Jim Fultz, Patricia A. Schoenrade: Distress and Empathy: Two Qualitatively Distinct Vicarious Emotions with Different Motivational Consequences. In: Journal of Personality 55 (1987), pp. 19–39; C. Daniel Batson: Altruism in Humans. New York 2011; William H. B. McAuliffe, Evan C. Carter, Juliana Berhane, Alexander C. Snihur, Michael E. McCullough: Is empathy the default response to suffering? A meta-analytic evaluation of perspective-taking's effect on empathic concern. https://psyarxiv.com/bwxm9/ (accessed 9/24/2019).

[31] Batson, Fultz, Schoenrade: Distress and Empathy (Note 30).

[32] Batson: Altruism in Humans (Note 30).

[33] C. Daniel Batson: Empathy-induced altruistic motivation. Draft of lecture/chapter for Inaugural Herzliya Symposium on »Prosocial Motives, Emotions, and Behavior«, March 24–27, 2008, p. 3.

[34] Batson: Empathy-induced altruistic motivation (Note 33), p. 8.

[35] Batson, Fultz, Schoenrade: Distress and Empathy (Note 30); Batson: Altruism in Humans (Note 30).

[36] Tania Singer, Olga M. Klimeck: Empathy and compassion. In: Current Biology 24 (2014), pp. 875–878, here p. 875; Janis H. Zickfeld, Thomas W. Schubert, Beate Seibt, Alan P. Fiske: Empathic concern is part of a more general communal emotion. In: Frontiers in Psychology 8 (2017) 723. doi: 10.3389/fpsyg.2017.00723 (accessed 9/24/

Moreover, many believe that the modern concept of empathy grew out of the concept of sympathy, which has been present in the philosophical thought at least since Ancient Greece. Stoics described sympathy as a power that enabled interaction between body parts of a single individual, between body and soul, as well as between many parts of the cosmos. The term was also used in medicine, most probably already in Hippocrates' (circa 460 BC–circa 370 BC) time. In the Renaissance, the social and moral dimensions of the concept of sympathy became more prominent. The 18th century philosophy, especially in works of David Hume and Adam Smith, established sympathy as one of the most important philosophical concepts.[37] It is evident that the modern use of the term sympathy lacks richness of the traditional concept. In the field of empathy research, sympathy is most often described as a sort of emotional reflection on the perceived or believed emotional states of the other. Unlike emotion matching – sometimes called affective empathy and described as »the vicarious sharing of an affect«[38] – sympathy needs not to be congruent with the other's emotion or situation. Rather, the sympathetic person reflects on the emotion of the other, i.e. she takes that emotion or situation as an object of her reflection and expresses concern for the other's well-being.[39] Thus, sympathy describes feeling for the other, not emotional-matching between individuals.[40] The unresolved issue here is whether sympathy includes one's reflection only on the sadness of the others[41] or on their happiness as well[42].

In an interest of providing a relatively comprehensive overview, a state known as emotional contagion has to be mentioned as well. The

2019); Martin Lamothe, Emilie Boujut, Franck Zenasni, Serge Sultan: To be or not to be empathic: the combined role of empathic concern and perspective taking in understanding burnout in general practice. In: BMC Family Practice 15 (2014), doi: 10.1186/1471–2296–15–15 (accessed 9/24/2018).

37 Zagorac: Bioetički senzibilitet (Note 14).

38 Karsten Stueber: Empathy. In: Edward N. Zalta (Ed.): The Stanford Encyclopedia of Philosophy. https://plato.stanford.edu/entries/empathy/ (accessed 9/24/2019).

39 Stueber: Empathy (Note 38); Heidi L. Maibom: Introduction: (Almost) everything you ever wanted to know about empathy. In: Heidi L. Maibom (Ed.): Empathy and Morality. New York 2014, pp. 6–50.

40 C. Daniel Batson: Testing the empathy-altruism hypothesis against egoistic alternatives. In: Lorraine L. Besser, Michael Slote (Eds.): The Routledge Companion to Virtue Ethics. New York 2015, pp. 385–400.

41 Stueber: Empathy (Note 38).

42 Maibom: Introduction (Note 39).

specificity of this emotional event is in its simplicity: emotional contagion describes the spread of an emotion across the group. Typical examples are newborn's reactive cry to the sound of other baby crying, the spread of panic, etc. One catches the emotion of the other, but experiences it as one's own emotion. Because of the lack of clear self-other distinction and the absence of conscious awareness (the process is automatic and involuntary), emotional contagion is often thought to be the most rudimentary form of emphatic relation.[43] In fact, given that this state typically occurs below the level of conscious awareness, authors who believe that empathy consists in both the cognitive and affective dimension should probably deny any empathic characteristics in emotional contagion. In this paper, I shall assume that empathy comes in different forms, i.e. that empathy is an umbrella term for different states that describe a variety of subject's emotional responses to the perceived or imagined situation of the other.

## 4. The role of empathy in intergroup relation programs

I shall now turn to the connection between forms of empathy, attitudes toward those in need, and helping behavior. The main aim of this section is to bring together the previous findings in order to examine the role a particular form of empathy might play in intergroup relation programs aimed to reduce prejudice or promote positive intergroup attitudes.

In their influential study, Batson et al.[44] concluded that »emotional strategy based on empathy« can be more successful in improving attitudes toward the stigmatized than cognitive or behavior strategies. According to authors, cognitive strategies rely on providing positive information about the particular stigmatized group, while behavior strategies are based on »cooperative, equal-status, personal contact« that is sometimes hard to achieve.[45] Empathy strategy, on the other hand, »induces the audience to feel empathy for one or a

---

[43] Maibom: Introduction (Note 39).

[44] C. Daniel Batson, Marina P. Polycarpou, Eddie Harmon-Jones, Heidi J. Imhoff, Erin C. Mitchener, Lori L. Bednar, Tricia R. Klein, Lori Highberger: Empathy and attitudes: Can feeling for a member of a stigmatized group improve feelings toward the group? In: Journal of Personality and Social Psychology 72 (1997), pp. 105–118.

[45] Batson et al.: Empathy and attitudes (Note 44), p. 117.

few members of the stigmatized group«.[46] Results indicate that the emotional strategy has advantages over other two strategies, mostly in terms of duration of its positive effects and its higher potential of generalizing positive emphatic feelings toward one member of stigmatized group to the whole group. Additional study showed that empathy has an effect on behavior as well, in terms that empathic feelings induce more helping behavior.[47] In this research, as well as in a previous one, the participants were asked to imagine how a needy individual felt about her own decisions and how they have affected her life. In other words, methodology focused on perspective taking. The same model of perspective-taking manipulation was used in other studies. In the study of Vescio et al., participants who were instructed to imagine how the member of a stigmatized group felt in a designed experimental situation subsequently reported more positive attitudes toward the particular group than the participants who were instructed to adopt an objective perspective. According to authors, empathy (together with situational attributions) was a mediator between perspective taking and intergroup attitudes.[48] Similar are the findings of Dovidio et al. who concluded that empathy can be in many ways important in intergroup relations and can significantly shape intergroup responses.[49] Given such findings, it is surprising that intervention programs aimed to reduce prejudice or promote positive intergroup attitudes in children and adolescent often neglected the role emotions played in the development of serious prejudice and discrimination.[50]

On the other hand, even though perspective taking seems to be a powerful tool in shaping more positive attitudes toward the vulnerable, it could also have other effects. In the previous analysis of the forms of empathy, it was pointed out that perspective taking might result in personal distress. As mentioned, personal distress is often described as a process different than empathic concern (sympathy,

---

[46] Batson et al.: Empathy and attitudes (Note 44), p. 105.
[47] C. Daniel Batson, Johee Chang, Ryan Orr, Jennifer Rowland: Empathy, attitudes, and action: can feeling for a member of a stigmatized group motivate one to help the group? In: Personality and Social Psychology Bulletin 28 (2002), pp. 1656–1666.
[48] Theresa K. Vescio, Gretchen B. Sechrist, Matthew P. Paolucci: Perspective taking and prejudice reduction: The mediational role of empathy arousal and situational attributions. In: European Journal of Social Psychology 33 (2003), pp. 455–472.
[49] Dovidio et al.: Empathy and intergroup relations (Note 10).
[50] Beelmann, Heinemann: Preventing prejudice (Note 10).

compassion).[51] Moreover, it would be intuitively described by many as non-empathic. Motivation based on personal distress might be perceived as cold, egoistic, and socially undesirable. Nevertheless, the thesis that our helping behavior is in fact motivated by selfish motives prevailed throughout the history of philosophy, with few respectful exceptions. Batson's empathy-altruism hypothesis, supported by empirical findings, opened up the possibility that altruism might exist and that individuals can be motivated by reasons other than selfishness. Recent research[52] on neural mechanisms added dynamics into the egoism–altruism debate by producing inconclusive results in favor of the thesis that empathic concern motivates altruism, while personal distress does not.

According to Batson's numerous experiments and follow-ups, both empathic concern (sympathy, compassion) and personal distress develop out of perspective taking. Perspective taking is a common method used for inducing positive attitudes toward the vulnerable. However, its utilization in anti-prejudice and anti-stigmatization programs has to be carefully prepared. As already mentioned, the instructions usually lead participants into imagine-other or imagine-self situation. Research findings suggest that the instruction »imagine how a person in need feels« mostly induces empathic concern, while »imagine how you would feel in the situation of the needy other« instruction results in a mix of empathic concern and personal distress which can further evoke egoistic motivation.[53] Stephan and Finlay cautioned about the additional pitfalls of empathy induction in intergroup relation programs.[54] One possibility is that empathy-strategies produce undesirable outcomes; such are negative attitudes, confirmation of stereotypes, increased tension and hostility, etc. It is possible that the subjects due to induced form of empathy change their attitudes toward the particular group, but remain unaware that they themselves share the responsibility for the very suffering that has triggered their empathizing. Another risk the authors warn

---

[51] Singer, Klimeck: Empathy and compassion (Note 36), p. 875.
[52] Oriel Feldman Hall, Tim Dalgleish, Davy Evans, Dean Mobbs: Empathic concern drives costly altruism. In: NeuroImage 105 (2015), pp. 347–356.
[53] C. Daniel Batson, Shannon Early, Giovanni Salvarani: Perspective taking: Imagining how another feels versus imaging how you would feel. In: Personality and Social Psychology Bulletin 23 (1997), pp. 751–758.
[54] Stephan, Finlay: The role of empathy (Note 10), pp. 738–740.

against is that empathizing might turn into fear for oneself.[55] This tendency was noted as early as in Aristotle's (384 BC–322 BC) *Rhetoric:* pity turns into fear when danger comes too close to us.[56] Induced empathetic response might lead to the identification with the sufferer, make the threat feel closer, and result in defensive avoidance. Instead of the attitude change, the existing negative attitudes toward the sufferer might even get stronger.[57] Finally, the question remains of whether empathizing with the sufferer translates into helping the sufferer. Research shows that empathy, at least in the form of empathic concern, induces more helping behavior.[58] However, helping behavior is not a necessary consequence of empathizing: broadly speaking, the empathic response is defined as such based on the elicited emotions and its overall other-orientation. Helping behavior is not a prerequisite of empathy either. One might even speculate that the social or self-imposed expectance of helping behavior might push the subject further away from the vulnerable.

## 5. Conclusion

In my previous studies on the concept of vulnerability,[59] I have reached the conclusion that both scientific community and policy makers are still unsure about many aspects of the very concept of vulnerability and what it entails. Interestingly, at the same time they seem to be sure that some groups, for example children or refugees and asylum seekers, are indeed vulnerable and in need of protection. In the discussions on vulnerability, the terms often used are duties and obligation, but also empathy and compassion. The underlying premise seems to be that if we cannot clearly formulate our duties and obligations towards the vulnerable,[60] then we should act guided by

55 Stephan, Finlay: The role of empathy (Note 10), pp. 738–739.

56 Aristotle: Rhetoric, book II, part 8. Translated by W. Rhys Roberts. http://classics.mit.edu/Aristotle/rhetoric.2.ii.html (accessed 9/24/2019).

57 Stephan, Finlay: The role of empathy (Note 10), p. 739.

58 Batson et al.: Empathy and attitudes (Note 44).

59 Ivana Zagorac: How Should We Treat the Vulnerable? Qualitative Study of Authoritative Ethics Documents. In: Journal of health care for the poor and underserved 27 (2016), pp. 1656–1673; Ivana Zagorac: What Vulnerability? Whose Vulnerability? Conflict of Understandings in the Debate on Vulnerability. In: Facta Universitatis, Series: Law and politics 15 (2017), pp. 157–169.

60 Zagorac: How Should We Treat the Vulnerable? (Note 59).

our compassion and empathy. However, I have already shown that the most famous predecessor of the modern concept of empathy – Hume's concept of sympathy/humanity – represents an insufficient means of protecting the weak.[61] On the other hand, there are some differences between the modern concept of empathy and the philosophical concept of sympathy as understood by Hume. In this paper, I have dealt with the modern concept of empathy. I pointed out that not every form of empathy is a suitable choice for attitude change. Other-oriented perspective taking seems as the most promising approach in programs designed to promote positive intergroup attitudes or reduce prejudice. It seems reasonable to conclude that the careful implementation of perspective taking exercises in anti-prejudice and anti-stigmatization programs has a great potential for inducing a positive change in attitudes toward the particular group. However, there is no guarantee that greater empathizing will motivate helping behavior.

[61] Ivana Zagorac: Hume's humanity and the protection of the vulnerable. In: Diametros 44 (2015), pp. 189–203.

*Katharina Fürholzer*

# Narration without borders. Migration, narrative medicine, and témoignage in the public work of Médecins Sans Frontières (Doctors Without Borders)

Abstract

Experiences of flight can be beyond words even in our mother tongue. After arrival in another country, the psychological language barrier refugees might be faced with can be exacerbated by the need to use a foreign language. This poses a challenge for medicine, where successful communication is a prerequisite for patient care. However, language barriers can lead to hierarchical communication structures, where patients are rather talked about than fostered to find their own voice. In contrast to that, raising awareness for patient stories is a central goal of the humanitarian NGO Médecins Sans Frontières (MSF; Doctors Without Borders). Methodologically based on a narratological analysis, this paper examines the representation of refugees in MSF public relations texts, focusing on a) mode of speech and b) type of text (narrative vs. report). It will be seen that the texts correspond both to the ideas of narrative medicine and the policy of témoignage (»bearing witness«). As I will argue, this results in a form of communication that can be defined as narrative témoignage.

## 1. Introduction

»A physician's science kills his humanity.«[1] The criticism German physician Ernst Schweninger (1850–1924) expressed in 1926 still remains valid today: A health care system purely based on scientific facts and figures ignores that a physician's task comprises not only the treatment of diseases but also to build a human connection with his or her patients. Some 50 years later, Schweninger's thought was taken up by George L. Engel (1913–1999): The American psychiatrist stressed the need for a holistic understanding of medicine, which requires the health care system to focus not merely on biological – e.g.

[1] Ernst Schweninger: Der Arzt. Radeburg 1926, pp. 45–46 [translated by Katharina Fürholzer].

genetic or biochemical – factors, but to take into account that health and disease are the results of a complex interplay of biological, psychological, and social dimensions.[2]

The holistic approach advertised by physicians like Schweninger or Engel is a basic feature of today's narrative medicine. This medical approach draws its ideas from the conviction that issues of illness, pain or dying should not only be approximated on the basis of objective, scientific facts as for example provided in medical reports. Instead, narrative medicine stresses the significance of personal accounts of illness, e.g. by patients, relatives or health care providers. American psychiatrist Arthur Kleinman (* 1941), one of the founding fathers of narrative medicine, elucidates the concept and effect of such illness narratives as follows:

> Patients order their experience of illness (…) as personal narratives. The illness narrative is a story the patient tells (…) to give coherence to the distinctive events and long term course of suffering. The plot lines, core metaphors, and rhetorical devices that structure the illness narrative are drawn from cultural and personal models for arranging experiences in meaningful ways and for effectively communicating those meanings.[3]

The cause of narrative medicine seems also relevant when providing health care for patients who had to flee their home countries due to severe crisis, for example due to war, natural disasters, hunger or violence. Experiences made before, during, and after migration can cause psychological and physical stress and pose a threat to refugees' health. As successful communication is a basic prerequisite for patient care, putting such experiences into words is both of help for the refugees and the medical team. However, times of crisis can be beyond words even in one's mother tongue. Having to seek for help in a different culture can cause a spectrum of additional sociocultural, psychological or biomedical challenges. Also, the need to use a foreign language may impair the communication and, in consequence, the relationship between patients and the medical team. Health care provided for refugees thus requires particular awareness for the barriers and effects of language as well as for alternative ways of communicating.

---

[2] George L. Engel: The need for a new medical model. A challenge for biomedicine. In: Science 196 (1977), pp. 129–136.

[3] Arthur Kleinman: The Illness Narratives. Suffering, Healing, and the Human Condition. New York 1988, p. 49.

An organization where issues of migration and medicine are an integral part of its work is Médecins Sans Frontières (MSF; Doctors Without Borders). The basic goal of this humanitarian and medical non-governmental organization (NGO) is to provide medical assistance to people affected by conflict, epidemics, natural disasters or exclusion from health care.[4] Founded almost 50 years ago by a group of French doctors and journalists, MSF consists today of 24 national offices worldwide. There are currently over 45.000 people working for MSF, most of them physicians, nurses or other health care professionals, who are deployed in over 460 projects in approximately 70 countries.[5] MSF's work entails taking care for migrants and refugees both at their points of arrival and during their journeys, inside and outside their home countries.[6] In light of its longstanding expertise in global patient care, MSF can be attributed a particular awareness for linguistic and intercultural challenges health care providers and patients may be faced with.

Against this backdrop, this paper examines and discusses the technical and ethical dimensions of MSF public relations texts from the viewpoint of Medical Humanities. Methodologically based on a narratological text analysis, the paper focusses on a) speech representation of refugees as well as b) type of text chosen to represent refugees in MSF's work (narrative vs. report). I will rest my analysis on two text samples by the German MSF association Ärzte ohne Grenzen: 1) an online project presentation on psychosocial help for asylum seekers in Germany, and 2) a book edited by MSF on the occasion of 40 years of MSF.

## 2. Voicing migration

MSF has laid down its operational guidelines and professional code of ethics of MSF in its own charter.[7] Its core working principles are 1) to

---

[4] Médecins Sans Frontières: About MSF. https://www.msf.org/ (accessed 9/24/2019).

[5] Médecins Sans Frontières: International activity report 2017. Geneva 2018.

[6] Médecins Sans Frontières: Refugees, IDPs and people on the move. https://www.msf.org/refugees-idps-and-people-move (accessed 9/24/2019).

[7] Médecins Sans Frontières: The MSF Charter. https://www.msf.org/who-we-are (accessed 9/24/2019); Médecins Sans Frontières: Chantilly Principles. Who are the Médecins Sans Frontières; Médecins Sans Frontières: La Mancha Agreement. 25 June 2006, Athens.

work independently, meaning to preclude any political, religious or economic factors when it comes to decision making, 2) to be strictly impartial, providing medical aid solely on the basis of need, with no acceptance whatsoever of for example ethnical, political or economic aspects, 3) to be neutral, meaning that MSF does not want to be considered part of any particular political side, and 4) to work transparently and accountable with regard to MSF choices and actions.[8] With regard to specific issues of communication there is also a fifth principle that is key for the work of MSF, which is 5) the principle of témoignage: The French verb *témoigner* literally translates as to witness or to testify. In the context of MSF, the term is used in the meaning of speaking out both privately and publicly when witnessing extreme acts of violence or exclusion from lifesaving medical care. In consequence, MSF has published a series of reports after missions in regions of crisis to make publicly aware of the hardship their patients may face.[9] When MSF was awarded the Nobel Peace Prize in 1999, James Orbinski (* 1960), MSF International Council president, expressly underlined the importance of témoignage in his Nobel lecture:

> Silence has long been confused with neutrality, and has been presented as a necessary condition for humanitarian action. From its beginning, [MSF] was created in opposition to this assumption. We are not sure that words can always save lives, but we know that silence can certainly kill.[10]

The policy of témoignage also carries weight in the context of migration and medicine: When extreme or traumatic events before, during or after migration go beyond a patient's words, speaking out on behalf of the people concerned is an essential part of MSF self-understanding.

### *2.1 Mode of speech representation*

A project that is of particular interest when dealing with issues of medicine, migration, and narrative is the project »Psychosocial help

---

[8] Médecins Sans Frontières: The MSF Charter (Note 7).

[9] Médecins Sans Frontières: About MSF. http://speakingout.msf.org/ (accessed 9/24/2019).

[10] James Orbinski: Nobel Lecture. Oslo, December 10, 1999. https://www.nobelprize.org/prizes/peace/1999/msf/lecture/ (accessed 9/24/2019).

for asylum seekers«. The project that has been started in March 2017 as a cooperation between Ärzte ohne Grenzen and St. Josef Hospital Schweinfurt aims at offering psychosocial help to asylum seekers of the arrival center in the German city of Schweinfurt, and to detect and react at an early stage to mental stress the asylum seekers might be faced with due to war, crisis, and migration. The project is presented on the MSF website via a press release,[11] a feature article,[12] and three patient stories.[13] Both the texts and paratexts – i. e. elements surrounding the main texts like headlines or pictures – are dominated by the voices and perspectives of the asylum seekers, e. g. in form of text type classifications like »patient story« in the tab titles, the use of direct quotes in tab and main titles (e. g. »I am not safe in Afghanistan«; »It helps if someone is listening«) or photographs showing private patient-counselor situations. The articles' teasers are designed as short biographical introductions giving insight into the psychosocial dimensions of refugees' possible experiences (e. g. fear, anxiety):

> The family of Hamdi G. (name changed) fled civil war in Somalia, he himself was born in Yemen. After a war broke out there, he was imprisoned for months in a prison where the inmates were severely abused. Under dramatic circumstances, he fled across the Sahara and the Mediterranean to Germany. He is afraid to be deported to Italy and end up on the street.[14]

Due to their focus on patients' hardships of war, prison, and flight, the quotes can also be seen as expression of MSF's ethical policy of témoignage.

Like the teasers, also the main patient stories, written as short first-person accounts, focus on what had happened to the refugees before, during, and after migration. The autobiographical representa-

---

[11] Stefan Dold: Modellprojekt für psychosoziale Hilfe für Asylsuchende in Schweinfurt gestartet. https://www.aerzte-ohne-grenzen.de/modellprojekt-psychosoziale-hilfe-asylsuchende-deutschland (accessed 9/24/2019).

[12] Ärzte ohne Grenzen: »Für euch habe ich drei Ohren« – Psychosoziale Hilfe für Asylsuchende in Schweinfurt. https://www.aerzte-ohne-grenzen.de/schweinfurt-psychosoziale-hilfe-asylsuchende (accessed 9/24/2019).

[13] Yassin E. [pseudonymized by MSF]: »Es hilft, wenn mir jemand zuhört«. https://www.aerzte-ohne-grenzen.de/schweinfurt-psychosoziale-hilfe-yassin (accessed 9/24/2019); Hamdi G. [pseudonymized by MSF]: »Man versucht immer, zu lachen und zu vergessen«. https://www.aerzte-ohne-grenzen.de/schweinfurt-psychosoziale-hilfe-hamdi (accessed 9/24/2019); Bachodur M. [pseudonymized by MSF]: »Ich bin nicht sicher in Afghanistan«. https://www.aerzte-ohne-grenzen.de/schweinfurt-psychosoziale-hilfe-bachodur (accessed 9/24/2019).

[14] Hamdi: »Man versucht immer, zu lachen und zu vergessen« (Note 13).

tion of patients' perspective sets itself apart from communication patterns common in the context of health care: Medical texts – from scientific articles to referral letters – are usually written from the viewpoint of medical experts (physician, scientist), causing patients to be represented by the voice and perspective of another person, who has made a pre-selection of what seems important and how this should be represented. As the patients' perspective is usually paraphrased, they have no or only limited possibilities to add their own way of seeing and saying the situation in question and, consequently, can hardly strengthen, broaden or maybe also correct the medical experts' depiction. The use of paraphrases thus corresponds to a hierarchy between the active role of the physician assuming the right to represent and the passive role of the patient spoken about. In contrast, by the use of autonomous direct speech as it is the case on the project website, refugees are given the opportunity to speak and represent themselves in front of a broad audience, which, in the long end, can be seen as a token of respect for their autonomy.

### 2.2 *Type of text*

In the MSF presentation of its projects, the voice and perspective of migrants is reinforced by the specific type of text: When looking for example at its brochures, leaflets or other forms of publications, one will notice that MSF usually does not only resort to factual reports, but integrates personal narratives of the people they care for. To summarize the differences between report and narrative very briefly: Reports are mainly objective, technical, focused on common experiences instead of what these mean for a single person. In contrast, narratives help us understand a situation unknown to ourselves, to re-live it, and to empathize and identify more easily, as we are not given insight into an abstract situation of anonymous people but are allowed to share the personal story of a concrete person.[15]

Reports and narratives can cause different effects which can exemplarily be shown through the following passage taken out of a

[15] Kleinman: The Illness Narratives (Note 3); Lars-Christer Hydén: Medicine and Narrative. In: David Herman, Manfred Jahn, Marie-Laure Ryan (Eds.): Routledge Encyclopedia of Narrative Theory. New York 2005, pp. 293–297; Rita Charon: Narrative Medicine. Honoring the stories of illness. Oxford, New York 2006.

book by MSF, in which a report written by a staff member on the travelling plight of refugees is juxtaposed by a quote in which a woman later on treated by MSF tells about her own experiences in this regard:

> [*MSF:*] Women and children are at particular risk, and sexual violence is common. A Congolese woman describes her way through the desert as follows:
>
> [*integrated patient quote:*] We travelled on foot. To do that, you have to be very strong. There was sand everywhere. If you are travelling with young children, it is very difficult. We barely had water and only a few cookies. A group of men approached us. They said, ›We need women‹. They hit me. They raped me for five days, five days! I cried for help, I prayed to God, but there was no miracle that helped me to escape. You wish for death, but death does not come either.
>
> [*MSF:*] People are severely traumatized after such experiences. Many have had bad experiences already before the decision to leave home. Because they usually flee due to war, violence or extreme poverty.[16]

The contrasting features of reports vs. narratives become apparent in the different ways sexual violence is spoken about in the text: In the initial report, the reader is informed in a neutral tone about sexual violence as a common risk for (female) refugees. This information is complemented by a quote of a women who had been raped herself. When telling about the incident she exclaims »They raped me for five days, five days!« The immediate doubling of the phrase »five days, five days!«, which corresponds to the rhetorical device of a so-called gemination, has an amplifying effect on the reader respectively listener, as it doubles the intensity of what is being said. One might just think of the well-known gemination in Jesus Christ's cry of dereliction »My God, my God, why have you forsaken me?«, where the repetitive syntax has become an epitome of the verbalization of a person's most desperate hour. Given in the text type of report, »sexual violence« has the character of a technical or legal term, whose inherent objectivity may create a distancing matter-of-fact stance towards act, actor, and victim. Given in the text type of narrative, however, rape is depicted in a way that reminds that sexual violence is not an abstract fact but a personal calamity, a terrible emotion.

---

16 Anonymous: Migranten und Flüchtlinge. In: Ulrike von Pilar (Ed.): 1971–2011. 40 Jahre MSF. Berlin 2011, pp. 104–106, here p. 105 [translated by Katharina Fürholzer].

The concreteness of the situation is reinforced by the woman's use of pronouns, which in the context of narratives can be full of camouflaged information. In the short quote, the woman uses three different personal pronouns when telling her story: »I«, »we« and »you«. When describing the phase of travelling, the woman speaks in first-person plural – »we travelled«, »we barely had water« – which can be interpreted as an emphasized feeling of togetherness and/or solidarity, both honoring the shared experience of migration and indicating a feeling of being part of a group that might help to handle the extremeness of flight. When the woman starts talking about having been raped, the first-person plural changes to singular: »They hit me. They raped me for five days, five days! I cried for help, I prayed to God, but there was no miracle that helped me to escape.« There is no longer a feeling of being part of a group, no sense of belonging, no shared identity – instead, being raped is depicted as an experience of solitude, as abandonment by a former collective (»we«), by anyone who could help, by humankind and humanity, even by God. When switching from the outer to the inner experience of being raped, the pronoun changes again: »You wish for death«. The abrupt reversion from the first-person singular can be understood in a twofold way: When understanding »you« as synonym for the impersonal third-person »one«, the switch suggests that some events are so extreme to handle, so extreme to bare that the person affected is not or no longer willing or able to identify with it. In contrast, when understanding »you« in the sense of a second-person personal pronoun, the reader can get the impression of being directly addressed and, by extension, of being indirectly encouraged to take action, e.g. to empathize with the woman, to witness her situation in particular or of migrants in general or to take active steps like supporting the MSF cause. The second-person pronoun »you« hence prevents the reader from remaining in a passive, detached role, but admonishes him or her to accept some sort of responsibility.

## 3. Voicing migration

As can be seen from the example, MSF public relations texts feature two aspects: a) MSF's attempt to make aware not only of its own work in the field but also of the hardship of the people they care for, which can be related to their ethical policy of témoignage, and b) doing so not (only) through objective, paraphrased reports but also in form of personal narratives directly told by their patients, which resembles the approaches of narrative medicine.

### *3.1 Narrative medicine*

Due to its emphasis on the voice and perspective of patients, narrative medicine offers itself as an effective means to tackle some of the communicative challenges refugees and health care providers can be faced with. For patients, telling what has happened to them can support them in their recovery process. After all, as stated above, the process of narrating allows us to structure, make sense of and gain control over difficult, chaotic or traumatizing events.[17] Next to that, listening to the stories of refugees is also of importance for health care providers. After all, when caring for refugees, physicians, nurses and the like are faced with a heterogeneous patient collective, both due to different cultures and to individual reactions to conflict, disaster, violence, epidemics, exclusion from health care, migration, et cetera. In this context, patient narratives are valuable pieces of personal evidence helping health care providers to gain insight into the individual backgrounds and needs of patients.[18]

So, what is the value of narratives in the context of medicine and migration? Compared to the typical features of narratives resp. narrative medicine, the stories presented in this paper display one striking idiosyncrasy: Narratives usually comprise tropes such as images, symbols, similes or metaphors, which is also true for illness narratives. Not least due to the work of US-American writer and philosopher Susan Sontag (1933–2004), the meaning of metaphors in medicine is a widely discussed topic within research.[19] In contrast to that, with a few minor exceptions, the MSF patient stories presented above hardly displayed any figurative language. This comes as a surprise as

---

[17] Kleinman: The Illness Narratives (Note 3), p. 49.

[18] Vera Kalitzkus, Peter F. Matthiessen: Narrative-based medicine. Potential, pitfalls, and practice. In: The permanent journal 13 (2009), pp. 80–86.

[19] Susan Sontag: Illness as Metaphor. New York 1978; Susan Sontag: AIDS and its Metaphors. New York 1989; Neil Pickering: The metaphor of mental illness. Oxford, New York 2006; Judy Z. Segal: Health and the rhetoric of medicine. Carbondale 2008; Alan Bleakley: Thinking with metaphors in medicine. London 2017.

metaphors or other forms of tropes can be seen as a possible way to react or even overcome the limit and loss of language[20] – which seems particularly important in light of the spectrum of linguistic, sociocultural, psychological or medical challenges refugees can be faced with. Using tropes instead of literal speech can offer figurative assistance to denote an idea or emotion otherwise impossible to utter. Figurative speech can thus be understood as some kind of »alternative« language that can facilitate coping with stressful or traumatic experiences. At the same time, the use of tropes can also help others – e.g. physicians or therapists – to visualize and empathize more easily with the inner and outer world of another person: Tropes are clues to a patient's background, convictions, beliefs, fears, and hopes. They can help to adjust therapy on the patient's individual language and needs, to find mutual pictures even beyond language barriers and to build a bridge between the patient and the health care professional, eventually leading to a relationship marked by understanding and trust.

However, the strong figurativeness and vividness of metaphors and other forms of tropes, their potential to catapult us into a situation that might be highly emotional or even traumatic, gives reason to assume that they can also have a negative effect, in the sense that the use of figurative speech might cause the speaker to recall and re-suffer old traumata. When following this conjecture, the absence of figurative speech could consequently be understood as the result of an – unconscious – eschewal, that ought to protect the speaker from re-traumatization. The absence of tropes allows for a second hypothesis. While according to the first interpretation the absence of tropes is to be understood as an unwillingness to speak, their absence might also be caused by an inability to speak. Even though pointing at a moral obligation to cease speaking, Theodor W. Adorno's (1903–1969) proposition that there can be no poetry after Auschwitz[21] might indirectly be seen as a key to understand the absence of tropes in the here negotiated narratives of refugees: Some acts of violence, some crimes

[20] Ina Habermann: Reaching beyond silence. Metaphors of ineffability in English poetry – Donne, Wordsworth, Keats, Eliot. In: Monika Fludernik (Ed.): Beyond cognitive metaphor theory. Perspectives on literary metaphor. New York 2011, pp. 77–93; Kathlyn Conway: Illness and the limits of expression. Ann Arbor 2007.

[21] Theodor W. Adorno: Kulturkritik und Gesellschaft. In: Rolf Tiedemann (Ed.): Gesammelte Schriften. Vol. 10.1: Kulturkritik und Gesellschaft I: »Prismen. Ohne Leitbild«. Frankfurt am Main 1977, pp. 11–30, here p. 30.

against humanity are so extreme that they confront us with such a vast linguistic threshold we are neither literally nor figuratively able to vanquish.

The distinction between being unwilling or unable to speak holds different implications: Avoiding the use of tropes in order to protect oneself from re-traumatization implies that the verbal representation of what has been experienced is principally possible. The limit of language is not caused by external aspects but – consciously or unconsciously – by the speaker him- or herself. In contrast, according to the second interpretation, the event in question cannot be put into words because it exceeds human language. Even if willing to do so, the person concerned is devoid of words and must remain silent. The inability to speak reminds of the medical condition of mutism,[22] in that the absence of figurative language can be understood as a precursor to mutism or, more precisely, as figurative mutism. The analogy suggests itself not least due to the fact that in the literature traumatic experiences are instanced as possible cause for mutism in refugees.[23]

It goes without saying that it absolutely forbids itself in the context of this paper to propose any form of diagnosis: The bridging between the loss of tropes and the loss of speech is not to be understood in a medical, but solely in a narratological sense. Rather, the concept of a figurative mutism is itself a kind of image – a trope – to understand the particularities of the negotiated text samples; any medical deliberation requires independent empirical research. Whether one chooses to follow the here proposed hypotheses or not: The examples show that even the very absence of metaphors can become a potential key to the subjective meaning experiences before, during, and after migration may have for the person concerned. However, in contrast to reports, narratives convey messages not only on an explicit level of speech but also between the lines. In order to capture the message contained in a refugee's story – e.g. the psychosocial dimensions that inform about his or her specific condition and situation – as completely as possible, the story needs to be interpreted. In the context of medicine and migration, it is thus the physicians' task to – as Rita Charon puts it – »listen to the narratives of the patient,

[22] ICD-10: F94.0.

[23] Philippe Charlier, Philippe Duverger, Fabiola Bou Abdallah: Memory recall of traumatic events in refugees. In: The Lancet 392 (2018), p. 2170.

grasp and honor their meanings«, meaning to recognize, absorb, interpret, and be moved by the stories of their patients.[24]

### *3.2 Narrative medicine vs. témoignage*

The proposition to be moved by the stories of patients can be understood as an implicit foundation of MSF's policy of témoignage: Patient stories are supposed to move the treating physicians to bring atrocities to the public eye, with the purpose that in turn the readers are moved and react as well. Although patient stories can be seen as a connecting link between narrative medicine and témoignage, the two approaches usually have no overlap: While the MSF policy of témoignage primarily concerns physician-public-communication, narrative medicine is first and foremost related to physician-patient-communication in private patient care. Not least due to their diverging addressees, témoignage and narrative medicine represent opposed objectives: While the former is focused on the well-being of a collective, i.e. an abstract group of patients, the latter aims at the well-being of a single patient.

In light of their apparent differences is has to be asked whether the ethical principles central to narrative medicine are actually compatible with those of témoignage: Narrative medicine is closely linked with the private sphere of patient care. In the context of this approach, working with the stories of vulnerable persons usually serves the goal to be to the benefit of the patient him- or herself. In contrast to that, témoignage is grounded on the idea to speak out when people are suffering extreme crisis or hardship – and to do so not only in private but also in public. Patient stories are a possible instrument to reach this goal, implying, in turn, that témoignage is indirectly based on the idea of making the vulnerability of patients public. In this regard, the reference to or usage of patient stories answers an external – e.g. political – purpose. In a way, stories of the vulnerable hence have to be understood less as an end in itself but rather as a means to an end. Accordingly, the policy of témoignage connotes a utilitarian stance: Patients and their stories are not referred to or used with the goal to serve one patient in particular but a greater patient collective.

[24] Charon: Narrative Medicine (Note 15), pp. 3–4.

### 3.3 *Narrative témoignage*

The way we present another person – e.g. with regard to the mode of speech representation or type of text – is closely linked with ethical deliberations. An example for this is the hierarchy communication structures can cause for the patient-doctor-relationship: MSF defines the policy of témoignage as »a willingness to speak on behalf *of* the people we seek to help«,[25] indicating that it is the responsibility not of the patients but of the physicians to bear witness for the greater good of patients. In this respect, the policy to »speak on behalf of« touches the paternalistic notion underlying the ancient Hippocratic principle of beneficence »salus aegroti suprema lex« (»the well-being of the patient is the supreme law«): With taking care for the patients' well-being as main motive, the physician assumes an active role, whereas the patient is represented by the eyes and language of an expert, remaining – in accordance to the term's etymology –[26] in a literally passive role (lat. *patiens, patior:* suffering, tolerating, bearing).

However, the text samples analyzed in this paper entailed both staff reports and passages where patients are narrators of their own stories, be it in form of an embedded quote or an independent patient story. This juxtaposition of staff reports and patient narratives can lead to a power shift of expertise: Instead of presenting health professionals as sole medical experts on disease and trauma, patients are given a platform where they can voice their stories, showing them as experts on their personal bio- and pathography. Even though issues of narrative medicine usually are not explicitly addressed by MSF, its public relations texts indicate a proximity to both general outlines of narrative medicine (fostering patients to narrate their stories) and témoignage (bearing witness to such stories), resulting, as I would argue, in a form of communication for which I would suggest the term narrative témoignage.

Combining narrative and témoignage yields some ethically relevant advantages for patients, physicians, and society. With regard to the patient, narrative témoignage meets the principles of post-Hippocratic ethics: When patients are enabled to speak for and of them-

---

[25] Médecins Sans Frontières: Speaking out case studies. https://www.msf.org/speaking-out-case-studies (accessed 9/24/2019).

[26] Julia Neuberger: Let's do away with »patients«. In: British Medical Journal 26 (1999), pp. 1756–1758.

selves, this can strengthen their autonomy, and, consequently, lead to a more equal relationship between patient and physician. As a result, the individual is not or no longer a utilitarian-motivated means to an end, i.e. instrument for the well-being of a greater patient collective, but an end in itself.

Moreover, combining staff reports and patient narratives corresponds with a re-allocation of interpretative and representative power. After all, the way a person or situation is represented influences the readers' notion of reality. Even allegedly objective, descriptive reports have a normative dimension: Reports are not written by inert machines but by human beings with individual sociocultural, historical, and biographical backgrounds and mindsets, which is why they may transport implicitly resonant ideas, attributions, and expectations.[27] In consequence, the way e.g. medical, cultural or political facts and events are – directly or indirectly – interlinked, represented, and assessed in a text can thus have an impact on how culture and crisis, medicine and migration are perceived within healthcare and society. However, when combining reports with quotes or stories by patients, these can strengthen or weaken, complement or correct medical experts' perspective, eventually strengthening patients' influence on medical, social, and individual notions of reality.

Last but not least, as mirrors and means of being moved, narratives appear as effective instruments to achieve the goals of témoignage: Objective reports are usually focused on the quantitative magnitude and meaning of witnessed atrocities (e.g. with regard to numbers of victims of persecution, sexual violence, hunger or disease). In addition to that, personal narratives provide insight into the qualitative magnitude and meaning of these facts and figures. Narrative témoignage has the potential to manifest itself both verbally and figuratively in this regard: As could be seen, even the mere absence of metaphors and other tropes can be understood as an *ex negativo*-indicator for psychological effects of experiences such intense that they go beyond words.

[27] Katharina Fürholzer: Das Ethos des Pathographen. Heidelberg 2019, p. 101.

## 4. Conclusion

Narrating is an essential part of being human. Consequently, allowing and fostering patients to voice their stories can be understood as a humanitarian act. When providing health care for refugees, sharing their personal stories either in private or public can be to the benefit of both the patients and their health care providers (narrative medicine) as well as the public (témoignage). Narratives and figurative speech like metaphors, symbols or similes help to recall and utter e. g. moods, stances or emotions towards experiences of war, violence, and migration. Due to their vividness and individuality, they might have both a positive (empathy, coping) and a negative effect (re-traumatization), which is why narrative communication in the context of migration and medicine requires special awareness and future research.

With regard to public relations texts on health care for refugees, the policy of témoignage can get into conflict with the principles of private patient care due to contrasting ethical premises. However, juxtaposing staff reports and patient narratives allows to combine approaches of narrative medicine with those of témoignage. Such narrative témoignage – as I would call it – can help safeguarding both the interests of a single patient and a patient collective. Texts designed after this concept unite personal experiences and interpretations as well as abstract facts and figures, the emotional and intimate as well as the rational and abstract, the inner world as well as the outer world, psychological and social factors of – potentially traumatizing – events as well as biomedical and political factors. Enabling refugees to speak out about what has happened to them before, during, and after migration both in private and in public can hence be seen as a comment or even correction of the perspectives of medical experts. In consequence, narrative témoignage may result in a power shift of expertise: Instead of showing health professionals as supposedly sole experts of disease and trauma, patients are given a platform to speak out as experts of their own stories, eventually strengthening them in their autonomy.

# II. Legal aspects

*Pedro A. Villarreal*

# Differential treatment in the International Health Regulations: towards a nuanced perspective

Abstract
This contribution deals, on the one hand, with the International Health Regulations (IHR) of 2005, an international law instrument adopted by the World Health Organization (WHO)'s Member States for the protection against the trans-border spread of disease; and, on the other hand, with the use of the concept of differential treatment regarding the IHR's capacity-building obligations. Differential treatment can be seen both as a point of reference in legal instruments, as well as an analytical tool ranging across several fields of international law. It is meant, inter alia, to acknowledge the unequal conditions between states for fulfilling certain obligations, while respecting the established principle of sovereign equality. The current wording of the IHR can be seen as incorporating differential treatment, since it provides for different possible timeframes in order to meet core capacity requirements. But beyond this point it does not allow, at first glance, for a more fine-tuned set of distinctions. The underlying complexities of national healthcare systems, and of the persistent challenges for pandemic surveillance and response, can be better tackled through a more nuanced perspective than the one currently enshrined in the IHR.

## 1. Introduction

The regulation of human health at the international level is divided across multiple thematic issues. Perhaps the oldest of them is the protection against the trans-border spread of communicable diseases, as signaled by the first International Sanitary Conference in 1851 in Paris. This regime ultimately evolved from a fragmented set of political statements, into what are currently the International Health Regulations (hereinafter IHR), approved by the World Health Assembly in 2005.

More recently, other dimensions of medicine and public health have also been addressed at the international level. The theory of epidemiologic transition states that, during the $20^{th}$ Century, non-communicable diseases displaced communicable ones at the top of the global burden of disease, both in terms of deaths and of impact in disability-adjusted life years. Certainly, this transition has not occurred at the same pace for all countries. This fact is directly related, among other factors, to the varying capacities of states to deploy strategies for communicable disease prevention and control.

The burden that communicable diseases represent for developing states with underperforming health systems has been documented elsewhere. In fact, communicable diseases have been labeled previously as »diseases of underdevelopment«.[1] But this does not mean they are a challenge only for states with comparatively limited capacities. To the contrary, communicable diseases have a potential for cross-border spread. The goal of the IHR is precisely to tackle such threats. In order to do so, the development of core capacities for disease surveillance and response in all WHO Member States has been highlighted as one of the central concerns. Nevertheless, as continuously stated in yearly reports, after more than twelve years of their entry into force, the capacity-building goals set in the IHR have yet to be fulfilled. The resulting gaps in pandemic preparedness are directly related to unequal degrees of development. As a caveat, this contribution does not address the topic of inequality between individuals, which has been discussed elsewhere in terms of »health inequities«.[2]

In light of the above, this chapter describes some of the persistent challenges for the IHR posed by the unequal capacities between WHO Member States. First, an overview of the concept of differential treatment in international law is provided. Notable instances of the historical background related to the division between developing and developed countries are discussed. Second, some of the obligations established by the IHR are described. Here, a critical perspective of the limitations of a rigid legal approach towards substantive inequality is fostered. Third, a brief appraisal of data from the WHO with regards to the fulfillment of surveillance and response requirements is undertaken. Lastly, concluding remarks underscore the persistent

---

[1] Arthur L. Reingold, Aubree Gordon: Infectious Diseases. In: Michael H. Merson, Robert E. Black, Anne J. Mills (Eds.): Global Health: Diseases, Programs, Systems and Policies. 3rd Edition. Burlington 2012, pp. 177–242, here p. 177.

[2] Frank Kressing: International diversity in healthcare. A critical review of the importance and handling of global health issues. In: Florian Steger (Ed.): Diversität im Gesundheitswesen. Freiburg, München 2019, pp. 112–113.

need for a differentiated approach towards states' obligations under the IHR in accordance with international law.

## 2. Framing Inequality Through International Law: Differential Treatment

Despite the increasing role of other actors as rights- and duty-holders,[3] states are still the core subjects of public international law.[4] As a result, the international legal regime of the protection against the cross-border spread of diseases is currently based on obligations for states. But, needless to say, not all states display the same conditions, particularly in economic terms. Consequently, the question of whether international obligations are formulated whilst taking the unequal positions of states into account comes to the fore. This is where the concept of differential treatment enters the scene. For this contribution, differential treatment is understood as a divergence in the scope and extent of states' obligations within one specific instrument of international law. The definition is broader than the similar one of common but differentiated responsibilities,[5] which is a term introduced in some treaties, resolutions and other instruments, particularly of international environmental law.[6] Other authors add a normative element to the term, by considering differential treatment as being limited to instances in which more substantive equality is sought for, or at the very least not actually hindered by the provisions in a legal instrument.[7] However, this normative dimension will not be

---

[3] Anne Peters: Beyond Human Rights. The Legal Status of the Individual in International Law. Cambridge 2016, pp. 58–59.

[4] Tom Sparks: State. In: Jean D'Aspremont, Sahib Singh (Eds.): Concepts for International Law. Contributions to Disciplinary Thought. Cheltenham, Northampton 2019, pp. 847–849.

[5] Ellen Hey: Common but Differentiated Responsibilities. In: Rüdiger Wolfrum, Frauke Lachenmann (Eds.): Max Planck Encyclopedia of Public International Law. Oxford 2011. https://opil.ouplaw.com/view/10.1093/law:epil/9780199231690/law-9780199231690-e1568, (accessed 9/24/2019).

[6] Sandrine Maljean-Dubois: The Paris Agreement: A New Step in the Gradual Evolution of Differential Treatment in the Climate Regime? In: Review of European Community & International Environmental Law 25 (2016), pp. 151–160, here p. 151.

[7] Philippe Cullet: Differential Treatment in International Law: Towards a New Paradigm of Inter-state Relations. In: European Journal of International Law 10 (1999), pp. 549–582, here p. 551.

taken in these lines as a condition for the existence of differential treatment.

The concept of differential treatment due to unequal capacities is by no means of recent origin. But, whereas sovereign equality is a consecrated principle of public international law,[8] differential treatment is haphazardly included throughout some instruments, and implicitly in others. It dates back to debates on the distinction between sovereign equality versus material or substantive inequality amongst states.[9] Historically, the issue became even more salient when a large group of states, with very unequal levels of economic development, became independent from former colonial powers and, in doing so, enlarged the international community.[10] With this in mind, accepting the elements of differential treatment does not entail depriving formal sovereign equality of its value, especially in political terms. Formal equality has been aimed at preventing the more powerful states from drafting and employing international rules to subjugate less powerful ones.[11] This is as valid now as it was when it emerged as a cornerstone of public international law.

International treaties incorporating differentiated treatment of states according to their capacities have been traced back to, at least, the beginning of the 20th Century.[12] The categories used more often in legal instruments are formulated for referring to developing economies. Alternative categories, with a political twist, include first world vs third world, as well as global north vs global south.[13] Unlike the categories of developed vs developing, the latter distinctions are scholarly and not strictly-speaking legal. They are nevertheless use-

---

[8] Ian Brownlie, James R Crawford: Brownlie's Principles of Public International Law, 9th Edition. Oxford, 2019, pp. 431–439.

[9] Cullet, Differential Treatment (Note 7), pp. 551.

[10] Bernard V. A. Röling: International Law in an Expanded World. Amsterdam 1960, pp. 5–6.

[11] United Nations General Assembly: Declaration on Principles of International Law concerning Friendly Relations and Co-operation among States in accordance with the Charter of the United Nations (A/8082), Resolution No. 2625 (XXV), 24 October 1970. https://www.un.org/ga/search/view_doc.asp?symbol=A/RES/2625(XXV) (accessed 9/24/2019); Juliane Kokott: States, Sovereign Equality. In: Wolfrum, Lachenmann: Max Planck Encyclopedia (Note 5), para. 10. https://opil.ouplaw.com/view/10.1093/law:epil/9780199231690/law-9780199231690-e1113 (accessed 9/24/2019).

[12] Ellen Hey: Common But Differentiated Responsibilities (Note 5).

[13] Bhupinder S. Chimni: International Law and World Order. 2nd Edition. Cambridge, New York, Melbourne 2017, pp. 15–18.

ful for critical debates on the issue of power and asymmetry in international law. Precisely on this point, longstanding disagreements in political negotiations related to international economic law and international environmental law have exposed the rifts between countries located within one of the two categories. The proposals spearheaded by the Non-Aligned Movement during the 1960s and 1970s, inter alia for a New International Economic Order (NIEO),[14] constitute landmark references. Even though they did not lead to the expected transformation of international law,[15] the claims stemming therein were nevertheless enshrined in multiple documents within the United Nations. The Charter of Economic Rights and Duties of 1974[16] and the ensuing controversy it ignited,[17] is an illustration of the historical divide between developed and developing countries.

On a different note, some authors consider that there has been an increase in the employment of differential treatment after the emergence of multiple environmental law instruments, such as the 1987 Montreal Protocol on Substances that Deplete the Ozone Layer.[18] This is also visible in Article 3, paragraph 1 of the United Nations Framework Convention on Climate Change (UNFCCC) of 1992.[19] Such binary distinctions have also been criticized due to their limitations, since, to this date, there is no universally accepted threshold for measuring development.[20] The IHR is a case in point, since this dis-

---

[14] Ingo Venzke: Possibilities of the Past: Histories of the NIEO and the Travails of Critique. In: Journal of the History of International Law 20 (2018) pp. 263–302, here pp. 277–290.

[15] Antony Anghie: Legal Aspects of the New International Economic Order. In: Humanity: An International Journal of Human Rights, Humanitarianism, and Development 6 (2015), pp. 145–158, here pp. 153–154.

[16] United Nations General Assembly: Charter of Economic Rights and Duties of States, Resolution No. 3281 (XXIX),12 December 1974. https://www.un.org/ga/search/view_doc.asp?symbol=a/res/3281(XXIX) (accessed 9/24/2019).

[17] The Charter of Economic Rights and Duties of States and the Deprivation of Foreign-Owned Wealth. In: The American Journal of International Law 75 (1981), pp. 437–475, here pp. 452–455.

[18] Daniel Barstow Magraw: Legal Treatment of Developing Countries: Differential, Contextual, and Absolute Norms. In: Colorado Journal of International Environmental Law and Policy 1 (1990), pp. 69–99, here p. 73.

[19] Christopher D Stone: Common but Differentiated Responsibilities in International Law. In: The American Journal of International Law 98 (2004), pp. 276–301, here p. 276.

[20] Philipp Dann: The Law of Development Cooperation. A Comparative Analysis of the World Bank, the EU and Germany. Cambridge, 2013, pp. 202–205.

tinction is seen throughout the Preamble and Article 44.2(c), though there is no definition offering further clarification. By contrast, more recent instruments of environmental law are more nuanced. A noteworthy example is the inclusion of common but differentiated responsibilities in accordance with national capacities in Article 2.2 of the Paris Agreements of 2015. This effectively overcomes the UNFCCC's binary approach, which divided countries across Annex I (developed) and Annex II (developing).[21]

At the same time, differential treatment in certain areas is not uncontroversial, whether due to its substance or to its form. In terms of substance, international trade law is one example, both before and after the establishment of the World Trade Organization in 1994. The differential treatment of certain countries through the generalized system of preferences (GSP)[22] was viewed by some analysts as particularly disruptive.[23] Here, the differentiation per se is the problem. Conversely, in terms of form, the criteria used when assigning qualities to states has also been criticized. For example, in an attempt to offer more objective yardsticks for assessing countries' economic circumstances, multiple mechanisms have been devised within international financial institutions. The Development Assistance Committee of the Organization for Economic Cooperation and Development,[24] or the World Bank's International Development Association,[25] are bodies which assess the features of states on a case-by-case basis. Their decisions on which countries are »eligible« for Official Development Assistance or preferential loans have a direct impact in the corresponding countries, including projects related to global health.[26] Considering that they are based exclusively on formal, abstract criter-

---

[21] Lavanya Rajamani: Guiding Principles and General Obligation (Article 2.2 and Article 3). In: Daniel Klein, María Pía Carazo, Meinhard Doelle, Jane Bulmer, Andrew Higham (Eds.): The Paris Agreement on Climate Change: Analysis and Commentary. Oxford, New York 2017, pp. 131–140.

[22] Andrew Lang: World Trade Law after Neoliberalism: Reimagining the Global Economic Order. Oxford 2011, pp. 45.

[23] Çaglar Özden, Eric Reinhardt: Unilateral Preference Programs: The Evidence. In: Simon J. Evenett, Bernard M. Hoekman (Eds.): Economic Development and Multilateral Trade Cooperation. Washington 2006, pp. 192–193.

[24] Organisation for Economic Cooperation and Development: DAC in Dates – The History of OECD's Development Assistance Committee. Paris 2006.

[25] World Bank: What is IDA? History. 2018. http://ida.worldbank.org/about/history (accessed 9/23/2019).

[26] Devi Sridhar, Janelle Winters, Eleanor Strong: World Bank's financing, priorities,

ia –be it Gross National Product (GNP) or Gross National Income (GNI) per capita– they have also been subjected to criticism.[27] In this setting, underlying formal issues of differential treatment, and not substantial ones, are at stake.

Other legal instruments may not include differential treatment explicitly, but the way in which their obligations are devised or implemented can be interpreted as such. As for the latter, perhaps the most challenging formulation of differential treatment consists of looking beyond the wording of legal provisions, in order to verify the distinctive impact they have on each signatory state.[28] The drawback is that the nature of legal obligations would be strictly dependent on their effects.[29] On one hand, this could provide for a possibility to adjust legal texts to factual reality. But herein lies an epistemological challenge, since it would require an ex post analysis of empirical data in order to determine whether and to what extent a certain subject has an obligation. Besides, the inevitable subjectivity and limited information used for assessing specific facts taking place at the national level would ultimately render it a problematic endeavor.

## 3. Differential Treatment and the IHR

At the 58th World Health Assembly in 2005, the time was ripe for WHO Member States to approve the revised IHR. It represented a major overhaul in comparison to the previous 1969 version. The then-recent experience with the SARS outbreak of 2003 was a catalyst for creating sufficient consensus within states.[30] Their concerns focused on the need to promptly notify all public health events with epidemic potential to the WHO, an aspect which had been much more

and lending structures for global health. In: British Medical Journal 358 (2017), pp. 1–4, here pp. 2–3.

[27] Dann: The Law of Development Cooperation (Note 20), pp. 203–205.

[28] Stone: Common but Differentiated Responsibilities (Note 19), pp. 277.

[29] Matthias Goldmann: Relative normativity. In: Jean D'Aspremont and Sahib Singh (Eds.): Concepts for International Law. Contributions to Disciplinary Thought. Cheltenham, Northampton 2019, pp. 740–759, here p. 755.

[30] David Heymann, Guénaël Rodier: SARS: A global response to an international threat. In: Brown Journal of World Affairs 10 (2004), pp. 185–197, here pp. 189–190; David Fidler: From International Sanitary Conventions to Global Health Security: The New International Health Regulations. In: Chinese Journal of International Law 4 (2005), pp. 325–392, here p. 325.

restricted in the previous IHR of 1969, which by 2004 only applied to cholera, plague and yellow fever.

The new IHR came into force on 15 June 2007, imposing a series of obligations on states. Two of them can be highlighted here. Firstly, under Article 6 IHR, notifying the WHO of all events taking place in a state's territory which might constitute a public health emergency of international concern, and not just those included in a specified list of diseases, is mandatory. Secondly, obligations to enhance surveillance and response capacities were also introduced in Article 5, whereas they were not present in the IHR of 1969. Both of these points are inextricably linked, since detecting an epidemiological event occurring in a state's territory and then notifying it requires having the technical capacity to do so. This contribution focuses on the second of these two sets of obligations.

During the discussions leading to the IHR, a recurrent question was how its obligations would be applicable to countries with less-developed public health infrastructures.[31] The first paragraph of Article 5 of the IHR foresees a five-year period for countries to achieve the development of core surveillance and response capacities. The possibility of granting two-year extensions, in addition to this initial period, is foreseen in the second paragraph of Article 5 IHR. Yet, unlike other instruments of public international law, there is no list of countries that would qualify as developing countries in need of a special status. The differential treatment in the IHR is not sufficiently nuanced, since the process of capacity stocktaking did not undertake a deeper assessment of material conditions. It can be inferred that such a task would have surpassed the WHO's technical possibilities.

Core capacity obligations for states according to Annex 1.1 consist, broadly speaking, of developing capacities for »surveillance, reporting, notification, verification, response and collaboration« as well as general activities involving airports, ports and ground crossings.[32] In Annex 1.2, states also commit themselves to self-assess their capacities, in order to inform of their progress for meeting the IHR's minimum requirements. Core capacities have been enumerated as: (i) national legislation, policy and financing; (ii) coordination and national

[31] Fidler, From International Sanitary Conventions (Note 30), pp. 372–374.

[32] World Health Organization: IHR core capacity monitoring framework: questionnaire for monitoring progress in the implementation of IHR core capacities in States Parties. 2017 Questionnaire. Geneva 2017.

focal point communications; (iii) surveillance; (iv) response; (v) preparedness; (vi) risk communication; (vii) human resources; and (viii) laboratory. Emphasis is placed on those public health events which are or might constitute a public health emergency of international concern, as defined by Article 1 of the IHR. Within these areas, states persistently report a lack of resources as a reason for not meeting the IHR's goals.

The actual infrastructure required for fulfilling obligations is embedded in the general healthcare setting. There is no requirement to build parallel institutions to those that already provide medical care to the population. The only additional obligation, under Article 4 IHR, consists of designating National IHR Focal Points, which then communicate with the WHO itself. Usually, these consist of offices at the national level already addressing issues of public health.[33] Though this choice is left to states, the actual act of designating a National IHR Focal Point is crucial for the proper implementation of the IHR. Otherwise, the central obligations of notifying the WHO would turn moot.

Despite the binding nature of the IHR, sanctions for non-compliant states are not provided for. Failing to fulfill the goals set in its provisions does not lead to follow-up measures by either the WHO or other Member States. But, contrary to claims in the opposite sense,[34] this does not mean they are not legally binding or ›soft law‹. Under Article 56 of the IHR, there is a possibility for a state to request dispute settlement with another state, though this requires the explicit acceptance of both to submit an issue to binding arbitration. The lack of compliance by state A could be used as an argument by state B, in case it has led to damages in the latter. This, however, remains a theoretical issue, since to this date there have been no disputes based upon the IHR.[35] One may also wonder whether there would be any benefit to opting for this approach.

---

[33] World Health Organization: National IHR Focal Point Guide. https://www.who.int/ihr/publications/nfp/en/ (accessed 9/24/2019).

[34] James Balcius, Thomas Novotny: New approaches to global health governance: The evolution of public-private partnerships. In: Journal of Commercial Biotechnology 17 (2011), pp. 233–240, here p. 234.

[35] Leonie Vierck: The Case Law of International Public Health and Why its Scarcity is a Problem. In: Leonie Vierck, Pedro A. Villarreal and A. Katarina Weilert (Eds.): The Governance of Disease Outbreaks. International Health Law: Lessons from the Ebola Crisis and Beyond. Baden-Baden 2017, pp. 113–142, here p. 117.

According to Annex 1, part A, second paragraph of the IHR, states have an obligation to self-assess and report their progress in developing core capacities to the WHO. National authorities are seen as best suited to do so. The Director-General conveys the collected information to the maximum decision-making body of the organization, the World Health Assembly, composed by Member States meeting in annual sessions. There are yearly reports on progress undertaken by states in the implementation of the IHR.[36] As seen in the most recent documents on the subject matter,[37] the issue of gaps due to uneven capacities, particularly of those countries with fragile health systems, is a constant concern. It has remained so since the initial five-year period expired in 2012.[38]

The WHO recognizes the differentiated status of states with specific features by referring to the term »special-context«, a category including »small island countries, Federal States, countries in conflict and overseas territories«.[39] Although the inclusion of federalism could be considered a strange fit, the category is meant to highlight factors justifying a differential approach instead of a uniform one. The referral to a set of circumstances can be useful for explaining the pace at which states comply with their obligations. But, to date, there has been no further action in this field.

On the one hand, enhancing surveillance and response capabilities will allow for the more effective notification of public health events with a potential for cross-border spillover. Therefore, developed states may foster the strengthening of health systems in other

---

36 World Health Organization: Implementation of the International Health Regulations (2005): five-year global strategic plan to improve public health preparedness and response, 2018–2023, World Health Assembly Decision WHA71(15), 2018. http://apps.who.int/gb/ebwha/pdf_files/WHA71-REC1/A71_2018_REC1-en.pdf#page=1 (accessed 9/24/2019).

37 World Health Organization: Annual Report on the Implementation of the International Health Regulations, Provisional agenda item 11.2, A72/8. Geneva 2019, paras. 10 and 35.

38 World Health Organization: Implementation of the International Health Regulations (2005). Report of the Review Committee on Second Extensions for Establishing National Public Health Capacities and on IHR Implementation. Provisional agenda itm 8.3, 16 January 2015, para. 3. https://apps.who.int/iris/handle/10665/251717 (accessed 9/24/2019).

39 World Health Organization: Annual Report (Note 37), para. 9.

countries from a perspective of enlightened self-interest.[40] By quelling hazardous events, e.g. disease outbreaks, in their places of origin, third states may ensure that the negative effects will not reach their borders. In order to do so, capacities for immediate response need to be present.

Additionally, the requirements of the IHR are not operative in isolation from other issues related to healthcare. Needless to say, ensuring the proper functioning of a healthcare system in the face of new challenges posed by demographic and technological changes represents a conundrum even for the most developed economies.[41] Given the costs related to core capacities for surveillance and response, least-developed and developing states would carry a higher burden if obligations were uniform. Simultaneously, the delay in the development of core surveillance and response capacities by some states hampers the effectiveness of the IHR to this day.[42] In the case of communicable disease outbreaks, the necessary requirements for surveillance and response are not exclusive to monitoring human activity. To the contrary, there are overlapping obligations with regards to animal health, particularly in light of diseases with zoonotic potential. Similar arguments have been raised in disputes at the World Trade Organization, where diverging capacities to monitor disease in animals may limit the legal grounds for imposing trade-restrictive measures of e.g. poultry products at risk of spreading avian influenza.[43]

Ultimately, the threshold for achieving core surveillance and response capacities has not been clearly established to this date. It is

---

[40] Obijiofor Aginam: Global Health Governance. International Law and Public Health in a Divided World. Toronto, 2005, p. 124.

[41] Walter Ricciardi, Stefania Boccia: New challenges of public health: bringing the future of personalised care into focus. In: European Journal of Public Health 27 (2017), pp. 36–39, here p. 39.

[42] Fidler: From International Sanitary Conventions (Note 30), pp. 390–391; Sara E. Davies, Adam Kamradt-Scott, Simon Rushton: Disease Diplomacy. International Norms and Global Health Security. Baltimore 2015, p. 112.

[43] World Trade Organization, India-Measures Concerning the Importation of Certain Agricultural Products. Report of the Appellate Body (4 June 2015), WT/DS430/AB/R. https://www.wto.org/english/tratop_e/dispu_e/cases_e/ds430_e.htm (accessed 9/24/2019); James Nedumpara, Ashish Chandra, Garima S. Deepak: India-Agricultural Products: Defending India's First SPS Dispute. In: Abhijit Das, James J. Nedumpara (Eds.): WTO Dispute Settlement at Twenty. Insiders' Reflections on India's Participation. New Delhi 2016, pp. 213–232.

assumed that states will continue to submit reports to the WHO, informing of their progress in the questionnaires. Given the uneven reporting by states so far, as well as the lack of means to enforce the obligation, any estimates of fully achieving the IHR's purported objectives could only be far-fetched.

## 4. Harmonizing Compliance with the IHR through Capacity-Building

If international law obligations are appraised in binary terms of compliance vs non-compliance, there is not much room for leeway. Failure to meet the five-year deadline, plus the two ensuing two-year extensions, would be understood as non-compliance. But this should not be seen as precluding further capacity-building activities, including implementation schedules. In terms of the WHO's mandate, this is challenging in so far as it requires looking beyond the IHR's text as it stands.[44] A different doctrinal perspective can be useful for the purpose of enhancing the effectiveness of this legal instrument.[45]

The lack of compliance, due to both inability and unwillingness,[46] with the core capacities for disease surveillance and response mandated by the IHR became manifest in the aftermath of the 2009 H1N1 Influenza Pandemic, as well as the 2014–2016 West African Ebola crisis. The IHR Review Committees constituted after each event repeatedly found that several countries failed to meet their core capacities, underscoring the dire state of some healthcare systems as an aggravating factor.[47] In addition, external factors also play a role in

[44] Susan Erikson: The Limits of the International Health Regulations: Ebola Governance, Regulatory Breach, and the Non-Negotiable Necessity of National Healthcare. In: Vierck, Villarreal, Weilert (Eds.): The Governance of Disease Outbreaks (Note 35), pp. 368–371.

[45] Armin von Bogdandy, Matthias Goldmann, Ingo Venzke: From Public International to International Public Law: Translating World Public Opinion into International Public Authority. In: The European Journal of International Law 28 (2017), pp. 115–145, here p. 125.

[46] Davies, Kamradt-Scott, Rushton: Disease Diplomacy (Note 42), pp. 111–136.

[47] World Health Organization: Implementation of the International Health Regulations (2005): Report of the Review Committee on the Functioning of the International Health Regulations (2005) in relation to Pandemic (H1N1) 2009. Report by the Director-General, 64$^{th}$ World Health Assembly, A64/10. Geneva 2010, p. 13–14; World Health Organization: Report of the Review Committee on the Role of the Interna-

justifying a need for differentiated approaches. Variations in prevailing challenges for surveillance and response can be assessed both through interregional and intraregional perspectives. The interregional dimension can be exemplified by how, according to data presented by the WHO's Director-General in May 2019, of the six regions, the African one reports the highest number of epidemiologic events (40 % of the global total).[48] And, as for the intraregional dimension, even within the countries in the African region, there is a visible disparity in terms of reported health infrastructure relevant for pandemic preparedness and response. Deeper analyses of intraregional governance structures have shown how this translates into a leadership role undertaken by countries with more developed economies, such as Nigeria in the case of the West African governance framework.[49]

Within the existing frameworks, there is no strong obligation under international law for developed economies to provide aid to other countries.[50] The scope and reach of solidarity, which underpins international assistance, is open to debate. The legal regime related to the prevention of epidemics and pandemics is no exception. In Article 44.2(c) of the IHR, States Parties commit themselves to technically and financially »support developing countries in building, strengthening and maintaining« disease surveillance and response capacities. But there is no further stipulation of which countries qualify as developing, nor what exactly the support will be. It is a legal provision without further means of implementation.

Despite the lack of strong obligations in the matter, there are financing initiatives aimed at enhancing disease surveillance and response across the globe. The Global Health Security Agenda stands out in the subject of pandemic preparedness and response. Instituted through donations by governments, international organizations and non-state actors, this partnership provides direct financial assistance

---

tional Health Regulations (2005) in the Ebola Outbreak and Response. Report by the Director-General, 69th World Health Assembly, A69/21. Geneva 2016, pp. 20 and 24–25.

[48] World Health Organization: Annual Report (Note 37), p. 1.

[49] Edefe Ojomo: Fostering Regional Health Governance in West Africa: The Role of the WAHO. In: Leonie Vierck, Pedro A. Villarreal and A. Katarina Weilert (Eds.): The Governance of Disease Outbreaks. International Health Law: Lessons from the Ebola Crisis and Beyond. Baden-Baden 2017, pp. 293–296.

[50] John Tobin: The Right to Health in International Law. Oxford 2012, pp. 340–343.

to states. Moreover, it has developed the Joint External Evaluation Tool in collaboration with the WHO, which is aimed at assessing the fulfillment of the IHR's core capacities along three lines: prevention, detection, and response.[51] The Tool is employed on a voluntary basis. Consequently, it cannot be affirmed that international assistance is non-existent overall. Nevertheless, overarching global financing gaps remain. And, also as a result of their soft nature, resources for assistance are heavily dependent on national political will, which makes their flow even more uncertain than if they were based on hard legal obligations.[52]

Still another factor relevant for grasping the uneven fulfillment with the IHR's core capacities obligations is the heterogeneous nature of health systems. Research has shown the disparities in national legislation implementing the IHR, the level of political and logistical coordination between health-related entities, or even the technological features of a determined healthcare infrastructure.[53] The obstacles can be underscored by having a glimpse at the numerous iterations. Given how uniformity is not feasible, taking a more contextualized approach would be of great use for the purposes of the IHR.

## 5. Conclusion: Towards A More Nuanced View of the IHR

The world in which the IHR were approved in 2005 has changed in significant ways. Medical technologies for surveillance and response continue to evolve, giving way to ever more sophisticated and effective tools. At the same time, challenges posed by rampant disparities in economic development between countries continue to be unsettled. As a result, the possibilities to fulfill international law obligations in the field of the protection against epidemics are stunted. A more cali-

---

[51] World Health Organization. Joint External Evaluation Tool. International Health Regulations (2005). Geneva 2016, p. 2. https://apps.who.int/iris/handle/10665/204368 (accessed 9/24/2019).

[52] Sophie Harman, Sara E. Davies: President Donald Trump as global health's displacement activity. In: Review of International Studies 45 (2019), pp. 491–501, here pp. 497–500.

[53] Amitabh B. Suthar, Lisa G. Allen, Sara Cifuentes, Christopher Dye, Jason M. Nagatae: Lessons learnt from implementation of the International Health Regulations: a systematic review. In: Bulletin of the World Health Organization 96 (2018), pp. 110–121E, here pp. 113–115.

brated set of goals in line with actual capacities would contribute immensely to the prevention of epidemics and pandemics. Originally, it would have required a more differentiated framing of the IHR's obligations, by taking into account additional circumstances. At the outset, its current either/or wording would, in principle, not allow for leeway. As empirical data shows, the limited compliance by groups of states is a testament to the continuous shortcomings in the process of strengthening IHR core capacities. In a more formalist legal sense, these delays could be interpreted as a breach of public international law. However, as argued above, the binary approach towards obligations does not go far in terms of improving pandemic preparedness and response. Instead, this contribution has argued for more nuanced perspectives. Adopting more gradual yardsticks for assessing capacity-building could provide a clearer path forward. After all, sufficiently robust healthcare systems cannot be built overnight. The five year-period, plus postponements, established in the IHR were a chimera from the very beginning.

## Acknowledgement

The author would like to thank Prof. Dr. Florian Steger, Dr. Marcin Orzechowski, as well as the participants of the BMBF Symposium, »Migration as a challenge for medicine. A comparison of ethical, juridical, and social aspects in Germany, Croatia and Austria«, which took place at the University of Ulm in March, 2019, for the valuable input provided.

*A. Katarina Weilert*

# The human right to health in public international law with particular reference to asylum-seekers, refugees, and migrants and its reception in German law*

Abstract
When international law speaks of a right to health, it means those services, measures, and facilities that can help a person to maintain or restore one's health. Moreover, the human right to health is conceptualized as »inclusive right«, meaning that it also embraces an array of socio-economic rights that enable a healthy lifestyle. This article aims at adding on the proper normative understanding of the human right to health in international law and its impact on the German law system. The right to health is especially relevant for vulnerable groups. Special attention is given to the situation of refugees, asylum-seekers and undocumented migrants.

## 1. Introduction

The human right to health is guaranteed in various international legal documents and recognized by all states in at least one treaty.[1] When international law speaks of a right to health, it means those services, measures, and facilities that can help a person to maintain or restore one's health. Health itself can never be guaranteed because it depends on the individual circumstances and conditions of the par-

---

* This article is partly a translation of A. Katarina Weilert: Das völkerrechtliche Menschenrecht auf Gesundheit und seine Umsetzung in Deutschland. In: Gesundheits- und Sozialpolitik 72 (2018), pp. 55–61 and A. Katarina Weilert: Das völkerrechtliche Menschenrecht auf Gesundheit und seine Implikationen für das nationale Recht. In: A. Katarina Weilert (Ed.): Gesundheitsverantwortung zwischen Markt und Staat – Interdisziplinäre Zugänge. Baden-Baden 2015, pp. 65–76. Some findings are traced back to A. Katarina Weilert: The Right to Health in International Law – Normative Foundations and Doctrinal Flaws. In: Leonie Vierck, Pedro A. Villarreal, A. Katarina Weilert (Eds.): The Governance of Disease Outbreaks. International Health Law: Lessons from the Ebola Crisis and Beyond. Baden-Baden 2017.

[1] World Health Organization (WHO): The Right to Health. Fact Sheet No. 31. Geneva 2008, p. 1.

ticular person.[2] In international law, the human right to health is conceptualized as »inclusive right«, meaning that it goes beyond immediate health care and is understood as an array of socio-economic rights that enable a healthy lifestyle.[3] This article aims at adding on the proper understanding of the human right to health in international law and its impact on the German law system. Public international law is a hybrid of different forms of »soft law« on the one hand and »hard law«, especially in form of treaties and conventions on the other hand. While soft law as well as political claims and aspirations help to develop international law, only the latter is binding for states. In particular, the right to health is normatively difficult because it combines elements of an individual right and a mere ›objective‹ state obligation. The right to health is especially relevant for vulnerable groups who are most likely to suffer from poor health conditions due to a lack of adequate socio-economic conditions. This article argues that the precise content of the right to health depends on the health system of the particular state. The key words here are »respect« and the »absence of discriminatory practices«. Discrimination is to be understood as unequal treatment without any solid reason. Despite criticism of the UN Committee on Economic, Social and Cultural Rights, German law is in accordance with the international right to health in respect to its legal provisions on access to health care for asylum-seekers and undocumented migrants.

The article will first focus on the development on the human right to health in international law and give deeper insight on how the most relevant norm in this matter, Article 12 of the International Covenant on Economic, Social and Cultural Rights (ICESCR), is to be interpreted. Special attention is paid to the question of vulnerable groups, in particular refugees, asylum-seekers and undocumented migrants. In the next step, we put forward the question of whether the human right to health is an actual human right in the sense of an individual right or whether it is a mere obligation of the states to strengthen their public health policy. The article goes on to explain how international law fits in the German legal system before it gives

---

[2] World Health Organization: The Right to Health (Note 1), p. 5.

[3] World Health Organization: The Right to Health (Note 1), p. 3; Alicia Ely Yamin: The Right to Health Under International Law and Its Relevance to the United states. In: American Journal of Public Health 95 (2005), pp. 1156–1161, here p. 1156.

more information on the current challenges in the German health system. Summarising remarks conclude the article.

## 2. The development of the human right to health

The underlying idea of a human right to health, its philosophical underpinnings and its social-historical development cannot be traced back here.[4] However, the content of the international human right to health will be shown on the basis of the respective international documents and their interpretation and reception by the actors of international law.[5]

### *2.1 The WHO and its impact on the human right to health*

In the founding treaty of the World Health Organization's (WHO) of 1946 (in force since 1948), the member states presented a broad definition of health. Health was defined as »a state of complete physical, mental and social well-being and not merely the absence of disease or infirmity«. The signing parties recorded that »the enjoyment of the highest attainable standard of health is one of the fundamental rights of every human being«.[6] The notion of a right to health being a human right was entirely new at the time and it is not clear whether the member states were aware of the dimension of this claim.[7] The broad definition of the right to health as put forward in the WHO constitution has been criticized to this day. The complete physical, mental and social well-being of every human being cannot be guaranteed by any state, and, moreover, has a dimension that could even allow the state

[4] For an overview of the history see John Tobin: The Right to Health in International Law. New York 2012, pp. 14–43.

[5] On the normative anchors of the human right to health compare also the overview given by Michael Krennerich: Das Menschenrecht auf Gesundheit. Grundzüge eines komplexen Rechts. In: Andreas Frewer, Heiner Bielefeldt (Eds.): Das Menschenrecht auf Gesundheit. Normative Grundlagen und aktuelle Diskurse. Bielefeld 2016, pp. 57–92, here pp. 58–66.

[6] United Nations World Health Organization Interim Commission, Preamble of the Constitution of the World Health Organization, Official Records of the World Health Organization No. 2, New York, Geneva 1948, p. 100.

[7] Brigit Toebes: The Right to Health as a Human Right in International Law. Antwerp 1999, p. 32.

to restrict the freedom of human beings in the name of the promotion of health. However, the definition correctly points out that health is not merely a physical state but highly dependent on many other factors.

Subsequently, the WHO organized a series of conferences which further substantiated the claim of global health promotion and the definition of health. Of particular importance was the Alma Ata Declaration, which was adopted at a conference organized by the WHO in September 1978, with representatives from 134 countries and 67 international organizations. The declaration, which sees primary health care as a an important resource for all, affirmed that health is a »fundamental human right« in the sense of »complete physical, mental and social well-being«. The Ottawa Charter, adopted in 1986, focused on developing a »healthy public policy«, creating »supportive environments« for health, strengthening health-related »community action«, developing »personal skills« in dealing with health and reorienting health services.[8] Thus, special attention was paid to the »objective and subjective possibilities of self-control«.[9] The Ottawa Charter was recognized as »source of guidance and inspiration for health promotion« in the preamble to the Jakarta Declaration. The Jakarta Declaration (1997)[10] also identified the determinants of health, including peace, appropriate housing, education, social security, nourishment, skills and a stable ecosystem. Poverty was classified as the biggest threat to health. The last global health promotion conference was held in November 2016 in Shanghai, China.

## 2.2 *The right to health in the International Covenant on Economic, Social and Cultural Rights*

The first binding recognition of health as a human right was accomplished by Article 12 of the International Covenant on Economic, Social and Cultural Rights (ICESCR) of 1966,[11] which reads as follows:

---

[8] World Health Organization: Ottawa Charter for Health Promotion, 1986.

[9] Rolf Rosenbrock: Die Umsetzung der Ottawa Charta in Deutschland. Berlin 1998, p. 4.

[10] World Health Organization: Jakarta Declaration on Health Promotion into the 21st Century, 1997.

[11] International Covenant on Economic, Social and Cultural Rights, adopted and

1. The states' Parties to the present Covenant recognize the right of everyone to the enjoyment of the highest attainable standard of physical and mental health.

2. The steps to be taken by the states' Parties to the present Covenant to achieve the full realization of this right shall include those necessary for: (a) The provision for the reduction of the stillbirth-rate and of infant mortality and for the healthy development of the child; (b) The improvement of all aspects of environmental and industrial hygiene; (c) The prevention, treatment and control of epidemic, endemic, occupational and other diseases; (d) The creation of conditions which would assure to all medical service and medical attention in the event of sickness.

Article 12 para 1 ICESCR stipulates the highest attainable standard of health[12] to be recognized by the states' Parties. A general comment was issued by the Committee on Economic, Social and Cultural Rights (CESCR) in 2000 in order to interpret Article 12 ICESCR.[13] The general comments of this Committee are not formally binding but highly regarded. The Committee shed light on the vague right to health and substantiated it by deriving more concrete rights. Whether the Member states of the ICESCR wanted to commit themselves to this extent or whether the Committee was going beyond the actual will of the states could be a separate topic in itself.

The broad definition of the right to health according to the preamble of the WHO constitution was not adopted by the ICESCR.[14] However, the Member states agreed in the ICESCR that a right to health goes beyond health care and that health is determined predominantly by many socio-economic factors.[15] The Committee on Economic, Social and Cultural Rights understood the right to health as »inclusive right« that includes not only medical treatment but also factors such as healthy living conditions, clean water, sanitary facil-

---

opened for signature, ratification and accession by General Assembly resolution 2200A (XXI) of 16 December 1966, entry into force 3 January 1976.

12 Tobin: The Right to Health (Note 4), pp. 121–174.

13 Committee on Economic, Social and Cultural Rights (CESCR): Substantive Issues Arising in the Implementation of the International Covenant on Economic, Social and Cultural Rights, E/C.12/2000/4 from 11. August 2000 (General Comment No. 14).

14 For the historical development of the definition of health compare Ben Saul, David Kinley, Jaqueline Mowbray: The International Covenant on Economic, Social and Cultural Rights. New York 2014, p. 980.

15 Committee on Economic, Social and Cultural Rights: Substantive Issues (Note 13), para 4; Saul, Kinley, Mowbray: International Covenant (Note 14), p. 984.

ities, safe food, and safe working conditions as well as health education.[16] The Committee acknowledged that the right to health cannot be a »right to be healthy«[17]. The individual biological health as well as the individual freedom to an unhealthy and risky lifestyle should be considered.[18] Rather, the right to health means that devices, services, goods, and conditions necessary for health should be made accessible to all. Above all, health care facilities and other health related services and goods should meet four main requirements, the so-called »AAAQs«: (1.) availability, (2.) accessibility (non-discriminatory, physical accessible and affordable), (3.) acceptability (»respectful of medical ethics and culturally appropriate«, and (4.) quality.[19] The issue of the insurance system (private, public or mixed) is not determined by the international right to health; however a system of insurance should be affordable for all.[20]

Human rights law has developed a doctrine of threefold state obligations, which are also applicable to the right to health: The states shall respect, protect und fulfil the right to health (tripartite obligation).[21] The obligation to respect means that the states must refrain from violation of the body and health of the individual. The obligation to protect obliges the states to protect the individual from violations done by third parties (e.g. drugs control) and requires the states »to adopt appropriate legislative, administrative, budgetary, judicial, promotional and other measures towards the full realization of the right to health«.[22] The latter includes measures pertaining to health care, such as programmes against contagious diseases, equal access to

---

[16] Committee on Economic, Social and Cultural Rights: Substantive Issues (Note 13), para 4, 11.

[17] Committee on Economic, Social and Cultural Rights: Substantive Issues (Note 13), para 8.

[18] Committee on Economic, Social and Cultural Rights: Substantive Issues (Note 13), para 9.

[19] Committee on Economic, Social and Cultural Rights: Substantive Issues (Note 13), para 12.

[20] Committee on Economic, Social and Cultural Rights: Substantive Issues (Note 13), para 36.

[21] Committee on Economic, Social and Cultural Rights: Substantive Issues (Note 13), para 33.

[22] Committee on Economic, Social and Cultural Rights: Substantive Issues (Note 13), para. 33.

the underlying determinants of health such as safe food and water as well as an affordable health care system.[23]

The Committee on Economic, Social and Cultural Rights acknowledges that the right to health can be realized progressively.[24] Article 2 Abs. 1 ICESCR obliges each »State Party, to take steps, (…) to the maximum of its available resources, with a view to achieving progressively the full realization of the rights recognized in the present Covenant by all appropriate means, including particularly the adoption of legislative measures«. This leaves much room for interpretation. However, the states are immediately obliged to eliminate any form of discrimination and to undertake steps for the full realization of the right to health *(»immediate effect«)*.[25] From the manifold obligations of the right to health of Article 12 ICESCR, the Committee has identified so-called core obligations,[26] which the states are obliged to respect, protect and fulfil, disregarding a potential lack of resources.[27] They include, amongst other things, »access to health facilities, goods and services on a non-discriminatory basis, especially for vulnerable or marginalized groups«, »minimum essential food«, »basic shelter, housing and sanitation, and an adequate supply of safe and potable water«, and the provision of essential drugs.

A further interpretation of the right to health is given in the reports of the Special Rapporteur on the right of everyone to the enjoyment of the highest attainable standard of physical and mental health. The mandate of the Special Rapporteur was established in 2002 by the Commission on Human Rights in Resolution 2002/31. The mandate was first given to Paul Hunt (2002–2008), followed by Anand Grover (2008–2014) and is currently exercised by Dainius

---

23 Committee on Economic, Social and Cultural Rights: Substantive Issues (Note 13), para. 36; Tobin: The Right to Health (Note 44), pp. 331–350.

24 Committee on Economic, Social and Cultural Rights: Substantive Issues (Note 13), para 30.

25 Committee on Economic, Social and Cultural Rights: Substantive Issues (Note 13), para. 30.

26 For the core obligations compare Committee on Economic, Social and Cultural Rights: Substantive Issues (Note 13), paras 43–44. Reaffirmed by CESCR, Duties of states towards refugees and migrants under the International Covenant on Economic, Social and Cultural Rights, 13 March 2017, E/C.12/2017/1, para 9.

27 Amrei Müller: Die Konkretisierung von Kernbereichen des Menschenrechts auf Gesundheit. Internationale Debatten zu »Minimum Core Obligations«. In: Andreas Frewer, Heiner Bielefeldt (Eds.): Das Menschenrecht auf Gesundheit. Normative Grundlagen und aktuelle Diskurse. Bielefeld 2016, pp. 125–168.

Pūras. The Special Rapporteur releases reports on different health relevant areas[28] such as mental health (2017)[29], unhealthy foods, non-communicable diseases, and the right to health (2014),[30] right to health in conflict situations (2013),[31] access to drugs (2013/2011/2010/2009),[32] as well as reports on vulnerable groups, such as migrant workers (2013),[33] adolescents (2016)[34] and older persons (2011)[35].

## 2.3 *Vulnerable groups and refugees, asylum-seekers and undocumented migrants in particular*

The care for marginalized groups or vulnerable members of society is a particular concern of modern international human rights law. Group-specific health protection can be found in the Committee on Economic, Social and Cultural Right's interpretation of the human right to health, according to Article 12 ICESCR and in further conventions that have been specifically adopted to protect vulnerable groups.[36] Group-related international treaties that provide for aspects of a right to health are the Convention on the Rights of the Child of

---

[28] United Nations Office of High Commissioner for Human Rights: Annual reports. http://www.ohchr.org/EN/Issues/Health/Pages/AnnualReports.aspx (accessed 9/24/2019).

[29] United Nations Human Rights Council (UNHRC): A/HRC/35/21 of 28 March 2017. https://undocs.org/A/HRC/35/21 (accessed 9/24/2019).

[30] United Nations Human Rights Council: A/HRC/26/31 of 1 April 2014. https://undocs.org/A/HRC/26/31 (accessed 9/24/2019).

[31] United Nations General Assembly (UNGA): A/68/297 of 9 August 2013. https://undocs.org/A/68/297 (accessed 9/24/2019).

[32] United Nations Human Rights Council: A/HRC/23/42 of 1 May 2013. https://undocs.org/A/HRC/23/42 (accessed 9/24/2019); United Nations Human Rights Council: A/HRC/17/43 of 16 March 2011. https://undocs.org/es/A/HRC/17/43 (accessed 9/24/2019); United Nations General Assembly: A/65/255 of 6 August 2010. https://undocs.org/en/A/65/255 (accessed 9/24/2019); United Nations Human Rights Council: A/HRC/11/12 of 31 March 2009. https://undocs.org/A/HRC/11/12 (accessed 9/24/2019).

[33] United Nations Human Rights Council: A/HRC/23/41 of 15 May 2013. https://undocs.org/A/HRC/23/41 (accessed 9/24/2019).

[34] United Nations Human Rights Council: A/HRC/32/32 of 4 April 2016. https://undocs.org/A/HRC/32/32 (accessed 9/24/2019).

[35] United Nations Human Rights Council: A/HRC/18/37 of 4 July 2011. https://undocs.org/A/HRC/18/37 (accessed 9/24/2019).

[36] World Health Organization: The Right to Health (Note 1), pp. 9 and 11–22.

1989 (Article 24)[37], the Convention on the Elimination of All Forms of Discrimination against Women of 1979 (Article 12)[38], the Convention on the Rights of Persons with Disabilities of 2006 (Article 25)[39], International Convention on the Protection of the Rights of All Migrant Workers and Members of their Families of 1990[40] (Article 28)[41] – Article 7 and 12 ICESCR is relevant here also –, and the Convention on Eradication of Racial Discrimination of 1965 (Art. 5 d iv).[42]

Against the background of an increasing number of people who are immigrants or asylum-seekers, special attention needs to be given to this group.[43] According to Article 1 of the 1951 UN Refugee Convention, modified by the 1967 Protocol, a refugee is a person who

> owing to well-founded fear of being persecuted for reasons of race, religion, nationality, membership of a particular social group or political opinion, is outside the country of his nationality and is unable or, owing to such fear, is unwilling to avail himself of the protection of that country.[44]

Within this sense of the Convention, economic migrants, internationally displaced persons, people suffering from a natural disaster or on the verge of an armed conflict are not to be classified as refugees.[45] People who are fleeing from an armed conflict or other serious violations of human rights can nevertheless become asylum-seekers.

---

37 Convention on the Rights of the Child. https://www.ohchr.org/Documents/ProfessionalInterest/crc.pdf (accessed 9/24/2019), Article 24 para 1 and paras 2–4.

38 Convention on the Elimination of All Forms of Discrimination against Women. https://www.ohchr.org/Documents/ProfessionalInterest/cedaw.pdf (accessed 9/24/2019), Article 12.

39 Convention on the Rights of Persons with Disabilities. https://www.un.org/disabilities/documents/convention/convoptprot-e.pdf (accessed 9/24/2019), Article 25.

40 International Convention on the Protection of the Rights of All Migrant Workers and Members of Their Families. https://www.ohchr.org/Documents/ProfessionalInterest/cmw.pdf (accessed 9/24/2019), Article 2 (1).

41 International Convention on the Protection (Note 40), Article 28. This Convention is not signed by Germany and most industrial countries.

42 International Convention on the Elimination of All Forms of Racial Discrimination. https://www.ohchr.org/Documents/ProfessionalInterest/cerd.pdf (accessed 9/24/2019), Article 5 d (iv).

43 Laura Smith-Khan, Mary Crock: ›The Highest Attainable Standard‹: The Right to Health for Refugees with Disabilities. In: Societies 9 (2019), p. 33.

44 UN Convention and protocol relating to the status of refugees. https://www.unhcr.org/4ae57b489.pdf (accessed 9/24/2019).

45 European Parliamentary Research Service Blog. https://epthinktank.eu/2015/10/27/refugee-status-under-international-law/ (accessed 9/24/2019).

The term asylum-seeker includes persons who formally apply for asylum, either because they are refugees or because they were forced to immigrate by any other reason.[46] Therefore, »[n]ot every asylum-seeker is a refugee, but every refugee is initially an asylum-seeker.«[47]

The Committee on Economic, Social and Cultural Rights has found in its general comment on the Right to health that:

> states are under the *obligation to respect* the right to health by, inter alia, refraining from denying or limiting equal access for all persons, including prisoners or detainees, minorities, asylum-seekers and illegal immigrants, to preventive, curative and palliative health services; abstaining from enforcing discriminatory practices as a state policy[48].

It is notable that the Committee understands the obligation to respect not only as a prohibition of the state to deny access to health services. If the emphasis was merely on what the state should not do, there would be no obligation for a positive act. The findings in the general comment are not always clear and stringent. It seems, however, that the obligation to respect means more than just a refrain from doing something. On the other hand, an obligation to respect can barely mean an obligation to fully (also financially) provide for health care. The exact meaning remains somewhat obscure and is open for political discussion and practice. In addition, it needs to be remembered at this point that the general comments of the Committee on Economic, Social and Cultural Rights are not a formally authoritative and binding interpretation. It is likely to assume that the precise meaning depends on the health system of the particular state. The key points here are respect and the absence of discriminatory practices.

The Committee on Economic, Social and Cultural Rights has reaffirmed its findings towards the right to health with special regard to

---

[46] In the literature, the terms are not always used coherently, see Hannah Bradby, Rachel Humphris, Dave Newall, Jenny Phillimore: Public health aspects of migrant health: a review of the evidence on health status for refugees and asylum seekers in the European Region. Copenhagen: WHO Regional Office for Europe. Copenhagen 2015 (Health Evidence Network synthesis report 44), Annex 2 Definitions of refugees, asylum seekers and migrants in the literature. http://www.euro.who.int/__data/assets/pdf_file/0004/289246/WHO-HEN-Report-A5-2-Refugees_FINAL.pdf (accessed 9/24/2019).

[47] Paola Pace: Migration and the Right to Health: A Review of International Law. In: International Migration Law 19 (2009), p. 2.

[48] Committee on Economic, Social and Cultural Rights: Substantive Issues (Note 13), para 34.

refugees and migrants in a more recent statement from March 2017.[49] The Covenant rights shall apply to »all people under the jurisdiction of a state«, including not only asylum-seekers and refugees, but also irregular migrants.[50] In this statement, the Committee has also further elaborated in how far states must grant the same access to the Covenant's rights without any discrimination on grounds of nationality or legal status and where a different treatment might be justifiable. Distinctions are possible under certain conditions:

> Any distinction, exclusion, restriction or preference, or other differential treatment on grounds of nationality or legal status, should therefore be in accordance with the law, pursue a legitimate aim and remain proportionate to the aim pursued. A difference in treatment that does not satisfy such conditions should be seen as unlawful discrimination prohibited under Article 2 (2) of the Covenant.[51]

The Committee on Economic, Social and Cultural Rights has given further insight on how it interprets Article 12 ICESCR in its recommendations on the periodic state's reports (according to Article 16 and 17 of the ICESCR). Within the context of these recommendations, the Committee has understood Article 12 ICESCR as demanding the states to also provide access to health care for refugees and asylum-seekers and undocumented migrants.[52]

In addition to that, the Committee has found in its general comment on »Non-discrimination in economic, social and cultural rights« (concerning Article 2 para 1 of the ICESCR) that:

> The ground of nationality should not bar access to Covenant rights, e. g. all children within a state, including those with an undocumented status, have a right to receive education and access to adequate food and affordable health care. The Covenant rights apply to everyone including non-nationals, such as refugees, asylum-seekers, stateless persons, migrant work-

[49] Committee on Economic, Social and Cultural Rights: Duties of states towards refugees and migrants under the International Covenant on Economic, Social and Cultural Rights, 13 March 2017, E/C.12/2017/1. https://undocs.org/E/C.12/2017/1 (accessed 9/24/2019).

[50] Committee on Economic, Social and Cultural Rights: Duties of states (Note 49), para 3.

[51] Committee on Economic, Social and Cultural Rights: Duties of states (Note 49), para 5.

[52] Committee on Economic, Social and Cultural Rights: Concluding observations on the fifth report of Germany submitted under Articles 16 and 17 of the Covenant from 12 July 2011, E/C.12/DEU/CO/5, para. 13.

ers and victims of international trafficking, regardless of legal status and documentation.[53]

The Committee on Economic, Social and Cultural Rights speaks of affordable health care, which makes clear that health care does not necessarily have to be for free. If a person has no income or other financial means and if the state provides free health care for its citizens in need, the principle of non-discrimination could argue in favour of free access to basic health care.

Moreover, in the Article 23 of the Geneva Refugee Convention[54], most states have committed themselves to grant to refugees »lawfully staying in their territory the same treatment with respect to public relief and assistance as is accorded to their nationals«. This rule only applies to those who have been acknowledged as »refugee« by the respective state.[55]

It needs to be noted here that according Article 2 para 1 ICESCR, states have to provide mutual assistance with respect to their obligations of the Treaty. This finding is strengthened by the general comment on the right to health provided by the Committee on Economic, Social and Cultural Rights:

> states parties have a joint and individual responsibility, in accordance with the Charter of the United Nations and relevant resolutions of the United Nations General Assembly and of the World Health Assembly, to cooperate in providing disaster relief and humanitarian assistance in times of emergency, including assistance to refugees and internally displaced persons.[56]

The owed international humanitarian assistance is not limited to the countries of origin but can be understood as to include assistance for those countries who have opened their borders for asylum-seekers. Refugees are not only to be regarded as the problem of the country of arrival or reception but the international community as a whole is

---

[53] Committee on Economic, Social and Cultural Rights: General Comment No. 20, E/C.12/GC/20, https://undocs.org/E/C.12/GC/20 (accessed 9/24/2019), para 30 (2 July 2009) on »Non-discrimination in eco-nomic, social and cultural rights« (Article 2, para. 2, of the International Covenant on Economic, Social and Cultural Rights).

[54] Convention Relating to the Status of Refugees from 28 July 1951 (in force since 22 April 1954) and Protocol relating to the Status of Refugees from 31 January 1967 (in force since 4 October 1967).

[55] Winfried Kluth: Gesundheitsdienstleistungen nach dem Asylbewerberleistungsgesetz. In: Soziale Sicherheit (2018), pp. 32–38, here p. 35.

[56] Committee on Economic, Social and Cultural Rights: Substantive Issues (Note 13), para 40.

called upon to help one another in case of humanitarian emergencies (including the care for refugees). The recent large flows of migrants and refugees have caused the Committee to elaborate on this issue. In its statement of March 2017, the Committee argued that the realization of the Covenant rights is a »common objective of all states parties« who need to »cooperate in fulfilling this aim«. As some states have a »heavier burden than others« the Committee »sees any measure that states parties adopt to support the realization of the Covenant rights on the territory of other states as contributing to the aims of the Covenant«.[57]

## 3. Is the right to health an individual right?

The international right to health combines elements of an individual right (right of freedom as well as a social right) and a mere »objective« state obligation which cannot be claimed as such by an individual.[58] Historically, the public-health approach predated the understanding of the right to health as a right of the particular individual.[59] This is not surprising if one considers that the idea of subjective rights is a quite recent one in international law.[60] Public health refers to the population and to groups and thus concentrates on group-related considerations instead of focussing on the individual person. It is a policy-oriented approach, which looks at human health with a comprehensive and interdisciplinary perspective, including the agreement of socio-economic and environmental conditions. From a law perspective, public health focuses above all on the objective obligation of the state to care for its population and does not grant individual rights to persons. An individual right to health is taking on a subjective point of view. It is about possible claims of a person, which help him or her to stay healthy or to restore one's health. The Committee on Eco-

---

[57] Committee on Economic, Social and Cultural Rights: Duties of states (Note 49), para 18.

[58] Weilert: The Right to Health (Note 1); Timothy Goodman: Is there a Right to Health? In: Journal of Medicine and Philosophy 30 (2005), pp. 643–662; P. Hunt: Interpreting the International Right to Health in a Human Rights-Based Approach to Health. In: Health and Human Rights Journal 18 (2016), pp. 109–130; Toebes: The right to health (Note 7); Tobin: The right to health (Note 4).

[59] Thérèse Murphy: Health and Human Rights. Oxford, Portland 2013, p. 30.

[60] Anne Peters: Jenseits der Menschenrechte. Tübingen 2014, p. 473.

nomic, Social and Cultural Rights interprets Article 12 ICESCR in a way that combines individual rights aspects and public health elements. Often the borders between both are blurred. This adds to the confusion about the proper understanding of a right to health.

## 4. The nature of international law and how it fits in the German law system

While German law is comprised of legal norms and additional procedural laws, which enable effective law enforcement, international law is characterized by binding law and non-binding agreements, the so-called soft law. Most statements by international organizations are non-binding. Agreements are more likely to be made at state conferences if they are non-binding, and this tends to be forgotten when referring to those agreements as though they were indeed binding.

There has been much confusion about the differences of soft law and formally binding law. A recent example is the Global Compact for Safe, Orderly and Regular Migration (GCM).[61] In December 2018, the Compact was adopted by the majority of UN Member states and a few days later adopted via a resolution of the UN General Assembly. In Germany, there has been a debate around the question whether Germany is bound by this Compact. The wording of the contract is explicit as to this question: In its preamble (para 7) it makes clear that the Compact »presents a non-legally binding, cooperative framework« and in para 15 lit b of the Compact it reads: »The Global Compact is a non-legally binding cooperative framework«. The adoption by the UN General Assembly does not change its status under international law, as its resolutions are generally non-binding. Although the compact is not legally binding, it is, however, politically imperative. When states adopt a non-binding compact, they present their intentions and their political outlooks and opinions. The format of a convention, even if legally non-binding, is powerful and goes far beyond the declaration of a singular state. In addition to that, the Migration Compact includes a whole section on »implementation« (paras 40–47). The states »commit themselves to fulfil the objectives and commitments … by taking effective steps at all levels«. There are

[61] United Nations General Assembly (UNGA): A/RES/73/195. https://www.un.org/en/ga/search/view_doc.asp?symbol=A/RES/73/195 (accessed 9/24/2019).

no specific duties, yet, these provisions present a strong political statement. Therefore, NGOs and other groups can point to state's failures with regard to the Compact which results into political pressure.

The distinction between hard and soft law is blurred by the fact that binding international law, such as Article 12 UN ICESCR, also suffers from an enforcement deficit and that there are monitoring systems also for soft law.[62] The individual complaint procedure as provided for in an additional protocol to the ICESCR, which itself also has only moderate enforcement mechanisms, has not yet been signed by Germany. The mandatory states' reports according to Article 16 and 17 of the ICESCR are supposed to contribute to the effective implementation of the pact. In fact, the evaluation of a state's report by the Committee on Economic, Social and Cultural Rights eventually leads only to rather toothless criticisms as well as suggestions and recommendations. It would be particularly effective for the individual if one could sue the obligations under Article 12 ICESCR directly in one's country. However, international law is not automatically part of national law. Rather, each state determines itself how it transfers international law into national law. Under German constitutional law, international treaties are transferred into the national legal sphere by the enactment of a federal law (Article 59 Abs. 2 GG).[63] This means that international treaties only have the status of a federal law and are not on the same legal level as (or even higher than) constitutional law. However, the German Federal Constitutional Court (*Bundesverfassungsgericht*) held that German constitutional law is to be interpreted in light of international treaty law.[64] In this way, international law can gain legal impact in a German courtroom. However, this does not mean that Article 12 ICESCR would form its own basis of entitlement (subjective right). Again, every state decides itself, whether international law after it is transferred into the national legal sphere, is »directly applicable«, i.e. whether a norm of international treaty law is sufficiently precise in order to form a legal basis for claims in the

---

[62] World Health Organization: The Right to Health (Note 1), pp. 31–39; Saul, Kinley, Mowbray: International Covenant (Note 14), pp. 1038–1083.

[63] International Covenant on Economic, Social and Cultural Rights (ICESCR). In: Bundesgesetzblatt (BGBl) 1976 II, p. 428.

[64] BVerfGE (Law Reports of the German Federal Constitutional Court) 111, 307 (317).

courtroom.[65] The question whether a norm of international law can be relied on in a case before a national court becomes less relevant if the content of the treaty-law is already provided for in national law. With regard to the right to health, German laws provide a system that – generally speaking – meets the standards of international law. Questions have primarily been put forward with regard to refugees and asylum-seekers.

## 5. Current challenges in the German health system

A major challenge for the German social system including the health care system is the high number of refugees and asylum-seekers who were and still are taking residence in Germany.

### *5.1 Health protection of refugees and asylum-seekers and undocumented migrants*

The German Federal Constitutional Court (*Bundesverfassungsgericht*) found in its ruling from July 2012 that all persons who are residents in Germany (no matter whether German nationals or foreigners) are entitled to claim state benefits in order to meet their basic needs with respect to their physical existence (i. e. food, clothing, housing, hygiene and health) as well as with respect to a minimum level of participation in social, cultural and political life.[66] This ruling also includes asylum-seekers.[67] The Court has derived this right from the human right to human dignity and thus given it the highest rank and authority possible in the German law. According to this ruling, the parliament has to enact laws which ensure theses rights.[68]

The UN Committee on Economic, Social and Cultural Rights has given only a few remarks on health-related issues in its »concluding observations« on the fifth periodic report of Germany under Article 16 and 17 of the ICESCR (from 2008).[69] Of particular interest is

---

[65] A. Katarina Weilert: Transnationale Unternehmen im rechtsfreien Raum? In: Heidelberg Journal of International Law 69 (2009), pp. 883–917, here pp. 903–904.

[66] BVerfGE 132, 134 (Note 64), p. 160.

[67] BVerfGE 132, 134 (Note 64), pp. 161–162.

[68] BVerfGE 132, 134 (Note 64), p. 160.

[69] Fifth periodic report submitted by Germany under Articles 16 and 17 of the Cove-

the Committee's call to provide asylum-seekers with equal access to health care. This should go beyond the (then already existing) emergency care.[70] The Federal Republic of Germany has replied to this position of the Committee in its sixth periodic report of 2016 (submitted to the Committee in February 2017). It referred to the situation of asylum-seekers that »although in principle the entitlement only covers services relating to the treatment of acute illnesses or pain (Section 4 (1) of the Act on Benefits for Asylum Applicants – ABAA – AsylbLG), it is also supplemented by ›other services‹, if these are essential to safeguard health or required to meet children's particular needs (Section 6 (1) of the ABAA)«.[71] The person who requires health treatment under these conditions needs to apply for this at the local municipal social security office (kommunale Sozialbehörde). This can lead to delays. This delay is avoided in those Federal states (Bundesländer), in which an electronic health card is introduced also for asylum-seekers.[72]

After 15 months of staying in Germany, asylum-seekers receive almost all benefits under the statutory health insurance (section 264 para 2 ScB V in conjunction with section 2 ABAA), and although they are not formally insured, they have the same access to medical services as all other insured persons there. German law passed in October 2015 (Asylverfahrenbeschleunigungsgesetz – Act on the Acceleration of Asylum Procedures) improved the situation for refugees, who have not yet reached the 15-month limit. Section 264 para 1 Social Code V (SCB V) was amended and now enables asylum-seekers to get free health care if there has been an agreement between the statutory health insurance and the Bundesländer (or subsidiary districts – Landkreise/kreisfreie Städte). The access to free health care for asylum-seekers during their first 15 months of being in Germany

---

nant from 16 September 2008, E/C.12/DEU/5. https://www.institut-fuer-menschenrechte.de/fileadmin/user_upload/PDF-Dateien/Pakte_Konventionen/ICESCR/icescr_state_report_germany_5_2008_en.pdf (accessed 9/24/2019).

[70] Committee on Economic, Social and Cultural Rights: Concluding observations (Note 52), para 13.

[71] Sixth periodic report submitted by the Federal Republic of Germany under Articles 16 and 17 of the International Covenant on Economic, Social and Cultural Rights 2016. https://www.institut-fuer-menschenrechte.de/fileadmin/user_upload/PDF-Dateien/Pakte_Konventionen/ICESCR/icescr_state_report_germany_6_2016_en.pdf. (accessed 9/24/2019).

[72] Kluth: Gesundheitsdienstleistungen (Note 55), pp. 36–37.

is, however, not uniform within Germany as this is an issue, which is not in the competence of the Federation (Bund).

The UN Committee on Economic, Social and Cultural Rights gave its »final remarks« on the sixth period report of Germany in November 2018[73] and herein again referred to the situation of asylum-seekers within the first 15 month of their stay in Germany. The Committee expressed its concerns that »under the Act on Benefits for Asylum Applicants, asylum-seekers' access to health care is restricted to acute and painful conditions for the first 15 months« and that the additional »other essential health-care services« as provided under the Act are not clearly defined«.[74] The Committee recommends changes in the respective laws in order to ensure »that all persons in the State party, including asylum-seekers, have equal access to preventive, curative and palliative health services, regardless of their legal status and documentation«.[75] These findings of the Committee are not taking into consideration that Germany, being a country with a high quality health system, wants to prevent people from crossing the borders only for reasons of free high-end health treatment.[76] This is one reason for the lack of a clear definition of »other essential health-care services« under Section 6 (1) of the ABAA.[77]

In addition, the German system is primarily funded by insurance premiums of the insured persons, which leads to a higher quality of health services than in countries with a purely tax-funded system. Health care is tax-funded only for those who cannot afford to contribute to the system.[78]

With respect to migrant's health, the Committee has expressed its concerns about section 87 (2) of the Residence Act (AufenthG) which »obliges public authorities to report undocumented migrants to immigration authorities«. This can »deter irregular migrant workers from seeking services, such as health care, that are essential for the

---

[73] Committee on Economic, Social and Cultural Rights: Concluding observations on the sixth periodic report of Germany, 27 November 2018, E/C.12/DEU/CO/6. https://undocs.org/E/C.12/DEU/CO/6 (accessed 9/24/2019).

[74] Committee on Economic, Social and Cultural Rights: Concluding observations (Note 73), para 58.

[75] Committee on Economic, Social and Cultural Rights: Concluding observations (Note 73), para 59.

[76] Kluth: Gesundheitsdienstleistungen (Note 55), p. 35.

[77] Kluth: Gesundheitsdienstleistungen (Note 55), p. 35.

[78] Kluth: Gesundheitsdienstleistungen (Note 55), p. 35.

enjoyment of their rights«. Therefore, the Committee »recommends that the State party establish a clear separation (›firewall‹) between public service providers and immigration enforcement authorities, including through repealing section 87 (2) of the Residence Act, to ensure that irregular migrant workers can access basic services without fear.«[79]

The addressed problem is a factual obstacle for undocumented migrants (also called »irregular migrants«)[80] to get access to public service providers because of their fear of being reported. Undocumented migrants are people who came to Germany without any residence permit and do not have a »temporary suspension of deportation« (Duldung) under section 60 a Residence Act (Aufenthaltsgesetz). Asylum-seekers are not undocumented migrants. Undocumented migrants are those migrants who have no right to stay in Germany and could face deportation if the authorities are informed about them being in Germany. Like any other sovereign state, Germany can regulate migration and is allowed to enforce its laws. Therefore, the question arises whether there is a state obligation to provide access to health care also for those people who are unlawfully taking residence in a country. As mentioned earlier, the Committee on Economic, Social and Cultural Rights has stretched the right to health under Article 12 ICESCR also to illegal migrants.[81] Again, it is not clear how »refraining from denying or limiting equal access« within the obligation to respect the right to health is to be interpreted. *De iure* these persons have also access to basic health treatment, however, not to the full range of health treatments.[82] *De facto* they are excluded from making use of their rights to get free health care (except for emer-

---

[79] Committee on Economic, Social and Cultural Rights: Concluding observations (Note 73), paras 26–27.

[80] Ibrahim Kanalan, Markus Krajewski: Medizinische Versorgung irregulärer Migranten aus menschenrechtlicher Sicht. In: Zeitschrift für europäisches Sozial- und Arbeitsrecht 10 (2017), pp. 418–426, here p. 419.

[81] Committee on Economic, Social and Cultural Rights: Substantive Issues (Note 13), para 34. See also the Recommendations as given on the periodic state reports: Committee on Economic, Social and Cultural Rights, Concluding observations on the sixth periodic report of Germany (Note 73), paras 26–27; Concluding observations on the sixth periodic report of the United Kingdom of Great Britain and Northern Ireland, 14 July 2016, E/C.12/GBR/CO/6, para 56; Concluding observations on the second periodic report of Greece, 27 October 2015, E/C.12/GRC/CO/2, paras 25–26.

[82] Section 1 No. 5 Act on Benefits for Asylum Applicants (AsylbLG); Kanalan, Krajewski: Medizinische Versorgung (Note 80), pp. 419–420.

gency cases[83] and cases of serious illnesses as a serious illness may form a »temporary suspension of deportation« (Duldung) according to section 60 a Residence Act (Aufenthaltsgesetz)[84]) because of the fear of having to leave Germany as the price for health treatment. It would of course be possible to get health treatment if a person paid for the treatment. However, unlawful immigrants usually have only low or no income and cannot afford health care. Non-governmental initiatives are set up to help them to get access to health care. Section 87 (2) of the Residence Act (Aufenthaltsgesetz) is not opposed to international law because people do not have a right to not being »detected« as illegal immigrants and states are allowed to decide upon immigration policies as long as they provide access to asylum-seekers and refugees.[85] However, the situation of undocumented immigrants is far from being satisfactory and might be unjust in a moral sense in some cases.

### 5.2 *Further fields of action*

Compared to many other countries, Germany has quite a high level of health care as well as the underlying determinants of good health. The health-related deficiencies with regard to Germany's treaty obligations that have been pointed out by the respective treaty bodies, concern predominantly rather marginal issues. Some issues also relate to highly debatable and ethical health issues. However, there are some deficiencies with respect to vulnerable groups such as children living in precarious circumstances and elderly people. The Committee on the Rights of the Child points out that children should be provided with better knowledge about the importance of physical exercise and the impact of healthy eating habits as well as a healthy lifestyle in general.[86] With regard to mental health, the Committee required Ger-

[83] Kanalan, Krajewski: Medizinische Versorgung (Note 80), p. 421.

[84] Kanalan, Krajewski: Medizinische Versorgung (Note 80), p. 422.

[85] But see also Kanalan, Krajewski: Medizinische Versorgung (Note 80), pp. 420–423 who argue that section 87 (2) of the Residence Act (Aufenthaltsgesetz) is contrary to international law.

[86] Committee on the Rights of the Child (CRC): Concluding observations on the combined third and fourth periodic reports of Germany, 25 February 2014, CRC/C/DEU/CO/3–4. https://undocs.org/en/CRC/C/DEU/CO/3-4 (accessed 9/24/2019), para 57.

many, inter alia, to pay more attention to »provide families with access to psychological counselling and emotional support« and »improve the diagnosis of mental health problems among children«.[87] The Committee on the Rights of the Child also calls for improving drug education for adolescents.[88]

The Committee on the Rights of Persons with Disabilities has requested Germany to repeal section 1905 BGB, a German law, according to which a custodian can give consent to a sterilisation of a person under his custodianship if the person is unable to give his or her consent.[89] In addition, the Committee has urged Germany to ensure that any forms of psychiatric treatment only take place under the condition of a free and informed consent of the patient.[90] Other than that, the Committee on the Rights of Persons with Disabilities has not specified any broader health related issues, but has only found that refugees and asylum seekers with disabilities do not have full access to health care.[91]

The Committee on Economic, Social and Cultural Rights has found already in its concluding observations on the fifth report of Germany in 2011 that the situation of older persons in nursing homes is not acceptable due to partly inhumane conditions and lack of qualified personal in these facilities.[92] Germany has replied to this criticism in its sixth periodic report (2016) in detail, and put forward the measures taken to improve the quality of nursing facilities and to overcome the shortage of qualified staff.[93] Demographic changes and changing family structures have led to a greater challenge for the whole care sector. In addition, after the periodic report of 2016, these problems have been on the political agenda in Germany. Therefore, the Committee has correctly repeated its concerns especially with re-

---

[87] Committee on the Rights of the Child: Concluding observations (Note 86), para 59.

[88] Committee on the Rights of the Child: Concluding observations (Note 86), para 61.

[89] Committee on the Rights of Persons with Disabilities: Concluding observations on the initial report of Germany, 13 May 2015, CRPD/C/DEU/CO/1, para 38.

[90] Committee on the Rights of Persons with Disabilities: Concluding observations (Note 89), para 38.

[91] Committee on the Rights of Persons with Disabilities: Concluding observations (Note 89), para 47.

[92] Committee on Economic, Social and Cultural Rights: Concluding observations on the fifth report (Note 52), para 27.

[93] Sixth periodic report submitted by the Federal Republic of Germany (Note 71), pp. 50–54.

spect to the »chronic shortage of qualified caregivers«.[94] The current measures can only be a first step in an area that is one of the big challenges for Germany in the near future.

## 6. Summarising remarks

The international right to health was first recognized in the preamble of the constitution of the WHO in 1946 and established as binding law with Article 12 ICESCR in 1966. Its specific content was shaped especially through the interpretation of the Committee on Economic, Social and Cultural Rights since its General Comment on the Right to Health, which was issued in 2000. Health issues especially endanger marginalized and vulnerable groups, i.e., asylum-seekers, refugees and undocumented migrants. Apart from core obligations, the Committee on Economic, Social and Cultural Rights has not provided for an absolute standard of health services and facilities that should be met by the state Parties. Rather, it has understood the right to health as to be provided in a non-discriminatory manner. As the costs for a high-quality health care system are one of the big challenges, even for industrial countries, the idea of unlimited access to free health care from the first day of being resident in a foreign country is difficult to achieve in a world which is still made up of nation states with different health systems (including different schemes of financing them) and different levels of quality of health services. Therefore, it may be well justified for a country, such as Germany, to make free access to health services dependent on the duration of the person's stay. However, as access to a basic health care (especially treatment of acute illnesses and pain) is a condition for a life with dignity, the state cannot exclude any person on the basis of nationality or legal status from such a basic care.

[94] Committee on Economic, Social and Cultural Rights: Concluding observations on the sixth report (Note 73), paras 48–49.

# III. Societal Aspects

*Frank Kressing and Maximilian Schochow*

# Aspects of migration, culture and health care in Germany's past and present

Abstract

Focussing on the actual state of health care in the present-day of Germany, it is pointed out that the country's health care system has neither been well prepared for the advent of refugees in the 21st century nor for specific health needs of migrants in the 20th century. The authors argue that the wide-spread neglectance of cultural diversity in Germany's contemporary health care system constitutes a surprising fact in regard of the country's intense historical experience with various migration movements, its colonial legacy and the multi-cultural composition of the country's pre World War I population. In an examination that is based both on anthropology and history, a careful usage of the term »culture« is advocated, transgressing the established notion of fixed ethnic, cultural and linguistic identities. These theoretical considerations result in practical suggestions for the improvement of cultural sensitive health care in hospitals in comtemporary Germany.

## 1. Introduction

According to 2017 figures, migrants and their descendants make up about 19 million people within Germany's population of roughly 83 million people, thus amounting to approximately 23 % of the country's residents.[1] Additionally, there is an unknown number of medical tourists looking for treatment in Germany which is either

[1] Statistisches Bundesamt: Mikrozensus – Bevölkerung mit Migrationshintergrund. Press Release No. 282, 1/8/2018. https://www.destatis.de/DE/Presse/Pressemitteilungen/2018/08/PD18_282_12511.html (accessed 9/24/2019); Bundeszentrale für politische Bildung: Migration. http://www.bpb.de/nachschlagen/zahlen-und-fakten/soziale-situation-in-deutschland/61621/migration (accessed 9/24/2019); Bundesamt für Migration und Flüchtlinge: Statistiken. http://www.bamf.de/DE/Infothek/Statistiken/statistiken-node.html (accessed 9/24/2019).

not available in their home countries, or available only at higher costs or lower quality.[2] Thus, the German health care system can be characterized by an increasing international composition of patients and health care providers, such as doctors and nurses, alike.[3] As recent results of health services research show, however, migrants can be counted among the vulnerable groups within the health care system.[4] Regarding pronounced cultural diversity within the German health care system often leading to the neglect of culture-specific needs in patients and raising ethical questions, the following hypotheses shall be put forward:

1. The German health care system is not prepared for the present extant of cultural diversity – even though Germany has a long history of migration and migrants as patients. Presently, there is an acute demand for cultural competence in health services.

2. If cultural diversity is at all taken care of, an essentialists, primordialist perception of the term culture is still prevailing. Therefore, the term culture needs to be put to a thoroughly, careful examination.

In support of these two hypotheses, we will first give an historical overview on migration to and within Germany, being followed by considerations relating to different concepts of culture in past and present. The last chapter of this paper is dedicated to conclusions linking experiences of migrations and concepts of culture to demands and challenges in health care.

---

[2] Frank Kressing: Aspekte kultureller Differenz im internationalen Medizintourismus. In: Michael Coors, Tim Peters, İlhan İlkılıç (Eds.): Umgang mit kultureller Differenz in der Gesundheitsversorgung. In: Ethik in der Medizin 30 (2018), pp. 251–262.

[3] Frank Kressing: Contested medical identities – migration of health care providers and Middle Eastern students at Western universities. In: İlhan İlkılıç, Hakan Ertin, Rainer Brömer, Hajo Zeeb (Eds.): Health, Culture and the Human Body. Epidemiology, Ethics and History of Medicine. Perspectives from Turkey and Central Europe. İstanbul 2014, pp. 113–124.

[4] Oliver Razum, Hajo Zeeb, Uta Meesmann, Liane Schenk, Maren Bredorst, Patrick Brzoska, Tanja Dercks, Susanne Glodny, Björn Menkhaus, Ramazan Salman, Anke-Christine Saß, Ralf Ulrich: Schwerpunktbericht der Gesundheitsberichterstattung des Bundes. Migration und Gesundheit. Berlin 2008.

## 2. Migration

### *2.1 Germany's modern nation-state (German Empire) since 1871 – A state of ethnically mixed composition with a colonial legacy*

There are numerous examples for prehistoric and historic migrations to the areas of present-day Germany.[5] In an outline of modern migrations within and into Germany, however, emphasis shall be given to the time after the founding of the German Reich in 1871. Although the German Empire of Bismarck's (1815–1896) and Wilhelmine times (1871–1918) was enthusiastically celebrated as the modern German nation-state, this state did not include many German nationals in the alpine and Danube areas of the then Austro-Hungarian Empire. The reason was the establishment of so-called Lesser Germany under Prussian leadership, excluding the Austrian territories (Kleindeutsche Lösung). Even though, the German Empire of 1871 was not as exclusively composed of Germans as its official representatives were prone to show. Instead, the Second German Reich hosted significant ethnic minorities such as speakers of French (approximately 200,000), Danish (140,000), Frisian (unknown number), Masurian (140,000), Kashubian (100,000), Lithuanian (100,000), Lusatian (Sorbs, approximately 90,000), and foremost Polish nationals (3 million) in the then Prussian provinces of Posen, Western and Eastern Prussia.[6] Today, these areas are roughly equal to the Polish voivodeships Greater Poland (Województwo Wielkopolskie) with the capital of Poznań, eastern Pomerania (Województwo Pomorskie) and Warmia-Mazury (Województwo Warmińsko-Mazurskie). These areas had been incorporated into the Kingdom of Prussia since 1701. The name of the Prussian Kingdom itself was derived from the Baltic speaking Old Prussians who had been the native inhabitants of the area between the rivers Vistula and Neman (Memel). Altogether, ethnic minorities within the Wilhemine German Reich amounted to some five million people out of a total population of 57 million in the year 1900, equaling roughly 9 % of German citizens at that time.[7]

---

[5] Helmut Castritius: Stammesbildung, Ethnogenese. In: Heinrich Beck, Dieter Geuenisch, Heiko Steuer, Rosemarie Müller (Eds.): Reallexikon der Germanischen Altertumskunde. Vol 29. Berlin, New York 2005, pp. 508–515.

[6] Michael Rademacher: Deutsche Verwaltungsgeschichte. Von der Reichseinigung 1871 bis zur Wiedervereinigung 1990. Osnabrück 2006.

[7] Rademacher: Deutsche Verwaltungsgeschichte (Note 6).

Besides the two dominant confessions of Protestant and Catholic Christianity, there were about 600,000 Jews living in Germany (1.04 %),[8] with the overwhelming majority of them being German citizens, and an unknown number of Sinti and Roma (so called Gypsies), being partly German citizens and partly foreigners.

By the year 1900, Germany's colonial possessions were third largest in size and fourth largest in regard of their population, being superceeded only by the U.K. and France and the Netherlands (population-wize). Estimations concerning the extent and population of pre-War I German colonies range from 2.6 to 2.9 million square kilometers, compared to 8.6 million square kilometers under British rule. The German colonies were populated by some 11 to 14 million native inhabitants, compared to 450 million people under British rule, 55 million under French and 53 million under Dutch rule.[9] The German-dominated territories, officially labelled protectorates (Schutzgebiete), roughly equal present-day Togo, the Cameroons, Namibia, Tanganyika, Burundi, Rwanda (German East Africa), Samoa, Nauru, Belau, the Federates States of Micronesia, the Marshall and northern Mariana Islands, Qingdao (Tsingtau) in China, the Solomon Islands, and the northeastern portion of New Guinea, called Kaiser-Wilhelm-Land at that time.[10] Within the modern state of Papua Nuigini, the Bismarck Archipelago still retains its colonial name, with the islands of New Mecklenburg and New Pomerania having been renamed New Ireland and New Britain in an ill-defeated act of linguistic decolonization. Only once in a while, this colonial legacy is present in 21st century German popular culture, with media coverage mostly centering on the Herero and Namaqua genocides of 1904 to 1908. In any case, Germany's $19^{th}/20^{th}$ century colonial endeavors cannot be regarded to be part of a collective memory in the sense of a *lieu de mémoire*,[11] despite the fact that Germany does have a colonial legacy – admittedly to a lesser extent than the U.K. and the neighboring countries of France, the Netherlands, and Belgium.

---

[8] Rademacher: Deutsche Verwaltungsgeschichte (Note 6).

[9] Heinrich Schnee (Ed.): Deutsches Koloniallexikon. Vol. 3. Leipzig 1920.

[10] Jürgen Petschull, Thomas Höpker: Der Wahn vom Weltreich. Die Geschichte der deutschen Kolonien. Hamburg 1986.

[11] Maurice Halbwachs: Les cadres sociaux de la mémoire. Paris 1952.

## 2.2 *Migration within Germany – prior to World War I*

The population of the German Reich rose from 41 million people in 1871 to 68 million in 1914.[12] Even though, there was surplus demand for – mostly unskilled – labor in the newly emerging industrial centers of the Empire such as the Rhine-Ruhr area, developing from the 18th century onward, and the Upper Silesia Industrial Area (Górnośląski Okręg Przemysłowy), developing from 1842 onward. This demand was mostly met by Polish migrants either from the Polish populated areas of Poznan, Silesia and Masuria or by Poles from abroad emigrating from the adjacent, Polish populated areas of the Russian Tzarist Empire. Shortly before World War I, about 1.2 million foreign migrant workers (*Wanderarbeiter*) were employed in Germany.[13] Descendants of these Polish migrants still form a significant portion of the present-day Rhine-Ruhr areas population within the German state of North-Rhine-Westphalia, as names like Horst Schimanski or the member's names of soccer team like Borussia Dortmund or Gelsenkirchen's Schalke 04 indicate.[14] Horst Schimanski is a fictional detective in the homicide department of the city of Duisburg who appears in a popular TV crime series and was portrayed by the actor Götz George (1938–2016). Concerning soccer, in 1934 the Warsaw based Polish sports magazine Przegląd Sportowy listed names of Schalke 04's soccer team like Emil Czerwinski (1905–1969), Ernst Kalwitzki (1909–1991), Ernst Kuzorra (1905–1990), Hermann Mellage (1906–unknown), Fritz Szepan (1907–1974), Otto Tibulski (1912–1991), Adolf Urban (1914–1943) und Ferdinand Zajons (1906–1987) to stress their obvious Polish origin.[15] A contemporary example for a German soccer star of Polish background is Łukasz

---

[12] Arnulf Scriba: Das Kaiserreich. In: Deutsches Historisches Museum: Lebendiges Museum Online. Berlin 2015. https://www.dhm.de/lemo/kapitel/kaiserreich (accessed 9/24/2019).

[13] Jochen Oltmer: Deutsche Migrationsgeschichte seit 1871. In: Bundeszentrale für politische Bildung (Ed.): Grundlagendossier Migration – Archiv. Bonn 2011. https://www.bpb.de/gesellschaft/migration/dossier-migration-ALT/56355/migration-1871-1950 (accessed 9/24/2019).

[14] Britta Lenz: »Gebürtige Polen« und »deutsche Jungs«. Polnischsprachige Zuwanderer im Ruhrgebietsfußball im Spiegel von deutscher und polnischer Presse der Zwischenkriegszeit. In: Diethelm Blecking, Lorenz Pfeifer, Robert Traba (Eds.): Vom Konflikt zur Konkurrenz. Deutsch-polnisch-ukrainische Fußballgeschichte. Göttingen 2014, pp. 100–113.

[15] N.N.: Mistrzostwo Niemiec w ręku Polaków! In: Przegląd Sportowy (30/06/1934).

Józef Podolski, born in Gliwice, Upper Silesia (Województwo Śląskie) in 1985.

Concerning the German protectorates (Schutzgebiete), there was not only migration to the colonies, with about 200,000 German settlers emigrating to Southwest Africa (Namibia), but also from the then German colonies. Early 20$^{th}$ century Germany saw Chinese laundries in Hamburg or Black ticket conductors in the Berlin tram.

### 2.3 *The Period after World War I to the end of World War II (1918–1945) – Migration, Deportation, Genocide*

During the German interwar period between 1918 and 1939, foreign labor migration into the country was not encouraged, and due to fear of unemployment within the domestic labor force and fear of competition, the market was more or less closed to immigrants from abroad. Even though, 100,000 to 300,000 foreign workers could be counted during the times of the Weimar Republic, with 375,000 foreign workers being employed under National Socialist rule in 1938.[16] As a result of a reduced size of the Reich's territory after World War I, a considerable number of German nationals found themselves outside of the Reich's borders, for example in Western Prussia, Wielkopolska (Poznań), or Upper Silesia. From such areas, about one million German nationals migrated to Germany, together with 600,000 Russian refugees from the early Soviet Union who mostly settled in Berlin, and 70,000 East European Jews. On a limited scale, Polish migration was still going on.

After the National Socialist Party gained power in 1933, half a million people fled the so-called Third Reich and found a temporary home in 80 different countries of the world.[17] Among these refugees, 280,000 people were of Jewish descent or assumed Jewish descent in the eyes of the National Socialist regime. Besides forceful deportations of Jews, Roma and Sinti, political and social dissidents to concentration camps for the purposes of workforce exploitation and genocide, even more people were deported from the newly occupied

---

http://buwcd.buw.uw.edu.pl/e_zbiory/ckcp/p_sportowy/1934/numer052/imagepages/image1.htm (accessed 9/24/2019).

[16] Oltmer: Deutsche Migrationsgeschichte (Note 13).

[17] Oltmer: Deutsche Migrationsgeschichte seit 1871 (Note 13).

territories in East and Central Europe as forced laborers, amounting to eight million people in the year 1944, among them two million Prisoners of War. This had a lasting effect in postwar times when a large number of Displaced Persons (between 10 and 12 million) found themselves in the four zones of Germany occupied by British, US-American, French and Soviet forces, besides another 12 million German nationals that had been expelled from eastern and central European countries like Poland, Czechoslovakia and the Soviet Union, and former Yugoslavia, Romania. In 1946, about 0.5 million Displaced Persons (heimatlose Ausländer) were still living in Germany,[18] including those who were not inclined to make their way back to Stalinist Russia out of fear of prosecution – about 150,000 repatriated Soviet citizens had been executed as collaborators during the last years of the war.[19] Especially members of national minorities within the Soviet Union such as Ukrainians, Crimean Tatars, and people from the Baltics chose to remain in the western zones of Germany to become the Federal Republic in 1948.[20]

### *2.4 Post World War II labor migration – West and East Germany*

A lot of the economic and social problems created by the displacement of German nationals from Central and Eastern Europe (Heimatvertriebene) was only solved in the course of the 1950ies during a period of prolonged economic growth in West Germany. This economic miracle is referred to as Wirtschaftswunder in German. In postwar Germany, about 2.7 million migrants and refugees had moved from East to West between 1949, when the Federal Republic of Germany was founded, and 1961, when the Berlin Wall was erected. These inner-German migrants met the expanded demand in workforce that was created by the economic miracle of the postwar years. But already starting in 1955, the West German government started migration agreements with Italy (1955), Spain (1960), Greece (1960), Turkey

[18] Oltmer: Deutsche Migrationsgeschichte seit 1871 (Note 13).
[19] Ulrike Goeken-Haidl: Repatriierung in den Terror? Die Rückkehr der sowjetischen Zwangsarbeiter und Kriegsgefangenen in ihre Heimat 1944–1956. In: Dachauer Hefte 16 (2000), pp. 190–209.
[20] Ukrainian Embassy in Germany: Ukrainisch-Deutsches Sprachenjahr/Ukrainer in Deutschland. Berlin 2017. https://germany.mfa.gov.ua/de/ukraine-de/ukrainians-in-de (accessed 9/24/2019).

(1961), Yugoslavia (1968), Tunesia, and Morocco to hire so-called guest workers (Gastarbeiter). These migrants were expected to return home after having spent a certain amount of time on their jobs in Germany. Between 1966 and 1989, the East German government hired approximately 0.5 million workers from allied socialist countries (Bruderländer) like Vietnam, Poland, Mozambique, or Cuba and granted asylum to several thousand political refugees from countries like Chile, Spain, or Greece. Contrary to the naïve expectations of the 1950ies and 60ies, the bulk of the foreign workers did not return home, with the foreign population in West Germany amounting to roughly 5 % already in 1970. In 1973, the number of foreign employees in FGR amounted to 2.6 million people.

### *2.5 Migration after the German reunification of 1990 – the refugee wave?*

Starting in the late 1970ies, the number of people asking for political asylum in West Germany was steadily increasing, amounting to more than 100,000 persons in 1980.[21] Since then, (West) Germany has become an internationally prime target of migration, be it politically or economically motivated, with asylum seekers and refugees coming mostly from countries of the southern hemisphere, but also from eastern, central and southeastern Europe (e.g. during the Balkan wars of the 1990ies). German policy, however, reacted rather reluctantly, with several changes of laws in regard of migration and asylum application, but not acknowledging the country's status as a destination of international migration (Einwanderungsland)[22] which only happened in the beginning of the 21st century. In the year 2017, Germany was the number 3 desired destination of international migration, after the U.S. and Saudi Arabia.[23] In the years before, 627,000 people had applied for asylum in 2014, 1.3 million in 2015 and 1.26 million in 2016, mostly coming from Syria, Afghanistan, Somalia and Iraq[24] due to war, oppressive regimes and genocide directed to

---

[21] Klaus J. Bade, Jochen Oltmer: Normalfall Migration (ZeitBilder 15). Bonn 2004.

[22] Martina Sauer, Heinz-Ulrich Brinkmann (Eds.): Einwanderungsgesellschaft Deutschland. Entwicklung und Stand der Integration. Wiesbaden 2016.

[23] United Nations Department of Economic and Social Affairs: International Migration Report 2017. New York 2017.

[24] Vera Hanewinkel: Fluchtmigration nach Deutschland und Europa: Einige Hinter-

certain ethnic and religious minorities like Aramaic-speaking Christians or Yazidis in these countries. Yazidis are Kurdish-speaking members of a non-Muslim and non-Christian religious community in Upper Mesopotamia who were subject to severe prosecution during the last decades, even in pre-Islamic State times, with the majority of the Yazidi population of Syria, Iraq and Turkey having fled to Western countries.[25] With more than a million people being granted access to Germany in the years 2015 and 2016 (Willkommenskultur), the country's political and social institutions were put under severe stress, leading the media to speak of a refugee crisis (Flüchtlingskrise) – a term that since then has developed into a common sense wording, implying that large scale migration to Germany constitutes a new, unknown and unfamiliar state of affairs.

Even though large scale migration of refugees from 2015 onward did provide a severe challenge to Germany's social, economic and also political system, it has to be stated in an historical perspective that large scale migrations are nothing new in German history. By the term migration, episodes of forced migration and deportation are included, especially in World War II and postwar times. However, the country's administrative, social, and health care institutions have failed to be prepared for migration in general and the mass movement of refugees specifically. When it comes to the question of how to integrate all these newcomers, the discussion is often centered on the term culture, implying that cultural differences constitute a major obstacle to integration, adaption and coping of migrants. According to official figures from the year 2017, 19.3 million out of 81.7 million inhabitants of Germany (23.6 %) are either migrants or at least descendants of one migrant parent (Migrationshintergrund). This fact provides another reason why the term culture deserves a closer examination.

---

gründe. In: Bundeszentrale für politische Bildung (Ed.): Dossier Migration – Archiv. http://www.bpb.de/gesellschaft/migration/flucht/265708/asylantraege-und-asylsuchende (accessed 9/24/2019).

[25] Jan İlhan Kızılhan: Behandlung traumatisierter Frauen in Deutschland. Transkulturelle Aspekte am Beispiel von 1.000 Jesidinnen aus dem Nordirak. In: Andreas Frewer, Lutz Bergemann, Caroline Hack, Hans G. Ulrich (Eds.): Die kosmopolitische Klinik. Globalisierung und kultursensible Medizin (Jahrbuch Ethik in der Klinik 10). Würzburg 2017, pp. 113–126.

## 3. Culture

### *3.1 Culture – a term with risks and side effects*

The phrase Risiken und Nebenwirkungen in German is meant to advise patients and drug consumers of being aware of unexpected or unwelcome risks and side effects while taking medical drugs. The commonly used term »culture« can also be regarded to be a term with Risiken und Nebenwirkungen,[26] referring to side effects when being used in labelling the background of certain population and their social behavior.

According to the classic definition given by Edward Burnett Tylor (1831–1917) who is considered to be one of the founding fathers of (evolutionist) anthropology,

> culture or civilization, taken in its wide ethnographic sense, is that complex whole which includes knowledge, belief, art, morals, law, custom, and any other capabilities and habits acquired by man as a member of society.[27]

By this definition, Tylor does purposely not refer to a narrow definition of culture as designation of high culture or elaborated culture including the fine arts, theatre, opera, or conventions of a cultivated-style of behavior.[28] Instead, Tylor uses culture in an inclusive and universal sense, referring to the variety of human behavior in toto, including language, tradition and self-assignment. In this sense, different cultures are a distinguishing factor, separating peoples, ethnic groups or religious communities from each other. Thus culture becomes a marker of ethnicity, with every nation and tribe presumably having a unique culture of its own, separating one ethnic group from the other. Furthermore, in a view that is heavily influenced by German Romanticism, a nation was perceived as a static, historically unaltered entity of its own destiny. A common language, a shared historical and also »racial« heritage, a shared territory or settlement

---

[26] Michael Knipper: Vorsicht Kultur! Ethnologische Perspektiven auf Medizin, Migration und ethnisch-kulturelle Vielfalt. In: Michael Coors, Tatjana Grützmann, Tim Peters (Eds.): Das Fremde verstehen. Interkulturalität und ethische Konflikte in Medizin und Pflege. Göttingen 2014, pp. 52–69.

[27] Edward B. Tylor: Primitive Culture: Researches into the Development of Mythology, Philosophy, Religion, Art, and Costum. Vol. 1, London 1871, p. 1.

[28] Adolph F. L. Freiherr von Knigge: Über den Umgang mit Menschen (On Human Relations). Hannover 1788.

area, and preferably a shared, common faith served as determining features of a given ethnic group (Volk). According to this viewpoint, a nation was regarded to be synonymous with a language group, and a language community would hold a fixed nature over time. Such ideas were mainly developed in in late 18th and early 19th centuries central Europe and were put forward by philosophers, poets, historians and linguists, examples being Johann Gottlieb Herder (1744–1803),[29] August Wilhelm Schlegel (1767–1845),[30] and Johann Gottlieb Fichte (1762–1814).[31] At that time, Britain, France and also Spain had already been established as firm nation states, whereas the central and eastern European nations (e.g. Germany, Italy, Poland, Hungary, and the Balkan peoples) were still in a process of formation, trying to gain their national independence during a series of violent uprisings and wars of liberation, e.g. the Greek War of Independence 1821–1830. The primordialist notion expressed in the writings of Fichte or Herder tended to claim that linguistic communities have a common racial origin. This view was expressed in popular depictions of the early 20th century, identifying speakers of Indo-European languages with the so-called Mediterranean or Caucasian race,[32] speakers of Hungarian or Finnic languages with the so-called North-Asian or Mongolian race. Even in the late 20th century, in an era of advanced genetic research, schemes of a common genetic-linguistic heritage of human populations have been published and widely popularized.[33] On the contrary, already centuries before the distinguished cultural anthropologist Franz Boas (1858–1942) had argued for race, language and culture being totally independent factors in shaping human communities.[34]

---

[29] Johann Gottfried Herder: Abhandlung über den Ursprung der Sprache. Berlin 1772.

[30] Friedrich Schlegel: Ueber die Sprache und Weisheit der Indier. Ein Beitrag zur Begründung der Alterthumskunde. Heidelberg 1808.

[31] Johann Gottlieb Fichte: Reden an die deutsche Nation. Berlin 1808.

[32] Johann Friedrich Blumenbach: Über die natürlichen Verschiedenheiten im Menschengeschlechte. Leipzig 1798.

[33] Luigi Lucca Cavalli-Sforza, Alberto Piazza, Paolo Menozzi, Johanna Mountain: Reconstruction of human evolution: Bringing together genetic, archaeological, and linguistic data. In: Proceedings of the National Academy of Sciences of the United States of America 85 (1988), pp. 6002–6006.

[34] Franz Boas: Race, Language, and Culture. Chicago 1940; Franz Boas: Kultur und Rasse. 2nd Edition. Berlin 1922.

### 3.2 *Multiple cultures – Shifting identities*

Models pertaining to the framework of culture, ethnicity, and identity that were developed in the second half of the 20th century skipped these static approaches,[35] stressing that acquisition and expression of culture should be viewed as dynamic processes which might be changed according to temporary conditions, challenges and circumstances during an individual's lifetime. Categorizing patients according to their heritage, mother language, nationality, ethnicity or religion might create a barrier, preventing health care workers from perceiving the individually based needs of their patients. On the other hand, stereotypes created by patients in their perception of the behaviour and the qualities of foreign doctors and nurses can be an obstacle to a mutually successful and satisfying interaction between patients and physicians. Therefore, some considerations regarding the dynamics of culture and identity might be useful at this point.

The Norwegian social anthropologist Frederik Barth (1928–2016) used shifting identities in Afghan tribal societies as an example to show how multiple ethnic, tribal and religious identities are negotiated in processes of ethnic separation and coalitions. A member of the Pashtun Ghilzai tribe, for example, might identify himself as a Ghilzai tribesman, as a member of the Pashtun people, or as a citizen of Afghanistan, depending on specific situations and circumstances. The same can be hold true for Yazidi refugees from Syria, Iraq or Turkey who, depending on the social setting, might identify as members of their religious community, as Kurds or as Iraqi, Syrian or Turkish citizens.[36] Within the Turkish-German community, the cartoonist Muhsin Omurca invented the Kanakmän character, illustrating the sudden change between a German and a Turkish identity (»Tags Deutscher Nachts Türke« – being German during daytime, being Turk at night).[37] Constructions of ethnicity and ethnic identiy have been a topic that has been highlighted by social and cultural anthropologists for decades, with many authors focussing on the relational aspects of identities and ongoing processes of negotiating eth-

---

[35] Frederik Barth: Ethnic Groups and Boundaries. The Social Organization of Culture Difference. Oslo 1969.

[36] Jan İlhan Kızılhan: Die Yeziden. Eine anthropologische und sozialpsychologische Studie über die kurdische Gemeinschaft. Frankfurt am Main 1997.

[37] Muhsin Omurca: Kanakmän. Ulm 2002. https://mussin.de/tags-deutscher-nachts-tuerke/ (accessed 9/24/2019).

nic, religious and national identities according to different social, political, and cultural contexts.[38] The construction of ethnic identities is often bound to religious affiliations, with religion serving as one among several markers of identity.[39] Obvious examples can be found in southeastern Europe, where Croatians identify as Roman Catholics, Serbs as Orthodox Christians, and Bosniaks as Muslims.[40] On the other hand, adherents of a specific faith may feel themselves belonging to different ethnic identies, like Alevi Muslims in Turkey identifying either as Turks, Kurds, or Zaza-speakers. Worldwide, numerous examples for multiple and shifting ethnic identities can be found, with recent publications highlighting shifting ethnic identities in classical antique and medieval times.[41]

Another striking example for multiple ethnic identities from modern times ($19^{th}$ to $21^{st}$ centuries) can be presented from the Balkans: Members of the small etho-linguistic community of the Vlahs or Aromanians are scattered throughout parts of Greece, Bulgaria, Albania, Romania and Serbia. They preserved a pastorilists, nomadic or semi-nomadic lifestyle until the mid $20^{th}$ century.[42] The Vlahs tended to assimiliate themselves to the dominant Greek, Bulgarian, Albanian, Romanian and Serbian cultures of their settlement areas and even fostered teaching their children in these foreign languages, but still maintained their Christian-Orthodox religious identity and their semi-nomadic traditions. Today, the Aromanians comprise between 0.3 and one million people, with their often hidden identity making exact numbering extremly difficult. As the British novelist Charles Eliot already wrote in the early $20^{th}$ century,[43] the Vlahs can be considered as a nation in disguise, revealing their true ethnicity only in the context of Church services, trade in livestock or veterinary services. Due to their pastoralist tradition, herding and dealing with

---

[38] Benedict Anderson: Die Erfindung der Nation. Zur Karriere eines folgenreichen Konzepts. Frankfurt, New York 1996.

[39] Shalina Randeria: Hindu-Nationalismus: Aspekte eines Mehrheits-Ethnizismus. In: Reinhard Kößler, Tilmann Schiel (Eds.): Nationalstaat und Ethnizität. Frankfurt am Main 1995, pp. 75–109.

[40] Cay Lienau, Ludwig Steindorff (Eds.): Ethnizität, Identität und Nationalität in Südosteuropa. München 2000.

[41] Erica Buchberger: Shifting Identities in Spain and Gaul, 500–700. From Romans to Goths and Franks. Amsterdam 2017.

[42] Thede Kahl: Ethnizität und räumliche Verteilung der Aromunen in Südosteuropa. Münster 1999.

[43] Charles N. E. Eliot: Turkey in Europe. London 1900, p. 409.

grazing animals still form favoured occupations among the Vlahs. In Albania, for example, Aromanians are over-represented among veterenarian doctors.[44]

Relational shifts in ethnic identities are often bound to situational linguistic code-switching,[45] indicating a person's temporarliy perceived identity by choice of language. Examples can be preferably found in small ethno-linguistic minorities and borderland communities such as Rhaeto-Romanians in the Swiss and Italian Alpes, Frisians in the Netherlands, Germany, and Denmark, or Hopi and Tewa in Arizona, U.S., to pick just a few arbitrarely drawn examples.[46]

## 4. Migration, Culture, and Health Care

### *4.1 Culture-bound conflicts in health care*

»I've caught a cold in my head – my bile's burst« read a headline in a regional southern German newspaper some ten years ago, implying that lack of correctly translating patients' complaints can cause to severe misdiagnoses[47] and shedding light on misunderstandings forming a routine part of hospital procedures. Within Germany, these perceived misconceptions mostly occur in patients of Muslim background, indicating a cultural gap in the way illness and disease are described and labelled due to a different cultural context. According to a commonly held opinion among hospital staff, it is usually Muslim patients who due to their presumably different cultural and religious background cause problems and disturb the usual medical routine, the reason being deviant expectations regarding food, medical care in general and care for deceased that are not always met, partially due to lack of inter-cultural understanding and knowledge.

Knowledge of restrictions concerning food and beverages in Islam (no pork, no alcohol) can be taken for granted. Less known is the fact

---

[44] Stephanie Schwandner-Sievers: The Albanian Aromanians' Awakening: Identity Politics and Conflict in Post-communist Albania. Flensburg 1999.
[45] John Gumperz: Dialect Differences and Social Stratification in a North Indian Village. In: American Anthropologist 60 (1958), pp. 668–681.
[46] Paul V. Kroskity: Language, History, and Identity. Ethnolinguistic Studies of the Arizona Tewa. Tuscon, London 1993.
[47] N.N.: »Kopf erkältet, Gallenblase geplatzt«. Sprachliche Missverständnisse können bei Migranten zu Fehldiagnosen führen. In: Südwestpresse Ulm (9/27/2008).

that many Muslim patients also abstain from medical remedies that are manufactured on base of pork lard or alcoholic liquids, e.g. cough syrup. Lack of knowledge is even more abundant when it comes to the demand that, due to Muslim rules, only running water should be used for ablution purposes, or regarding the required ritual obligations after the death of patients.

According to Muslim ritual, the last words of a patient who is about to die should be the creed (shahada) »la ilaha illa llah« – there is no God but the only One. After the patient has passed away, eyes and mouth should be shut and the deceased's head should be directed towards Mecca. The corpse should then be washed by a member of the same sex as the deceased. Western hospital staff is often surprised by spontaneous and very expressive mourning by the deceased's family members.

In case of an infaust prognosis, the patient's family members as well as interpreters show the tendency to hide this forecast, the reason being that the patient should not be troubled by the expectation of death, or that death should not be precipitated by talking too much about the end of life. Of course, this widespread behavior will often prevent diagnoses and prognoses being transmitted to the patient and does not meet the requirements of modern, 20th and 21st centuries accounts of patient autonomy.[48]

It was intended to give a few examples showing how important culture-bound conceptions of health, illness and disease can be, and to which extent they might not fit into established modes of treating patients and their families. Deviant, non-Western views of health do not only concern religiously sanctioned food-habits or adequate post-mortem behavior, but also the etiology of illness and disease, as is shown by the large number of culture-bound syndromes (CBS) in different cultures.[49] Examples for culture-bound syndromes are the evil eye (mal de ojo in Spanish), possession by jinn (in the Islamic World), susto (sudden fright, South and Central America), or latah

---

[48] Tom L. Beauchamp, James F. Childress: Principles of Biomedical Ethics. 7th Edition. Oxford 2013.

[49] William Sax: Culture Bound Syndromes Reconsidered. In: Katarina Greifeld, Wolfgang Krahl, Hans Jochen Diesfeld, Hannes Stubbe (Eds.): Grenzgänge zwischen Ethnologie. Medizin und Psychologie. Für Ekkehard Schröder zum 75. Geburtstag (Curare – Journal of Medical Anthropology 3–4). Berlin 2018, pp. 149–158.

(sudden shock, South-East Asia),[50] but also the premenstrual syndrome in the West. The existence of these different culture-bound syndroms lead medical anthropologists Arthur Kleinman and Peter Benson to speak of »the heterogeneity of explanatory models«[51] in disease and illness etiologies. Handling these non-Western explanatory models that do not fit into the system of biology-centered medicine certainly requires cultural sensibility as a part of medical diversity management, being aware of the existence of CBS, and accepting the patient's explanation of their causes according to a non-Western etiology.

### *4.2 Lost in translation*

A factor that is intervening between doctors' duty and their patients is the lack of communication that is prevailing on several scales in health care procedures. In Germany, like probably in most other countries of the world, difficulties in the verbal transmission of diagnosis, therapeutic suggestions, and prognoses do not only occur between doctors and patients of foreign background, but also between health care workers and patients of the same ethnic or linguistic group.[52] In the case of non-German or only slightly German-speaking patients and their family members, these problems are of course more severe. In spite of many serious attempts to fill the gap of professional interpreters in hospitals by hiring volunteers, the demand for qualified translation remains a severe problem in Germany's hospitals and clinics. In need of ad hoc interpreters, doctors and nurses often resort to family members, cleaning or kitchen staff of the respective nationality for translations services. Arbitrarely chosen phrases like »Agron, could you please tell us what the Albanian patient tries to tell us?« or »Svetlana, we do not understand this Russian patient« may serve as fictive examples to illustrate this kind of patients treatment implying no guarantee at all in regard of a correct, medically qualified and culturally sensitive transmission of messages.

---

[50] Anne Fadiman: The Spirit Catches You and You Fall Down: A Hmong Child, Her American Doctors, and the Collision of Two Cultures. New York 1997.

[51] Arthur Kleinman, Peter Benson: Anthropology in the Clinic: The Problem of Cultural Competency and How to Fix It. In: Public Library of Science Medicine 10 (2006), e294. doi:10.1371/journal.pmed.0030294.

[52] Kressing: Contested medical identities (Note 3), pp. 113–124.

Sometimes, younger bilingual family members, children or teenagers, are employed for interpretation, raising questions of translation quality, biased translations, and ethical responsibility. Demands that have recently been expressed by a number of committees[53] and widely published[54] envisage not only skillful translators, but culturally qualified community interpreters to be provided by hospitals on a compulsory base to avoid incidents like not translating end of life prognoses. A commonly used phrase like »we can't tell your grandfather – that is not part of our culture« or giving an religiously biased advice like »even when you're ill, you should fast during *Ramadan*« may again serve as arbitrarely drawn, fictive examples.

### 4.3 *The inter-cultural trap*

On the other hand, however, stressing the existence of culture-bound syndromes, etiologies, diagnosis, and therapies might prevent the doctor's or nurse's awareness of illness as an individually perceived experience that might be very different from patient to patient. Overemphasizing the cultural factor can easily cause an individual's cultural stigmatization and lead health care workers into the pitfall of perpetuating already existing stereotypes. In this sense, an overdose of culture as a term with risks and side-effects (*Risiken und Nebenwirkungen*) might cause the side effect of a well-intended, but ill-deceived othering and alienation of patients,[55] examples to be found from the early times of post-World War II labor migration (Gastarbeiter) to Germany: Not knowing how to handle formerly unknown, often very unspecific descriptions of illnesses by workers from Turkey, Greece, former Yugoslavia, Spain or southern Italy, doctors developed a coping strategy of their own, resorting to makeshift cul-

---

[53] Tim Peters, Tatjana Grützmann, Walter Bruchhausen, Michael Coors, Fabian Jacobs, Lukas Kaelin, Michael Knipper, Frank Kressing, Gerald Neitzke: Grundsätze zum Umgang mit Interkulturalität in Einrichtungen des Gesundheitswesens. Positionspapier der Arbeitsgruppe Interkulturalität in der medizinischen Praxis in der Akademie für Ethik in der Medizin. In: Ethik in der Medizin 26 (2014), pp. 65–75.

[54] N.N.: Geflüchtete und Asylbewerber. Ohne Sprachmittler funktioniert die Versorgung nicht. In: Deutsches Ärzteblatt 116 (2019), pp. A308–A313.

[55] Johana M. Metzl, Helena Hansen: Structural competency: Theoretisizing a new medical engagement with stigma and inequity. In: Social Science and Medicine 103 (2014), pp. 126–133, doi:10.1016/j. socscimed. 2013.06.032.

ture-bound syndrome labelling like Morbus bosporus, Mama-mia-syndrome or guestworker's ulcus as pseudo-explanations.[56]

What do we learn when we apply recent models emphasizing the dynamic character of culture and ethnicity to health services taking place in a multi-cultural setting? To a certain degree, ethically grounded conflicts occuring in patient's treatment and health care tend to be labelled as ethnic conflicts,[57] thus having found a comparatively easy excuse for not having to deal with individual demands of patients and/or their families. Thus, using the expression »Vorsicht Kultur« (be aware of culture)[58] again, it has to asked whether labeling conflicts in the multicultural setting of health care as intercultural conflicts – to a certain degree – reflects an overemphasize put on a cultural sensitive attitude in health services, intended to benefit the patients but in reality fostering ethnic stigmatization and segregation. Regarding migrants and people with a migration background in Germany it has to be pointed out that the individual life history of migration constitutes but only one aspect of an individual's health state, and maybe not the most important one. Thus, the status as a migrant patient does request mindfulness, attentiveness, and watchfulness on the side of the health care providers – but just in the same way as any kind of patient with specific, individual needs, expectations and his or her unique personality.[59]

There is no need to establish any kind of special migrant medicine dedicated to migrants to fulfill their specific needs. Instead, it should be regarded necessary to apply standards of an individualized medicine that have been developed in the course of medical diversity management for foreign background patients to apply to all patients. In this sense, the term medical diversity management has to be broadened, not just relying to cultural diversity, ethnic diversity, or religious diversity, but to diversity of sex, gender, age and sexual orienta-

---

[56] İlhan İlkılıç: Medizinethische Aspekte des interkulturellen Arzt-Patienten-Verhältnisses. In: Deutscher Ethikrat (Ed.): Migration und Gesundheit. Kulturelle Vielfalt als Herausforderung für die medizinische Versorgung, Berlin 2010, pp. 29–40.

[57] Christiane Imhof, Frank Kressing: Die ethnische Verlagerung von ethischen Problem- und Konfliktfällen. In: Michael Coors, Tatjana Grützmann, Tim Peters (Eds.): Das Fremde verstehen. Interkulturalität und ethische Konflikte in Medizin und Pflege. Göttingen 2014, pp. 70–80.

[58] Knipper: Vorsicht Kultur! (Note 26), pp. 52–69.

[59] Walter Bruchhausen: Interkulturalität als Thema der Medizinethik. In: Michael Coors, Tatjana Grützmann, Tim Peters (Eds.): Das Fremde verstehen. Interkulturalität und ethische Konflikte in Medizin und Pflege. Göttingen 2014, pp. 23–36.

tion as well. In this respect it has to be point out that the demand for diversity management and respect for diversity in health services does completely comply with the respective sections of the Hippocratic Oath and the Declaration of Geneva: I will not permit considerations of age, disease or disability, creed, ethnic origin, gender, nationality, political affiliation, race, sexual orientation, social standing or any other factor to intervene between my duty and my patient.[60]

## 5. Still many goals to be achieved

Even though the term culture and its possible implications in treating foreign background patients have to be treated very carefully, hospitals and surgeries in Germany still lack a convincing, non-discriminatory medical diversity management[61] that would be able to fulfill the needs of non-native and native patients alike. As was pointed out before, the concept of medical diversity should not just cover cultural or religious diversity, but patients' diversity in a broad sense, combined with attempts to implement personalized medicine and enhancing structural competence regarding the patient's sex, gender, age, socio-economic status, ethnicity, and value system.[62] Therefore, all members of the hospital and surgery staff, medical doctors and nurses, but also administration, kitchen and cleaning personnel have to undergo intercultural training, but also training in gender and age related medicine. In recent years, a number of working groups and committees have stressed the need to prepare medical students, nurses and all other medical staff members for the internationalisation of health care.[63] Despite obvious needs for an effective cultural diversity management in medical institutions, however, the education

[60] World Medical Association: Declaration of Geneva, 9th July, 2018, https://www.wma.net/policies-post/wma-declaration-of-geneva/ (accessed 9/24/2019).

[61] European Project Migrant Friendly Hospital: The Amsterdam declaration towards migrant-friendly hospitals in an ethno-culturally diverse Europe. Amsterdam 2014, http://www.mfh-eu.net/public/files/european_recommendations/mfh_amsterdam_de-claration_english.pdf (accessed 9/24/2019).

[62] Christine Binder-Fritz, Anita Rieder: Zur Verflechtung von Geschlecht, sozioökonomischem Status und Ethnizität im Kontext von Gesundheit und Migration. In: Bundesärzteblatt 57 (2014), pp. 1031–1037.

[63] Bundesvereinigung der Medizinstudierenden Deutschlands (bvmd): Kerncurriculum für die medizinische Ausbildung in Deutschland. Ein Vorschlag der Medizinstudierenden Deutschlands. Berlin 2006.

of medical students in central Europe still shows severe shortcomings in this respect,[64] even though »high-quality health care as a goal calls for the systematic internationalization of undergraduate medical education«.[65]

A decisive agenda on what topics should be incorporated in global health studies and how global health curricula should be structured is presently prepared by the working-group »Cultural Competence and Global Health« within the Association for Medical Education (GMA).[66] Due to their relevance to the routine of medical care, cultural competence and global health should be integrated into the standard curricula and required from all medical students to ensure that the basic human value of health equity be implemented for migrants and non-migrants alike. Health equity is defined as the recognition of »the enjoyment of the highest attainable standard of physical and mental health« and has been declared a basic human right according to article 12 of the International Covenant on Economic, Social and Cultural Rights (ICESCR).[67] On the contrary, »health inequities are systematic differences in the health status of different population groups. These inequities have significant social and economic costs both to individuals and societies.«[68] Thus, health equity constitutes a crucial requirement for a health care policy in respects of the patients' diversity – whether they happen to be migrants or not.

---

[64] Sabine Gabrysch, Philipp Jean: Germany must invest in its global health academic workforce. In: The Lancet 391 (2018), pp. 656–657, here p. 656.

[65] Claudia Mews, Sylvie Schuster, Christian Vajda, Heide Lindtner-Rudolph, Luise E. Schmidt, Stefan Bösner, Leyla Güzelsoy, Frank Kressing, Houda Hallal, Tim Peters, Margarita Gestmann, Linn Hempel, Tatjana Grützmann, Erika Sievers, Michael Knipper: Cultural Competence and Global Health: Perspectives for Medical Education. Position Paper of the GMA Committee on Cultural Competence and Global Health. In: GMS Journal for Medical Education 53 (2018), Doc28, pp. 1 and 5.

[66] Mews et al.: Cultural Competence and Global Health (Note 65).

[67] CESCR: General Comment 14, paras 11–12. http://www.refworld.org/pdfid/4538838d0.pdf, CESCR General Comment 14, paragraph 7 (accessed 9/24/2019).

[68] World Health Organization: 10 facts on health inequities and their causes, April 2017. http://www.who.int/features/factfiles/health_inequities/en/ (accessed 9/24/2019).

*Tamara Schwertel*

# Difficulties in the trajectories: an investigation of care structures for refugees suffering from tuberculosis in Germany

Abstract
This contribution focuses on the challenges faced in the treatment of TB-infected refugees in Germany. A wide range of problems arises when a refugee traverses his or her trajectory, while the involved actors search for and develop strategies to solve them. I provide a qualitative analysis of the challenges and the strategies to avoid them, which is based on interviews, which have been conducted and evaluated based on grounded theory. I draw on Strauss' concept of trajectories, which I built on the basic assumptions of symbolic interactionism. The qualitative sample consists of two actual care chains in Germany. It covers the inpatient treatment and the outpatient treatment as well as the health department, who organize transitions in the treatment.

## 1. Introduction

But in the first storey Hans Castorp suddenly stopped, rooted to the spot by a perfectly ghastly sound coming from a little distance off round a bend in the corridor. (…) It was coughing, obviously, a man coughing; but coughing like to no other Hans Castorp had ever heard, and compared with which any other had been a magnificent and healthy manifestation of life: a coughing that had no conviction and gave no relief, that did not even come out in paroxysms, but was just a feeble, dreadful welling up of the juices of organic dissolution.[1]

In his novel *The Magic Mountain* Thomas Mann describes a tuberculosis sanatorium; here, tuberculosis (TB) represents a source of creativity, as shown by the character of Hans Castorp, the intelligent and charismatic son of a merchant. However, in its final state the romanticized image of the illness collapses. In the quote, the patient disappears losing his status as a subject. Ultimately, he becomes reduced to

---

[1] Thomas Mann: The magic mountain. With a postscript by the author on the making of the novel. Translated from the German by Helen T. Lowe-Porter. London 1999.

just a cough, which remains as an indication of the death of the coughing person.

To this day, TB remains one of the most dangerous infectious diseases, causing 1.6 million deaths worldwide in 2017.[2] The World Health Organization (WHO) mapped out a strategy to eradicate TB by 2030. However, in an increasingly globalized world, approaches to stop TB cannot solely focus on medical treatment, but there is also a need for social approaches as is demonstrated by the increasing focus on sociological studies. Sociological research can help to shed light on social relationships beyond clinical factors in order to examine problems arising during treatment and in social interactions. This contribution focusses especially on the treatment of refugees suffering from TB. To begin with, I provide an overview of the previous research. A first set of studies covers the effectiveness of health monitoring and prevention programs by health authorities in general.[3] Another set of studies analyses the discourses surrounding TB, focusing on the governmental and medial interest to differentiate between persons suffering from TB in order to control the political and medical situation.[4] In this context, migrants are often characterized as disease carriers and potential danger in national discourses. According to Scott et al. »these categories achieve ›power effects‹ enacting governmentality through a set of laws, regulations and other socio-political practices«[5]. Other studies focus on the factors affecting the therapy of

---

[2] World Health Organization: Fact sheet. Tuberculosis (2019). https://www.who.int/en/news-room/fact-sheets/detail/tuberculosis (accessed 9/24/2019).

[3] Rodrigues R. Neves, Rubia dos Santos Ferro, Laura M. Vidal Nogueira: Access and link to treatment of tuberculosis in primary health care. In: Revista de Pesquisa. Cuidado é Fundamental Online 8 (2016), pp. 5143–5149; World Health Organization: Global Tuberculosis Report. Executive Summary (2018). https://www.who.int/tb/publications/global_report/tb18_ExecSum_web_4Oct18.pdf?ua=1 (accessed 9/24/2019); Penelope Scott, Dennis Odukoya, Hella von Unger: The Classification of »Migrants« as a Discursive Practice in Public Health. A Sociology of Knowledge Approach. In: WZB Discussion Paper SP III (2014). https://bibliothek.wzb.eu/pdf/2014/iii14-601.pdf (accessed 9/24/2019); Maren Mylius: Die medizinische Versorgung von Menschen ohne Papiere in Deutschland. Studien zur Praxis in Gesundheitsämtern und Krankenhäusern. Bielefeld 2016, pp. 197–252; Morag Bell, Tim Brown, Lucy Faire: Germs, genes and postcolonial geographies: Reading the return of tuberculosis to Leicester, UK, 2001. In: Cultural Geographies 13 (2006), pp. 577–599.

[4] Bell, Brown, Faire: Germs, genes (Note 3); Scott, Odukoya, von Unger: The classification of »Migrations« (Note 3), p. 12.

[5] Bell, Brown, Faire: Germs, genes (Note 3); Scott, Odukoya, von Unger: The classification of »Migrations« (Note 3), p. 12.

TB, emphasizing the importance of social environments and provider-patient relationships. They also highlight the impact of stigmatization and ignorance of symptoms on treatment and recovery.[6] These studies address fears and concerns especially among migrants, preventing access to the health care system, which often arise in the course of their migration experience. For example, Westaway[7] points out that the stigmatization by nurses and racial prejudice towards migrants often lead to treatment discontinuation. This demonstrates the need to provide better access to health care for migrants, as they face a greater risk of damaging their health due to delays in treatment and treatment discontinuation. These studies reveal the need to diminish prejudice and to support persons suffering from TB. After having compiled the most important scientific findings, I will outline the current situation in Germany, which helps to demonstrate the particular risks faced by refugees, who are migrants without a choice to migrate.

## 2. Situation in Germany

The rise of TB infections in Germany is the starting point for this contribution. While 4.526 people were diagnosed with TB in 2014, the number had increased to 5.915 in 2016.[8] Stadtmüller et al. demonstrate that 2015 marked an increase of 30 per cent compared to the previous year, which they trace to an increase in migration during 2015 by showing that 72.1 per cent of the new infections affect people

[6] Magaret S. Westaway: Knowledge, beliefs and feelings about tuberculosis. In: Health Education Research 4 (1989), pp. 205–211; Ernesto Jaramillo: Tuberculosis and stigma: Predictors of prejudice against people with tuberculosis. In: Journal of Health Psychology 4 (1999), pp. 71–79; Arthur J. Rubel, Linda C. Garro: Social and cultural factors in the successful control of tuberculosis. In: Public Health Reports 107 (1992), pp. 626–636; Martha J. Chinouya, Oyinlolu Adeyanju: A disease called stigma. The experience of stigma among African men with TB diagnosis in London. In: Public Health 145 (2017), pp. 45–50; Marylyn M. McEwen: Mexican immigrants' explanatory model of latent tuberculosis infection. In: Journal of Transcultural Nursing 16 (2005), pp. 347–355.

[7] Westaway: Knowledge, beliefs and feelings about tuberculosis (Note 6).

[8] Robert Koch-Institut: Bericht zur Epidemiologie der Tuberkulose in Deutschland für 2016. Berlin 2017, p. 24. https://www.rki.de/DE/Content/InfAZ/T/Tuberkulose/Download/TB2016.pdf?__blob=publicationFile (accessed 9/24/2019).

not born in Germany.[9] Among these, particularly refugees from Eritrea, Somalia, and Gambia were affected.[10] On the one hand, the increase can be explained by the origin of many refugees from high-prevalence countries. In addition, they are often exposed to outbreaks of active TB due to the physical and psychological strains such as post-migratory stressors in German facilities.[11] This new socio-demographic composition of patients poses specific challenges to the health care system.[12]

To make matters worse, the X-ray screening procedures currently applied when refugees enter the country are not uniformly organized across federal states; therefore, TB is often diagnosed at a very late state and when refugees stay already at an accommodation.[13] The situation is aggravated further, as symptoms during the initial stage are extremely inconspicuous and similar to flu symptoms.[14] Poor hygienic conditions and tight spatial conditions in the accommodation add to the risk of infection.[15] In addition, to these specifics, other

---

9 Sven Stadtmüller, Jette Schröder, Stefan Ehlers: Eine Schätzung der Prävalenz von Tuberkulose bei Asylsuchenden in Deutschland. In: Epidemiologisches Bulletin 43 (2017), pp. 487–491, here p. 487.

10 Robert Koch-Institut: Dem Robert Koch-Institut übermittelte meldepflichtige Infektionskrankheiten bei Asylsuchenden in Deutschland: Zusammenfassung und Bewertung (2018), p. 42. https://www.rki.de/DE/Content/Gesundheitsmonitoring/Gesundheitsberichterstattung/GesundAZ/Content/A/Asylsuchende/Inhalt/meldepflichtige_Infektionskrankheiten_bei_Asylsuchenden.pdf?__blob=publicationFile (accessed 9/24/2019).

11 Bundesverband der Ärztinnen und Ärzte des Öffentlichen Gesundheitsdienstes e. V. (BVÖGD): Tuberkulose bei Flüchtlingen und Asylbewerbern. Tuberkulose – Screening bei Einreise und Fallmanagement (2017). http://bvoegd.de/wp-content/uploads/2017/05/2017_05_23_STN_TBC_FA_IFS.pdf (accessed 9/24/2019).

12 Laura Frank, Rahsan Yesil-Jürgens, Oliver Razum et. al: Gesundheit und gesundheitliche Versorgung von Asylsuchenden und Flüchtlingen in Deutschland. In: Journal of Health Monitoring 2 (2017), pp. 24–47.

13 BVÖGD: Tuberkulose bei Flüchtlingen und Asylbewerbern (Note 11); Robert Koch-Institut: Thorax-Röntgenuntersuchungen bei Asylsuchenden gemäß § 36 Absatz 4 IfSG. Stellungnahme des Robert Koch-Instituts (2015). https://www.rki.de/DE/Content/InfAZ/T/Tuberkulose/Tuberkulose_Roentgen-Untersuchungen_Asylsuchende.html (accessed 9/24/2019).

14 Robert Koch-Institut: Untersuchung auf Tuberkulose bei asylsuchenden Kindern und Jugendlichen < 15 Jahren. Stellungahme des Robert Koch-Instituts. https://www.rki.de/DE/Content/InfAZ/T/Tuberkulose/Tuberkulose-Screening_Kinder.html (accessed 9/24/2019).

15 Robert Koch-Institut: Bericht zur Epidemiologie der Tuberkulose (Note 8); Sandra Beermann, Ute Rexroth, Markus Kirchner, Anna Kühne, Sabine Vygan, Andreas Gilsdorf: Asylsuchende und Gesundheit in Deutschland. Überblick über epidemiolo-

factors are important too: fear, refugee status, and language barriers reduce access to medical care and affect the health of refugees due to a lack of structural and personal support.[16] These factors help to explain the high percentage of fled TB patients and emphasize the need for sociological research. Finally, dealing with the actors involved in the treatment of fled TB patients is particularly problematic due to the social connotations of TB. While large parts of the German population believe due media campaigns that TB has come back to Germany due to refugees alone, it had in fact never entirely disappeared.[17] This perceived (imagined) change triggers fears and threatens communal identities, thus dealing with TB-infected refugees becomes symbolically charged.[18] As I will demonstrate later on, fear and uncertainly as well as a lack of knowledge are factors that negatively influence treatment.

## 3. Trajectories and the conception of TB

Before delving into the theoretical framework, the term refugee needs to be defined. This group is regarded to consist of forced migrants, which cannot take the protection of ›their own country‹ or return there.[19] Conceptually, I draw on Anselm Strauss' concept of trajectories in order to analyze the key problems that involved actors

---

gisch relevante Infektionskrankheiten. In: Deutsches Ärzteblatt 112 (2015), pp. 1717–1720.

[16] Didier Fassin: Das Leben. Eine kritische Gebrauchsanweisung. Frankfurter Adorno-Vorlesungen. 1st Edition. Berlin 2017; Theda Borde, Tanja Braun, Matthias David: Inanspruchnahme von Notfallambulanzen. In T. Borde (Ed.): Gut versorgt. Migrantinnen und Migranten im Gesundheits- und Sozialwesen. Frankfurt am Main 2003, pp. 43–81; Robert Koch-Institut: Bericht zur Epidemiologie der Tuberkulose (Note 8); Emil Zimmermann: Ausländische Patienten in der klinischen Praxis. In: Doron Kiesel, Sabine Kriechhammer-Yagmur, Hans von Lüpke (Eds.): Kränkung und Krankheit. Psychische und psychosomatische Folgen der Migration. Arnoldsheiner Texte. Frankfurt am Main 1994, pp. 13–24.

[17] Katharina Edtstadler: Narrating illness. Krankheit erzählen. Tuberkulose in Literatur und Medizin. Wien 2016, p. 108.

[18] J.-C. Diallo: Flucht und Krankheit. In: Kiesel, Kriechhammer-Yagmur, von Lüpke (Eds.): Kränkung und Krankheit (Note 16), pp. 105–109; Fassin: Das Leben. Eine kritische Gebrauchsanweisung (Note 16), p. 62.

[19] León Grinberg, Rebeca Grinberg: Psychoanalyse der Migration und des Exils. München 1990, here p. ix; UNHCR: Abkommen über die Rechtsstellung der Flüchtlinge vom 28. Juli 1951 (2015), p. 6.

face during the treatment process of refugees. Strauss' concept derives from symbolic interactionism and defines trajectories as follows: »I shall use trajectory in two ways: (1) the course of any experience as it evolves over time and (2) the actions and interactions, which contribute to its evolution«.[20] Consequently, the course of disease is characterized by a certain time course, the occurrence of unexpected events, the interaction with external influences, and the interaction of the participants.[21] As such, the concept is not limited to the perspective of the patient or to the progression of the disease but includes further areas. Therefore, patients as well as all other involved persons are participants.[22] I focus on the handling of uncontrollable situations and attempts to guide them. In addition, an emphasis is put on the fact that being involved is always linked to the actor's experience. In other words, involved actors on the trajectories experience loss of control, insecurity, and suffering, while having to learn how to cope with these factors. The trajectories include routinely or »relatively routinely«[23] work, but they are also shaped by unexpected incidents. Accordingly, a lack of knowledge can lead to highly problematic and exceptional situations and every new »contingency«,[24] regardless of its scope, requires a set of alternative approaches to master the trajectory.

I draw on a sociological understanding of TB, which assesses the disease not merely based on its physical effects. Instead, the interaction of the involved interaction partners is key, as TB gains its meaning through negotiations and interactions of the participants and cannot be reduced to its infectious characteristics and effect on the body. I analyze the practices in which the disease is embedded, since these are crucial for the attributed importance of the disease and its (cultural) interpretation in the convalescent circle. For example, the disease is treated as severe or meaningless based on the practices of the actors involved in the field. In conclusion, TB is not merely a physical con-

---

[20] Anselm L. Strauss: Continual permutations of action, communication and social order. New York 1993, pp. 53–54.

[21] Strauss: Continual permutations (Note 20), pp. 53–54; Gerhard Riemann, Fritz Schütze: »Trajectory« as a basic theoretical concept for analyzing suffering and disorderly social processes. In: David R. Maines (Ed.): Social organization and social process. Essays in honor of Anselm Strauss. New York 1991, pp. 333–357.

[22] Anselm L. Strauss: Social organization of medical work. Chicago 1985.

[23] Strauss: Social organization (Note 22), p. 9.

[24] Strauss: Social organization (Note 22), p. 26.

dition, but gains significance through the interactions of actors acting in the field and is socially produced through interactions. The treatment process is therefore a social process in which the interviewed actors are involved.

## 4. Methodology

The evaluation is based on 10 problem-centered interviews as defined by Witzel (1982),[25] covering all phases of the treatment. The focus is on barriers in the treatment and problems arising from the interaction between the involved actors. The problem-centered interview is a dialogical interview, which is based on a guideline used in the background to control the conversation content.[26] In the research process, the guideline functions as a clarification of the problem area by deepening its understanding and reflecting on its content. The guideline covers experiences in dealing with TB, the situation during the treatment phases, specific features of TB-infected refugees, possible improvements of the treatment, and the knowledge about the disease itself.

In order to address problems in the treatment, this contribution examines the different institutions, which TB-infected refugees traverse during their trajectory. These consist of inpatient and outpatient treatment as added by the health department.[27] Inpatient treatment is represented by two senior physicians and a nurse. For outpatient treatment, three social workers were interviewed. Finally, two TB experts and two public health officers of the health department, who monitors the infection protection law and processes organization during treatment, are part of the sample. The sample repre-

---

[25] Andreas Witzel: Verfahren der qualitativen Sozialforschung. Überblick und Alternativen. Frankfurt am Main 1982, p. 322.

[26] Witzel: Verfahren der qualitativen Sozialforschung (Note 25), p. 90; Cornelia Helfferich: Die Qualität qualitativer Daten. Manual für die Durchführung qualitativer Interviews. 4. Aufl. Wiesbaden 2011, p. 39.

[27] Uwe Flick: Design und Prozess qualitativer Forschung. In: Uwe Flick, Ernst von Kardorff, Ines Steinke (Eds.): Qualitative Forschung. Ein Handbuch. 12. Aufl. Hamburg 2017, pp. 252–275; Bernhard Borgetto, Karl Kälble: Medizinsoziologie. Sozialer Wandel, Krankheit, Gesundheit und das Gesundheitssystem. Grundlagentexte Soziologie. Weinheim 2007; Klaus Hurrelmann: Gesundheitssoziologie. Eine Einführung in sozialwissenschaftliche Theorien von Krankheitsprävention und Gesundheitsförderung. Grundlagentexte Soziologie. 7. Edition. Weinheim 2010.

sents two actual care chains in Germany. Due to lack of access, no interview could be conducted with a patient.

| **Phases of the treatment** | **Interviewed actors** |
|---|---|
| Inpatient treatment: hospital | Two senior physicians, one nurse |
| Health department | Two TB experts, two public health officers |
| Outpatient treatment: refugee accommodation | Three social workers, one volunteer |

Tab. 1: Phases of treatment and interview partners

The interviews are analyzed using the process-oriented research approach of grounded theory, which aims to grasp the viewpoints of the actors in order to understand interaction, process and social change.[28] Grounded theory is characterized as a research style to evaluate material with a methodological guideline and an abductive approach aiming at a continuous comparison.[29] This abductive evaluation logic is based on a circular logic, which generates hypotheses and repeatedly links them to the research process, reviewing and adapting them in order to develop and condense concepts.[30] Supportive questions are asked repeatedly, such as: What is the phenomenon? Who is involved? Which aspects of the investigated phenomenon are addressed? When? For what reason? Which intentions are clear? Which tactics, means, and strategies can be identified? Furthermore, an interpretation group has been consulted to ensure the quality of the interpretation and intersubjective comprehensibility. The analysis was further amended by memoing, and a constant comparative analysis was carried out.

---

28 Anselm L. Strauss: Basics of Qualitative Research. Techniques and Procedures for Developing Grounded Theory. 4thh Edition. New York 2015, p. 30.

29 Strauss: Basics of Qualitative Research (Note 28), p. 30.

30 Bruno Hildenbrand: ›Anselm Strauss‹. In: Uwe Flick, Ernst von Kardorff, Ines Steinke (Eds.): Qualitative Forschung. Ein Handbuch. 12. Aufl. Hamburg 2017, pp. 32–42; Jo Reichertz: Qualitative und interpretative Sozialforschung. Eine Einladung. Studientexte zur Soziologie. Wiesbaden 2016; Strauss: Basics of Qualitative Research (Note 28), p. 30.

# 5. Treatment Process and Problem Outline

## *5.1 Inpatient treatment*

Starting with inpatient treatment, this section introduces key problems in the treatment process and uncertainties arising from them. The diagnosis is the starting point for the treatment and for the subsequent trajectories of TB-infected refugees. In case of infectious TB, patients usually remain in inpatient treatment for 14 days, where they are provided with medical treatment by physicians and nursing staff. At this stage, uncertainties arising from the inconspicuous symptoms of TB are the key problems. This is further aggravated by a lack of interpreters who are needed to convey information on treatment and compliance, delays in treatment due to overbooked hospital beds, and limited time for inpatient treatment. These aspects can be sum up as lacking resources; this is also pointed out if social workers attempt to contact a physician. These, however, request an interpreter to be present during treatment but neither the clinics nor the accommodations have sufficient interpreters available. Besides a general lack of interpreters, there further obstacles for translation, namely incomplete or incorrect translation, as doctors often cannot ensure correct translation:

I: Concerning tuberculosis, are there any certain ideas that refugees have about the disease?
B: Um, if we have made the diagnosis and educate them about the diagnosis in the therapy, yes that- in fact, it is not uncommon under the restriction that I cannot talk directly to them but about interpreters and I do not know exactly what they translated exactly.[31]

Here, the translation causes problems, accordingly they are considered to be failed interaction by the actors involved, which lead to obstacles in the treatment such as a lack of compliance. However, the translation is often more complicated than physicians perceive. In most cases, caregivers do not only have to translate literally, but also have to calm down the patient and provide emotional support. At the same time, misunderstandings arise, which have to be addressed. As one caretaker explained: »Then you have to show it is against the sickness, not against the skin color or anything, not against the im-

[31] Interview 1, 26 Mai 2018. Difficulties in the trajectories. Frankfurt am Main.

migration, but the sickness is just so contagious and has to stay in a room.«[32] This shows a need for special sensitivity, in order to communicate the necessity of treatment and to provide treatment without causing feelings of discrimination. However, the necessary resources and competences are currently not available at the necessary scale. Accordingly, the actors involved are largely referring to obstacles of lacking resources.

### 5.2 *Transition*

The transition does also provide challenges for the treatment of refugees suffering from TB. Here, the health department is involved from the outset and works in parallel with the clinic in order to track the roots of infection through analyzing the environment of the patient. After the inpatient treatment, the health department delegates social workers to organize the transfer back to the accommodation. In this process, tasks are separated into organizational aspects (i. e. transfer from inpatient to outpatient treatment), educational aspects (i. e. informing social workers and volunteers), and security and control aspects (i. e. monitoring the course of illness). In the latter, the state of health as well as compliance to the medication is checked. The main challenge for the health department is to ensure compliance on the side of infected refugees.

> I think for the greater proportion of those who are not that willing to cooperate (.) values, origin, how they grew up, and cultural, religious backgrounds play a role. There are communication difficulties, but there is also a simple lack of compliance, which is simply there. These are very simple cultures and very different mentalities, that is, you can often explain to those with interpreters exactly how important and necessary that is, they just do not do it. They say yes and just do not do that (annoyed tone)? So that's very, very, very difficult, um very difficult.[33]

In contrast to the inpatient treatment of the clinics, interpreters are not seen as a resource to ensure compliance, as health department officials do not trace missing compliance to languages barriers but cultural barriers instead. Thus, the health department worked out a sanction-based and highly monitored strategy: If refugees are not

[32] Interview 2, 26 Mai 2018. Difficulties in the trajectories. Frankfurt am Main.
[33] Interview 4, 27 August 2018. Difficulties in the trajectories. Frankfurt am Main.

compliant, the health department initiates measures such as monitored medication in order to prevent further infections and avert dangers for the population. Another problem-solving strategy of the health department is a network that performs hard controls and monitors the therapy. Additionally, there is a need to conduct cross-site environmental surveys as is required by the infection protection law (IfSG).

Another challenge regarding the transition to the outpatient treatment is the maintenance of organizational and support structures. Here, different actors become involved which are not medically trained, such as social workers and volunteers. Occasionally, these actors withdrawn from their work at the accommodation, as they lack knowledge of TB, which fundamentally affects the treatment and the transition. Besides they have no concept how to handle TB patients properly and efficient. However, to establish and maintain organizational and support structures (social infrastructure), the health department has to introduce additional measures as office hours and informational events, as these structures are permanently endangered due to fear, overload, and stereotyping by social workers, volunteers, and the general population. These should aim to inform actors and raise awareness and reassurance, as quoted:

> The disease tuberculosis is burdened with such fears and even ignorance-(.). We even did some educational evenings for social workers and volunteers and so on, just a little bit about the disease, the (.) um incubation period, the um chance of infection, which is very low, and also how the ways of infection and so on, we have tried everything (.) uh tried to make it clear uh, that such fears (.) no longer exist (.).[34]

Finally, it can be stated that health authorities work differently depending on the structures they are in, which was already pointed out by Mylius.[35] For example, doctor's experience with rural health departments, which do not ensure the supply of medicines and ambulance and thus endanger the entire treatment. As one doctor explained, if a health department does not conduct the transition and provides no guidance to social workers, the therapy of refugees is jeopardized due to lack of correct medication.

---

34 Interview 7, 27 August 2018. Difficulties in the trajectories. Frankfurt am Main.

35 Mylius: Die medizinische Versorgung (Note 3).

Here it should be noted that if the organizational structure of the responsible health department is lacking, the whole trajectory is threatened. In such a case, other involved institutions, for example doctors, have to safeguard the transition. Obviously, this is a barrier in the treatment due to a lack of resources and time.

### 5.3 *Outpatient treatment*

At the accommodation, professional social workers and volunteers are involved in filing applications, for example for health insurance certificates, and are responsible for organizing transportation to and from the clinic. When refugees suffering from TB arrive at the accommodation, they have to be looked after and the infrastructure must be set up and maintained. This point lies at the intersection of administration and rehabilitation. Moreover, social workers are responsible for monitoring and controlling outpatient treatment. Here, they have to meticulously record the organizational structure and safeguard compliance. However, professional interpreters are often missing, and medical confidentiality prohibits physicians from disclosing a patient's illness, thus missing and incorrect communication are the result. Overall, social workers cannot react adequately, for example, social worker expressed his lack of knowledge due to the medical confidentiality as follows:

> I have heard (.) about nothing, until the day (.) when it was said that a conversation about tuberculosis in the context of a master thesis would take place. And it was only THEN that I realized that in my (.) house there had been a TB case, this was not communicated previously. it- yes so I do not know that there have been measures, at that time when the case occurred, I wasn't told anything either.[36]

This is further aggravated due to a lack of practical routines resulting in disoriented actions and uncertainties:

> On the one hand (.) there is always the question, to what extent am I protected myself. That was among other things what the nurse asked me: where are my protection devices and I said, how? What? What do you mean? And she said, your glove, mouth guard and something like that and

[36] Interview 5, 27 August 2018. Difficulties in the trajectories. Frankfurt am Main.

I said to her, that I did not have the information, what it is all about. I was just told to pick up somebody.[37]

In this instance, the social worker does not know how to deal with the information that patient is infected with TB. He asks for information and security for his co-workers, but the communication channels do not function, which is no exceptional case. This incident points to knowledge hierarchies during the course of the treatment. Social workers and other involved actors responsible for the treatment are often not specifically trained and sometimes lack any knowledge of the disease. It is important to know that the social workers are not trained and possess usually only makeshift information from the Internet. Although their knowledge is limited or entirely non-existent, they bear great responsibility for, as they have to react adequately when problems arise despite a lack established practical routines: »[T]here is no scheme or schemes, which could be applied, there is no such thing. The person was then sent to a doctor (.)«[38] Another social worker mentions an instance in which a colleague was infected with scabies, but their employer, despite the hoped-for support, failed to help them:

Er, even when the colleague was apparently really sick of scabies, that was (.) trivialized by the management, she could have contracted it outside of the work or somewhere maybe (.) At home in bed or no idea and it was – it was also for me at the moment, this is our team room, that was also so (.) weird, a very weird feeling, (.) because the employer has a certain care duty, I think and (.) he has not complied with it and instead of this the situation has been trivialized and he also pretended that it (scabies) could have come from elsewhere. Of course, there is a probability, but (.) I believe- (.) yes and I think that was bad for the person, right?[39]

A lack of knowledge, frustration, and feelings of excessive demands often drive providers to quit their jobs. Especially volunteers and infrastructure services providers like building contractors often cancel their support. The results show a need for further emotional, informational, and organizational support. Furthermore, social workers often struggle to maintain communication channels, preventing providers from resigning, ensuring the therapy, and the life in the ac-

37 Interview 6, 27 August 2018. Difficulties in the trajectories. Frankfurt am Main.
38 Interview 6, 27 August 2018. Difficulties in the trajectories. Frankfurt am Main.
39 Interview 6, 27 August 2018. Difficulties in the trajectories. Frankfurt am Main.

commodations. A social worker leading an accommodation for refugees impressively described how volunteers and the building contractors break away from her. On the one hand, she is confronted with keeping actors in the process, calming them and at the same time keeping the TB case secret due to the medical confidentiality. If she does not succeed in this balancing act, there is the need to inform the health department, which tries to stabilize the situation through information and reassurance.

Overall, the outpatient treatment features a range of crucial difficulties, which cause uncertainties. Starting with missing medical competences, insufficient information and communication processes, lacking of knowledge of the illness as well as the fear of being infected and the potential to cause feelings of discrimination on the side of TB-infected refugees. Many barriers arising in the inpatient treatment and in the transition can be found here to a greater extent, which amplifies the need supportive measures and structures.

## 6. Overall view of the situation

Uncertainties and problems during the treatment process can have very different causes. They endanger the treatment process, since they lead to delays and prevent adherence to defined processes. This inhibits actors from acting in line with their practical routines, who in turn lack an orientation for their actions. Here it should be noted that the treatment is further complicated with a growing number of involved actors, as more unforeseeable events and ambiguities occur. Lacking knowledge is a key concern, as uninformed actors or actors with insufficient knowledge cannot react properly to symptoms, thus leading to incorrect diagnoses and treatment. Consequently, support structures are threatened by collapse due to arising fears. Finally, the involved actors also ascribe a risk to the patients, which are said to introduce uncertainties into the treatment process. Lacking compliance is often ascribed to unsuccessful interactions and explained based on language and culture. Therefore, it is often not possible to convey information.

Overall, organizational and communication problems are added by resource scarcity (e.g. missing interpreters) and lacking infrastructure (e.g. bad hygienic conditions), which all increase the risk of infection and jeopardize the treatment. The following table sums up the main challenges interview partners identified in the treatment process.

| Diagnosis and inpatient treatment | Transition to outpatient treatment | Outpatient Treatment |
|---|---|---|
| Diagnosis often accidental | Pressure from health insurances, lack of proper explanation of medication, | Lack of interpreters, incomplete translations |
| Illness is difficult to detect but highly contagious | Partly insecure, scared, and uninformed social workers | Legal impediments lead to misinformation, a lack in communication and mistaken reactions |
| Lack of resources at the clinic | Insufficient compliance by refugees due to language or cultural barriers | Insufficient hygienic conditions |
| Language and cultural barriers, uncertainty of correct translation | | Weakened refugees become more easily infected |
| Delays and limited accessibility of physicians | | Missing instructions and missing knowledge of TB, lead to uncertainties |

Tab. 2: Problems in the treatment process

## 7. Anticipatory actions in response to uncertainties

As pointed out before, the infectious characteristics of TB promotes uncertainties which is further aggravated by a certain unawareness which illness is exactly present due to lacking knowledge of the disease (and its treatment) and inherent uncertainties in the treatment of the illness due to organizational and resource obstacles. This part highlights how the actors involved manage uncertainties in form of anticipatory actions. These anticipatory actions are woven very differently into the process and affect different actors. Among these were strategies to *control* the treatment process, efforts to *expand and maintain the support system* through education and reassurance as well as attempts of *emotional support*.

Based on grounded theory, several problem-solving strategies have been identified, which seek to organize treatment more consistently, efficient, thus providing stability. These strategies can be interpreted as trajectory schemes in the form of anticipatory actions, which try to counteract the inherent contingencies of trajectories and the illness treatment.

Anticipatory actions start already in the clinic by caring for and *controlling* medication. These actions are performed by nurses and organized by doctors, here the development of TB and medication are the focus of controls. Therefore, the doctors try to convey the importance of treatment and the correct intake of medication to the refugees. In doing so, they hope, that the patients will be show greater compliance.

The aspect of controlling is also important for the health department. In order to control the spread of the infection, the health department examines the accommodation, checking patients in regular intervals and monitoring the development of the TB. Throughout the process, its control tasks comprise everything for which the clinic is no longer responsible. Therefore, it also involves social workers, who fulfil the control tasks in the accommodations. Moreover, the health department develops strategies to evolve and maintain the support system. It tries to calm down social workers and other involved actors, who are afraid of the infectious characteristics of TB, and to inform social workers and volunteers about the correct behavior of TB appears.

Last but not least, the social workers accompany and organize large parts of the overall process and are expected to have a diverse competence profile. In their daily work, they carry out all the tasks the health department transfers to them, hence they are a part of different control strategies even if they did not develop them or realize they are part of it. Furthermore, they have to be attentive, recognize problems of the inhabitants, and react quickly and sensitively to them. If a case appears, they try to convey the important information without trying to causing feelings of discrimination. This behavior has an effect on compliance, as it helps refugees to overcome fears of acceptance. However, social workers sometimes overlook actual problems of sick refugees and start to execute commands without questioning them in order to meet all requirements.

Finally, the anticipatory strategies themselves do not complement each other, but are contradictory instead. This becomes clear when different anticipatory actions overlap. For example, controlling the disease and maintaining supportive structures creates a seemingly contradictory strategy. As pointed out before, refugees were frightened of TB (especially by TB experts), as they were told that the illness is extremely dangerous and a lack of cooperation could lead to their death. In the case of non-compliance, the TB expert calls the police, as the infection is considered to be too dangerous to remain untreated. Hence, refugees must take the illness seriously. This behavior can be interpreted as a way of dealing with anxiety. Hard controlling and forced compliance is emphasized in order to limit the illness and raise consciousness; however, this causes fear among refugees. The health department act similarly to safeguard compliance and to control the illness. To maintain the support system, the health department reassures, trivializes, but also educates social workers and volunteers in order to dispel fears. For example, health department staff refers to the low probability of infection thus reassuring social workers. In doing so, the TB expert tries to calm the social worker down and in the case of an interview tells them that there is no necessity to be examined, instead of providing an opportunity for a medical check-up. While the TB expert helps to relieve anxiety by trivializing the characteristics of the illness, this highlights a problematic gap in the support structure for social workers. Later in the interview, the social worker also states that she should not be afraid of the disease, as she would not be a good social worker otherwise. However, if social workers witness how infected refugees were threatened, they can be unsettled and require reassurance and education to dispel their fears. Finally, I will present, whom these strategies referring to. As non-specialists in medicine, social workers and volunteers constitute the greatest risk potential in the trajectories followed by the health department and the clinic. For this reason, many anticipatory actions aim at controlling the illness, as well as the refugees and volunteers. Most anticipatory actions affect the refugees to be treated. The greatest risk potential regarding uncertainties in the treatment is attributed to refugees.

Hence, the trajectories are characterized by a hierarchical knowledge structure, in which the clinic and the health department solely retain both key forms of knowledge regarding the illness. First, knowledge on the illness itself and, second, knowledge on treating and handling the illness. The clinic and the health department possess the first kind of knowledge, as it presupposes fundamental medical knowledge. Furthermore, the clinic and the health department also possess knowledge on treating and handling the illness, because they organize and structure the monitoring process to which social workers in the accommodations have to adhere. On the contrary, the anticipatory actions demonstrate that social workers and volunteers lack exact knowledge of the illness and how to act and help correctly, even though they were assigned key tasks in the treatment process for over six months. This hierarchical structure is reproduced through authority. The health department tries to counteract deviations and uncertainties by means of clear instructions and by reassuring social workers and volunteers.

Nevertheless, disruptions or deviations in such rigid systems are hardly bearable or sustainable for actors on the lower bound of the knowledge structure, like social workers, volunteers, and refugees. These uncertainties can cause enormous fear; this aspect is of great importance and requires further research.

## 8. Outlook

This contribution showed that the treatment of TB-infected refugees faces particular challenges, which lead to uncertainty. The anticipatory actions developed by the actors involved provide only a limited solution, but they often speed up treatment by making it more efficient. However, the results also point to a lack of understanding for the refugee patients. For instance, compliance issues are reduced to language or cultural barriers and are less often localized in the organization of treatment. Lack of knowledge and lack of time jeopardize the treatment, which poses the risk that actors may respond incorrectly to contagion. Other organizational structures are necessary to counteract inadequately sensitized personnel, communication difficulties, and time lost in treatment. This requires shorter communication channels as well as close cooperation between the different institutions and actors in order to combat TB efficiently but also humanely. In this case, intercultural competence is key to prevent fears and to convey the importance of the treatment. Education for dealing with TB and identifying possible fields of action can be stabilizing measures. This is not only a financial and political issue, but also a social and individual question. How should one act when treating patients who are exposed to completely new experiences and structures and who may not understand what is happening to them? Further research should also take the perspective of refugee patients into account.

*Robert Doričić*

# The challenges of the migration crisis in Croatia – the Primorje-Gorski Kotar County and the city of Rijeka example

Abstract
In the last quarter of 2015, the eastern part of Croatia encountered a large number of migrants moving to the West of Europe using the so-called Western Balkan route. The Croatian Government's response to the emerging migration crisis was in organizing a network of numerous organizations aimed at providing humanitarian assistance to migrants. One of them was the National Society of the Red Cross of the Republic of Croatia. In the upcoming period, the experience of the migrant wave raised the necessity to check the alertness of the Croatian standard operational forces, which are organizations prepared for possible crisis situations, stationed in different parts of the country. Such type of exercise was organized by the regional Red Cross Society in 2017 in the city of Rijeka, Primorje-Gorski Kotar County. The exercise held in Rijeka is an example of organizing a system of reception and assistance to a large number of migrants arriving by sea.

## 1. Introduction

In the late summer of 2015 Croatia faced the first large wave of immigrants who were passing via the so-called Western Balkan route, i.e. a corridor through Macedonia, Serbia, Croatia and Slovenia, attempting to reach their destinations in Western European countries, mostly in Germany, Austria and Sweden.[1] By the decision of the Croatian government, the State Headquarters for Coordination of Migrant Related Activities chaired by the Ministry of Interior was

---

1 Senada Šelo Šabić: Humanitarianism and Its Limits: The Refugee Crisis Response in Croatia. In: Melani Barlai, Birte Fähnrich, Christina Griessler, Markus Rhomberg (Eds.): The Migrant Crisis: European Perspectives and National Discourses. Münster 2017, pp. 93–106; Josip Esterajher: Iskustva zbrinjavanja prognanika i izbjeglica i suvremena izbjegličko-migrantska kriza u Hrvatskoj [Experience of accommodating displaced persons and refugees at the current refugee-migrant crisis in Croatia]. In: Političke analize 23 (2015), pp. 15–22.

established. According to the Croatian Act on International and Temporary Protection, migrants in transit through Croatia were treated as migrants under temporary protection.[2] The above-mentioned Act provides emergency medical care and appropriate health care for vulnerable groups in this category of migrants for a maximum period of three years. The organization of the health care for migrants came within the competence of the Ministry of Health, which was involved in the State Headquarters' Activities.

Although the main entry point was in the Municipality of Tovarnik, Vukovar-Srijem County of the Eastern Croatian territory, health care for migrants has been provided by coordinated activities of county departments of emergency medicine from the eastern and northwestern parts of Croatia. Medical teams from almost every Croatian county have been involved in providing health care in the Opatovac refugee camp, Vukovar-Srijem County.[3] On the 9 of March 2016, the Western Balkan route was closed.[4]

However, sporadic transits of smaller migrant groups occur to the present day. Due to its geographical position in the north Mediterranean and its vicinity to the economically developed EU countries, primary Italy, the regional administrative unit Primorje-Gorski Kotar County with its macro regional and administrative center, the city of Rijeka, has been seen as a potential transit point for larger groups of migrants and asylum seekers. On the other hand, the transit of smaller groups of migrants has been noticed and the media reported on several cases of immigrant smuggling in the area of this county, especially since the late summer of 2018.[5]

---

[2] Croatian parliament: Act on international and temporary protection »clean version«. Official Gazette (70/2015, 127/2017).

[3] Maja Grba-Bujević, Maja Dragosavac, Nataša Janev-Holcer, Damir Važanić: Odgovor zdravstvenog sustava Republike Hrvatske na migrantsku krizu u razdoblju od 16. rujna do 31. prosinca 2015 [Response of Croatian health care system to migrant crisis in the period from September 16 to December 31, 2015]. In: Liječnički vjesnik 138 (2016), pp. 99–103.

[4] Senada Šelo Sabić, Sonja Borić: At the Gate of Europe: a Report on Refugees on the Western Balkan Route. Zagreb 2016.

[5] Slavica Kleva: Masovno privođenje krijumčara ljudima u Rijeci. Jedan je u kombi uspio strpati čak – 61 migranta! [Massive arresting of people smugglers in Rijeka. One managed to squeeze 61 migrants in the van!]. In: Novi list (9/10/2018). http://www.novilist.hr/Vijesti/Crna-kronika/Masovno-privodenje-krijumcara-ljudima-u-Rijeci.-Jedan-je-u-kombi-uspio-strpati-cak-61-migranta (accessed 9/24/2019).

The European migration crisis, in particular its most intense migrant waves, has set for the countries on these routes demanding tasks of organizing humanitarian aid to migrants. The experience of the humanitarian crisis and the treatment of migrants on the territory of the Republic of Croatia during migrant wave 2015/2016 showed the preparedness of the involved stakeholders to deal with such a crisis.[6] On the other hand, it has become a starting point for testing organizational requirements and implementing such interventions in case new migrant wave emerges, taking into account the geographical heterogeneity of the Croatian state territory. The aim of this paper is to introduce through the exercise held in the city of Rijeka, Primorje-Gorski Kotar County, a system of measures and institutions related to the acceptance, registration, and care of migrants who, on an exceptional basis, would reach the Croatian territory by sea. The data were collected from interviews, reports and other organizational documents.

Primorje-Gorski Kotar County geographically belongs to the region of *Primorska Hrvatska* (Littoral Croatia) and is located on the northeast coast of the Adriatic Sea. The area of Primorje-Gorski Kotar County covers 6.3 % of the territory of the Republic of Croatia and is divided into three parts – the mountainous area, the coastal, and the island area. According to the analysis of the Croatian Chamber of Economy, Primorje-Gorski Kotar County is ranked among the most developed Croatian counties, along with the neighboring Istria County and the City of Zagreb.[7] The structure of the economy in the Primorje-Gorski Kotar County could be characterized using the number of employees in individual economic sectors. According to the rank, among the first three activities in Primorje-Gorski Kotar County are wholesale and retail trade; repair of motor vehicles and motorcycles (21.3 %), processing industry (19.6 %), and activities relating to accommodation service, preparing and serving food (12.8 %).[8]

---

[6] Maren Larsen, Elma Demir, Maja Horvat: Humanitarian Responses by Local Actors: Lessons Learned from Managing the Transit of Migrants and Refugees Through Croatia (IIED Working Paper). London 2016.

[7] Hrvatska gospodarska komora: HGK indeks gospodarske snage [CCE index of economic power]. https://www.hgk.hr/documents/hgk-indeks-gospodarske-snage-0720 1759803f707ec38.pdf (accessed 9/24/2019).

[8] Primorsko-goranska županija: Statistički podaci o gospodarstvu Primorsko-goranske županije [Primorje-Gorski Kotar County: Statistical data on the economy of

Rijeka is the third largest city in Croatia and it is the administrative center of Primorje-Gorski Kotar County. The largest Croatian port is located in Rijeka. According to the 2011 census, the city of Rijeka has 128,624 inhabitants.[9] In the 19th century, Rijeka became one of the largest European ports and a powerful industrial center. After the Second World War, Rijeka was significant as one of the most important financial centers of the former Yugoslavia. At the beginning of the nineties of the 20th century, industry collapsed and a sudden decrease in port traffic occurred. In the 21st century, Rijeka is turning to the development of tourism and the service sector. The city of Rijeka will be the European Capital of Culture in 2020.

The organized exercise »Migrants RI 2017«, held in Rijeka in the autumn of 2017 that will be presented here, was initially suggested by the Red Cross Society of the Primorje-Gorski Kotar County. The National Society of the Red Cross of the Republic of Croatia (Croatian Red Cross) is organized through the work and activities of 20 Red Cross legal entities and 111 Red Cross municipal and city societies. Guided by the fundamental principles of their organization (humanity, impartiality, independence, neutrality, voluntary service, unity, and universality), their work is clearly defined by international conventions (the Geneva Conventions) and regulated by the Law on the Croatian Red Cross. As part of the activities of the Croatian Red Cross, the Migration Service was organized. Red Cross activities towards international protection seekers and international and temporary protection applicants and towards other migrants in need are based on the Fundamental Principles of the International Red Cross and Red Crescent Movement as determined by the Migration Policy of the International Federation of the Red Cross and Red Crescent Societies. At the level of the Croatian Red Cross, three departments were established: the Department for assistance to migrants, asylum seekers, and displaced persons, the Department for integration of persons under international and temporary protection, and the Department for prevention of trafficking in persons and psychosocial support.[10] As one can read on the web pages of the Croatian national

---

the Primorje-Gorski Kotar County]. https://www.pgz.hr/Zupanijski_ustroj/Upravna_tijela/UO_gospodarstvo/Statisticki_podaci_o_gospodarstvu_PGZe (accessed 9/24/2019).

[9] Croatian bureau of statistics: Census of population, households and dwellings 2011. https://www.dzs.hr/default_e.htm (accessed 9/24/2019).

[10] Dejan Ajduković, Helena Bakić, Marina Ajduković: Psihosocijalna podrška u kriz-

society of the Red Cross and the Red Cross Society of the Primorje-Gorski Kotar County, the concept of so-called »operational forces of the Croatian Red Cross« foresees employees and volunteers of this society. They are organized into pivot crisis units, intervention teams, and support teams at the local, county and national levels. All these teams are involved in the implementation of activities throughout all the stages of the crisis, from crisis prevention to response generation, and crisis recovery efforts. At the local level, the team for disaster response and emergency situations is prepared through the training of city and county intervention teams. Each member adopts basic knowledge of first aid, psychosocial support, security, self-protection, and communication. After completing basic education, there are upgrading courses to carry out specific tasks from a certain segment of actions in case of crisis situations: for example, gaining additional knowledge in providing first aid, knowledge relevant to crisis assessment, job search, organization of reception and accommodation, or providing safe drinking water as well as minimum hygiene conditions. It can be pointed out that the best members of the intervention teams seek additional training to operate in international aid missions.[11]

## 2. Migrant Wave Experience in November 2015

Since they face crisis situations, the migrant wave 2015/2016 on the territory of the Republic of Croatia represented another challenge for the national organization of the Red Cross and its components. It was necessary to focus on the activities of equipping and training their own operational forces and to carry out the education for all age groups in the population.

During an interview with the current director of the Primorje-Gorski Kotar County Red Cross Society, Vesna Čavar, a former associate of the society, shared her experiences from the ground during the migration wave in Croatia.[12] Namely, the Croatian Red Cross has

---

nim situacijama velikih razmjera [Psychosocial Support in Large Scale Crisis Situations]. Zagreb 2017.

[11] Croatian Red Cross. http://www2.hck.hr/en (accessed 9/24/2019); Red Cross Society of Primorje-Gorski Kotar County. https://www.dck-pgz.hr (accessed 9/24/2019).

[12] Vesna Čavar, personal communication, 2/20/2019.

been empowered to co-ordinate all non-governmental organizations (for example, United Nations High Commissioner for Refugees (UNHCR), Caritas, and all other non-governmental organizations) who have come up with food, clothing and, together with emergency assistance, provide elementary health care for migrants. The Primorje-Gorski Kotar County Red Cross Society had a task to send an educated group of volunteers every three weeks on the ground to assist in a variety of activities for a one-week period. Most often, the activities included the psychosocial support since the Primorje-Gorski Kotar County Red Cross Society has been equipped with such staff. Mrs. Čavar stayed there for six days in November 2015. After the Croatian state had organized the reception of migrants, they were transferred by trains near the city of Slavonski Brod where a refugee camp was organized. Migrants were held there for several hours and were provided with some refreshments and clothes by volunteers. After that, they would continue their path towards Slovenia. The umbrella organization that ran all the activities was the Ministry of the Interior. A group of the Red Cross organization with whom Mrs. Čavar was, was responsible for the distribution of clothing, warm drinks, and for providing psychosocial support as well as the tracing service. The usual procedure was that when the train with migrants reached the station, the special police officers entered the train first to inform the migrants about further proceedings. There used to be 800–1000 migrants in every train. After the special police, the Red Cross volunteers would approach the passengers. Then, the migrants went to the registration point. After receiving refreshments and packages of food, they were directed to heated tents where they could rest and get some clothes, if they had not been dressed up for the winter conditions. Psychosocial support was provided that included assistance in situations where, for example, a child would be lost and did not know where the rest of the family was, or for women after their newborns had passed away. Among the memories during her stay at the refugee camp, Mrs. Čavar particularly mentioned the situation when a child came out of the train and ran barefoot through the snow and when an older man who had a stroke was driven in a wheelchair by his family. Mrs. Čavar noted that it was necessary to organize some type of psychosocial support on the ground for the members of the Red Cross Society as well.

Mrs. Branka Marečić, an expert associate in the Primorje-Gorski Kotar County Red Cross Society, did not have a personal experience of participation in assisting in the midst of the migrant wave in autumn 2015. However, in the interview she pointed out that the tracing service, provided by the national societies of the Red Cross on the migrant route, was run by the unique protocol as it is prescribed at the level of the International Committee of the Red Cross. According to her, one of the really important tasks of the Red Cross along the migratory routes is to try to keep the families together.[13]

The Mrs. Čavar's impression was that all those who had been involved in providing assistance were very well organized. To overcome language barriers, the Croatian Red Cross had volunteers of different nationalities, for example, there was a translator for the Pashtu language. Among the translators, there were Croatian citizens who knew foreign languages and offered their help. When asked whether the experience of mass migration that occurred during the Croatian War of Independence had contributed to the good organization in this aspect of migrant crisis, she answered that it had made a substantial contribution at the state level. The first contact with the migrant wave in Opatovac stirred up local population's memories of their own experiences during the war and encouraged them to assist migrants.

## 3. »Migrants RI 2017« Exercise

Conceptual creator of »Migrants RI 2017« exercise, the director of the Primorje-Gorski Kotar County Red Cross Society, Mrs. Čavar pointed out how the idea of implementing this action in Rijeka evolved. According to the current Law on civil protection system, the Red Cross has become the standard operational power, which, in other words, means that the law equates the Red Cross with the fire brigade, ambulance, mountain rescue service, civil protection, etc.[14] These organizations must be prepared for possible crisis situations of any kind, from elemental disasters to war or migrants. Each year, with all operating forces, different exercises are performed in the areas of a particular county. Encouraged by the stay in the midst of the migrant wave in the east of Croatia, in the refugees camp in Slavonski Brod in November 2015, Mrs. Čavar had proposed that the

---

[13] Branka Marečić, personal communication, 2/20/2019.

[14] Croatian parliament: Law on civil protection system. Official Gazette (82/2015).

scenario for the annual exercise in Rijeka might be the simulation of the reception of a large number of migrants who would come to Rijeka by boat.

Similarly, a demonstrative exercise involving illegal migrants was organized at the beginning of October 2016 in the city of Split, the capital of the Split-Dalmatia County, in the area of Lora, the military harbor. The demonstrative exercise in Split included two scenarios. The first involved the reception of a large number of migrants who were given the first aid, after which they were referred to a tent for registration. Another demonstration exercise was a simulation of an abduction of a merchant ship by 8 terrorists. The demonstrative exercises were organized by the Ministry of the Interior of the Republic of Croatia. In the exercise to rescue illegal migrants, besides the police force, the Red Cross volunteers have also been involved.[15]

As seen in the initial proposal of a demonstrative exercise in Rijeka, entitled »Ship with Migrants/Refugees in Rijeka Port«, the main objective of the exercise was to check the operational efficiency in the crisis situation of managing a large number of migrants/refugees from the ship entering the Rijeka port.[16]

Besides the main objective, the exercise included specific objectives. According to them, this exercise should:

1. check the readiness of each operational force to intervene in a crisis situation and 2. enhance the communication between all practitioners at the crisis level (between headquarters – the vehicle – the operational force).

The scenario exercise under this proposal included the berthing of a ship with a larger number of migrants/refugees in the port of Rijeka. It had been anticipated that 50 participants (markers) of all ages were included in the simulation. At one moment, the ship fired, and some of the panicked passengers jumped into the sea, swam to the shore and ran to the abandoned port warehouses. The second group of illegal immigrants/refugees came to the prepared vessel and set off to escape. Some of the migrants were injured and an outbreak was suspected.

---

[15] Al Jazeera Balkans: Split: Pokazna vježba prihvata nelegalnih migranata [Split: a demonstrative exercise of reception of illegal migrants] (10/11/2016). http://balkans.aljazeera.net/video/split-pokazna-vjezba-prihvata-nelegalnih-migranata?page=1&qtvideo_side_tabs=1&qtvideo_wide_tabs=0 (accessed 9/24/2019).

[16] Primorje-Gorski Kotar County Red Cross Society: Proposal of a demonstrative exercise in the crisis situation (internal organizational document) 2017.

According to the proposal, the exercise was supposed to be held in early September morning in the waters of the Rijeka port at three points: 1) the breakwater/Terminal; 2) Senj dock, and 3) Brajdica container terminal. An implementation of the exercise would involve numerous operational powers: the Primorje-Gorski Kotar County Red Cross Society, Headquarters and General Units of the Primorje-Gorski Kotar County Civil Defence, general troops of the Civil Defense of the City of Rijeka, Fire Board of the Primorje-Gorski Kotar County, Public Fire Brigade of the City of Rijeka, National Protection and Rescue Directorate – Regional Office for Protection and Rescue Rijeka (these institutions merged with the Ministry of Interior in early 2019), Department of emergency medicine of Primorje-Gorski Kotar County, Teaching Institute of Public Health of Primorje-Gorski Kotar County, Primorje-Gorski Kotar County Police Department, Harbormasters' offices in Rijeka, and the Croatian Mountain Rescue Service – Rijeka Station.

The initial proposal of the Primorje-Gorski Kotar County Red Cross Society was later elaborated in the final feasibility study drawn up by the Local office for protection and rescue, after which the Primorje-Gorski Kotar County Assembly adopted the study by its final name »Migrants RI 2017«.[17]

### *3.1 »Migrants RI 2017« Exercise Participants*

In the final study, the specific objectives of the exercise are described in detail in which the individual operational forces involved should check the specificities related to their own engagement in this type of crisis situation:

1. Headquarters of the Primorje-Gorski Kotar County Civil Defence (HCD PGC) similar to the organization of the Red Cross at the county level, the Primorje-Gorski Kotar County Civil Defence (CD PGC) is a part of the operational forces responsible for the protection and rescue of people, animals, material and cultural goods, and the environment in large accidents and disasters and for the elimination of consequences of terrorism and war destruction. The objective to its participation in the »Migrants RI 2017« was to check the competences

[17] Local office for protection and rescue: Feasibility study of the exercise (elaborate of the exercise) »Migrants RI 2017« (internal organizational document) 2017.

of mobilization and alignment of operational forces acting on the ground and the verification of communication between the participants;

2. Primorje-Gorski Kotar County Police Department (PD PGC) tested with the exercise the implementation procedures and plan(s) of the treatment of migrants;

3. Public Fire Brigade of the City of Rijeka had the purpose to verify the competence of the fire brigades in the intervention of the fire fighting on board, as well as verify the competence of the divers' team while rescuing the injured persons from the sea;

4. Primorje-Gorski Kotar County Red Cross Society (RCS PGC) aim was to check the capability of making reception points, check the procedure of registration, and care for the injured, as well as to test skills of the Red Cross water rescuers;

5. Croatian Mountain Rescue Service (CMRS) – Rijeka Station (CMRS-RI) is a volunteer, non-for-profit and public organization, specialized in rescuing in mountains, where rescuing requires application of special mountain-rescue skills and equipment.[18] The goal for CMRS-RI was to test their response in the event of an emergency rescue incident;

6. Special forces of the Primorje-Gorski Kotar County Civil Defence wanted to verify the effectiveness of specialized civil defense units in the case of providing support to other operational forces in the Primorje-Gorski Kotar County by using available human and material-technical resources;

7. Department of Emergency Medicine of the Primorje-Gorski Kotar County (DEM PGC) aimed at training triage, supply and transport of injured persons;

8. Teaching Institute of Public Health of Primorje-Gorski Kotar County (TIPH PGC) as part of the exercise aimed to test sea sampling methods, check the purity of drinking water, check the procedures in conducting epidemiological investigations, and train the coordination with other operational forces;

9. The Ministry of the Sea, Transport and Infrastructure of Republic of Croatia – the Harbormaster's office of Rijeka aimed to establish a review of operational procedures for sudden oil pollution by oil derivatives;

---

[18] Croatian Mountain Rescue Service. http://www.gss.hr/ (accessed 9/24/2019).

10. Primorje-Gorski Kotar County Operational Centre (COC PGC), a competent body at the county level, is responsible for the implementation of procedures and measures for predicting, preventing, restricting, and readiness according to the Intervention plan and for operational participation in the implementation of national and sub-regional contingency plan.[19] This center aimed to check the response in case of accidental sea pollution and the coordination with Headquarters of Primorje-Gorski Kotar County Civil Defense and other operational forces;

11. Dezinsekcija Ltd. is a company, which provides services in the field of the sea protection in the Republic of Croatia.[20] The company set the goal of verifying the plan of action at the request of the County Operations Centre and its competence in case of marine pollution.

### *3.2 The Exercise Scenario*

The final report contains a detailed description of the exercise scenario. For some of the above-mentioned exercise participants the abbreviations of the organization names will be used. The Captain of catamaran while entering the port of Rijeka reports to the control center (Harbor Control Centre) that an undetermined number of people are discovered on board, he assumes they are migrants. The Harbor inspector general informs the competent services and the county civil defense. The police force and the RCS PGC come first to the ship. Based on the request of the RCS PGC for additional assistance, an activation of Special Forces of the CD PGC is required. The Red Cross Society's volunteers start preparing reception points for migrants. It should be pointed out that the employees of the TIPH PGC monitor sanitary hygiene in shelters for migrants. The supervision includes an accommodation, sanitary facilities and food for migrants. There is an explosion on the ship approaching the mainland and 4–5 migrants in a panic jump into the sea, among them are also non-swimmers (one

[19] Primorje-Gorski Kotar County: Activities of the County operational centre for marine protection. https://www.pgz.hr/Zupanijski_ustroj/Upravna_tijela/Upravni_odjel_pomorstvo_promet_turizam/Promet/Rad_Zupanijskog_operativnog_centra_za_zastitu_mora (accessed 9/24/2019).

[20] Dezinskekcija Ltd. http://www.dezinsekcija.hr/ (accessed 9/24/2019).

manikin in the role of a drowned person). The rescue action of the non-swimmer is led by the team of the Red Cross water rescuers and the public fire troops with divers aiming to save the drowned. Rescued landless detainees were accepted by the members of civil defense units and follow them together with the police to the preassigned reception center (reception and processing points for TIPH PGC, PD PGC, DEM PGC). The first information that the civil defense officer receives from the police officers, who entered the ship after the tug, says that the situation on the ship is complex; migrants are upset and aggressive, probably injured and possibly ill.

At the same time, the procedure of examining and registering migrants from the ship is carried out by the members of the police, firefighters and civil defense units. During the disembarkation of the migrants from the ship, smoke is detected on the ship and the fire is spreading. The firefighter team approaches the ship to tackle a blaze and inspect the ship, and the members of civil defense units under the supervision of police take migrants to the reception center.

As a result of the explosion and fire, the oil pollution is observed in the sea around the ship. The coordinator at the site informs the HCD PGC. The headquarters informs about the COC PGC, which activates Dezinsekcija Ltd. The employees of the Dezinsekcija Ltd. go out on the field, set up the bar and access to the collection of pollution.

At the same time, the PD PGC conducts the identification of persons in the reception center, after which the DEM PGC conducts triage of injured persons, the TIPH PGC conducts an epidemiological survey, and the RCS PGC provides a care for a vulnerable group of migrants. They provide the psychosocial support and hand out clothes to the migrants. They register the members of separated families and thus provide the tracing service. After the registration one migrant leaves, i.e. runs away from the reception center. He climbs to the nearby harbor crane. At this point, the CMRS-RI is engaged.

### *3.3 Volunteers-Migrants*

It was envisaged that a total of 50 markers would be involved in the role of migrants, out of which 49 members of the RCS PGC. The types and number of simulated injuries have been agreed between the DEM PGC and the RCS PGC. For the most credible scenario, the markers playing migrants should speak English or another foreign language or be silent. Funding the simulation of detonation and fire on board according to the study should have been provided by the Public Fire Brigade of the City of Rijeka.

The heterogeneous group of markers consisted of adult men and women, younger and older people, properly trained and carrying their luggage in which were some clothes, food and a couple of knives. Out of a total of 47 people, 10 suffered injuries. The injuries included heavy burns, light burns, burns of the air gastropods, broken ribs, closed forearm fracture, open fracture of the lower leg, casualties of the arcade with brain concussion, and forearm loss. Markers played the role of migrants who were very weak and in deep unconsciousness. Additionally, two migrants were pregnant, one of whom was in a high stage of pregnancy i.e. in labors; one migrant was in a wheelchair due to a stroke; one was a deaf person with developmental difficulties. One woman migrant was deaf-mute and travelled alone; the other one was mute and illiterate and she was separated from her husband. Two migrants were mothers. They had puppets mimicking little children.

### *3.4 »Migrants RI 2017« Location*

Six work points were established to perform the exercise that was determined to be held on the port side of the harbor, which is called the Sušak breakwater. The location of the exercise included: 1. location – acceptance center, 2. location – catamaran, 3. location – contaminated sea, 4. location – crane, 5. location – injured at sea and 6. location – the HCD PGC.

At the first point of work – the acceptance center, the most operational forces were engaged. The RCS PGC was in charge of securing and setting up the necessary infrastructure (tents), while the members of the PD PGC at work point 2, the catamaran, did the examination of the migrants and their belongings, and were engaged in their rescue. The members of the police department were doing the identification at the reception center point. The DEM PGC carried out a triage of injured persons on board. Triage was also carried out in the reception center. At the same place, the transfer of the injured to the hospital was organized. For the emergency team it was necessary to prepare a large tent provided by the Red Cross Society and set up by the CD PGC. Tasks of the TIPH PGC, which participated in the action, were to conduct an epidemiological survey of migrants with the aim of detecting signs of possible acute infections or signs of contagious diseases. In the cases of acute infections, the exercise participants from the teaching institute had a task to determine an isolation of patients accompanied by the representatives of the PD PGC. Since the scenario of exercise anticipated marine pollution as the result of a ship's explosion, one of the tasks of the team coming from the TIPH PGC was to approach sampling of the contaminated sea. That was possible after setting up a dam and cleaning the pollution that was carried out by the Dezinsekcija Ltd.

At the first operating point, the Red Cross Society had the task to organize tracing service and provide accommodation for the members of separated families. According to the elaboration, in charge of the securing of the reception center from the entrance of the unauthorized persons as well as controlling of the exit were the PD PGC and the Harbormaster's office of Rijeka in cooperation with the Port of Rijeka captain.

At the point 6, a location of the HDC PGC, was intended to be the center for the coordination of operational forces on the field.

### *3.5 Structure and Number of Exercise Participants*

In the exercise, 13 operational forces were involved and 218 participants, 17 vehicles and 7 vessels were provided. The following human resources and technical equipment of the operational forces were included in the exercise: staff members CD PGC (12 members), RCS PGC (80 persons, 3 vehicles, 2 boats, 2 tents, rescue equipment, 3 sets of tables and benches and 2 booths), PD PGC (20 persons, 3 vehicles, 1 vessel), public fire troops (20 persons, 4 vehicles, 1 boat), DEM PGC (12 persons, 4 vehicles), TIPH PGC (4 persons, 1 vehicle, protective suits and masks), CMRS-RI (5 persons, 1 vehicle, height-saving technical equipment), specialized unit CD PGC for rescue from ruins (20 members) and specialist unit CD PGC for logistics (20 members), COC and Harbor captain Rijeka (8 persons, 1 vehicle), harbor administration (6 persons), Dezinsekcija Ltd. (6 persons, 2 yachts), Jadrolinija – liner shipping company (catamaran), and the National protection and rescue directorate – regional office for protection and rescue Rijeka (5 persons).

The largest number of participants in the exercise was hired by the Red Cross Society. The medical team, which was scheduled for implementation of the triage, involved 12 persons, while an epidemiological survey and other tasks assigned to the TIPH PGC were scheduled to 4 persons.

### *3.6 Schedule*

According to the elaboration, the implementation part of the exercise should have lasted 4 hours. It was scheduled to begin on September 9, 2017, at 9.00 am, by the report of the ship captain and his discovery while entering the port, of an undocumented number of migrants on board and finish the same day at 14.00. The operating part of the exercise was to start an hour after captain's discovery of migrants.

As for the media and invited guests, it was foreseen that they attend the exercise one hour after the beginning of the operational part of the exercise. As a protocol part of the exercise, reception of guest speakers and journalists was planned. The general public had been informed about the exercise via the media one week before the exercise.

## 4. Results and Evaluation

The exercise evaluation was conducted 15 days after the exercise had been held. At the joint meeting, the exercise »Migrants RI 2017« was evaluated by the members who participated in the organization of the exercise and/or in its realization. At the end of 2017, the conclusions of the joint evaluation were accepted by the Headquarters of the Primorje-Gorski Kotar County Civil Defense.[21]

The improvements achieved in relation to the previous joint operational exercises included among other things: an improvement in preparation (organization) and exercise implementation; more effective use of means of communication; better coordination of all operational forces; professionally (in accordance with defined procedures)

[21] Headquarters of the Primorje-Gorski Kotar County Civil Defence: Meeting report 11/20/2017 (internal document) 2017.

all prescribed activities were executed. The markers, who tried to imitate migrants more realistically, were in particular praised.

At the meeting of operational forces, proposals that could be used to improve future exercises were also presented. Among other things, they implied: raising the level of communication/joint operational action of emergency services (police, fire brigades, emergency assistance) in terms of harmonizing the treatment of major accidents; the participants of the exercise should not be familiar with exercise scenario before its beginning; striving to keep the scenario as realistically as possible following the course (time plan) of the exercise.

### *4.1 Results and Evaluation at the Red Cross Society*

On the web pages of the Primorje-Gorski Kotar County Red Cross Society in the report of the activities carried out in 2017, the implementation of the »Migrants RI 2017« exercise is mentioned. The exercise was attended by 63 representatives of the Primorje-Gorski Kotar County Red Cross Society: one member in headquarters (Vesna Čavar, the director), 15 members of the intervention team and 47 volunteers in a realistic presentation of injuries and the role of migrants. The Primorje-Gorski Kotar County Red Cross Society, besides being an initiator and a member of the Primorje-Gorski Kotar County exercise organizer, had several tasks in the exercise. Some of them were: the provision of equipment and preparation of the reception center (large and small tents for the needs of operational forces participating in the exercise); participation of the members of the water rescue team in difficult conditions; provide first aid, provide psychosocial support and the tracing service; the realistic presentation of injuries; provide markers who were willing to act as migrants.[22]

The Primorje-Gorski Kotar County Red Cross Society evaluated the operational force cooperation positive. However, there were also some omissions. According to the observations of the markers, the following omissions were noticed: upon arriving of the ship, regarding the atmosphere on board and the behavior of the actors, some of the rescuers were not immediately aware of the injured; some mar-

---

[22] Primorje-Gorski Kotar County Red Cross Society: Report for the activities carried out in 2017. http://www.dck-pgz.hr/wp-content/uploads/2016/06/Izvje%C5%A1%C4%87e-o-radu-DCK-PG%C5%BD-u-2017.pdf (accessed 9/24/2019).

kers believed that there had been too much unnecessary physical contact; the baggage was not checked at checkpoint; some markers were not registered or even inspected.

During an interview, the director of the County Red Cross Society pointed out that the role of migrants had caused a strong emotional reaction in some volunteers.[23]

## 5 »Migrants RI 2017« Exercise and Its Impact in Media

According to the protocol, the Primorje-Gorski Kotar County has informed the general public about the performance of the exercise. The exercise has had a great publicity. The national and local media included reports about it via the mass media and the electronic media.[24] News caused numerous comments on social networks. As the director of the Red Cross added in an interview, all the operational forces, which had participated in the exercise, were unpleasantly surprised by the number of negative reactions. On social networks, there were negative comments about the exercise itself and migrants in general. For example, one of the comments was that migrants were indeed coming, because otherwise the operational forces would not have been preparing themselves for their arrival, they just did not want to say it.[25] According to the Director of the Primorje-Gorski Kotar

[23] Čavar, personal communication (Note 12).

[24] Hina: U Rijeci održana vježba sustava civilne zaštite »Migranti RI 2017« [In Rijeka held the civil defence system exercise – »Migrants RI 2017«]. https://www.index.hr/vijesti/clanak/u-rijeci-odrzana-vjezba-sustava-civilne-zastite-migranti-ri-2017/993434.aspx (accessed 9/24/2019); Croatian Radio-television: Vježbe operativnih snaga »Migranti RI 2017« [Exercises of operational forces »Migrants RI 2017«]. https://vijesti.hrt.hr/404393/vjezbe-operativnih-snaga-migranti-ri-2017 (accessed 9/24/2019).

[25] Rijecan. In: RIJEKA SE PRIPREMA ZA DOLAZAK MIGRANATA! U subotu u riječkoj luci vježba civilne zaštite PGŽ – »Migranti RI 2017« [Rijeka is preparing for migrants arrival! On Saturday, the PGKC civil defence exercise in the port of Rijeka – »Migrants RI 2017«]. http://rijecanin.rtl.hr/rijeka-se-priprema-za-dolazak-migranata-u-subotu-u-rijeckoj-luci-vjezba-civilne-zastite-pgz-migranti-ri-2017/ (accessed 9/24/2019); Marinko Kleva: Spašavanje migranata u riječkoj luci vježba snaga civilne zaštite zabrinula Riječane [Rescue of migrants in the Port of Rijeka. The PGKC civil defence exercise worried residents of Rijeka]. In: Novi list (9/9/2017). http://www.novilist.hr/Vijesti/Rijeka/SPASAVANJE-MIGRANATA-U-RIJECKOJ-LUCI-Vjezba-snaga-civilne-zastite-zabrinula-Rijecane (accessed 9/24/2019).

County Red Cross Society, this had been a completely different reaction from the situation in autumn and winter of 2015.[26]

## 6. Conclusion

The migrant wave, which Croatia faced on the East of the country, ended in spring 2016 and hired the national force operating system. Certainly, the timeliness of such humanitarian crises with an experience of active participation in assisting migrants motivated the organizing of the demonstration exercise in the area that was not directly affected by migrant wave. Choosing a geographical location that was not directly on the main migrant route in Croatia could be at the same time a challenge in planning and carrying out such an exercise. The operational forces involved in the »Migrants RI 2017« exercise held in Rijeka showed a high degree of preparedness for such crisis situations. In the cases of real facing such a humanitarian crisis, this presented example of the exercise points to the importance and necessity of good coordination of the involved operational forces. Because of the negative impact of the exercise on the social network, for future reflection remains only an incentive to make an effort to raise awareness of migration-related issues within the local community.

## Acknowledgements

I would like to take this opportunity to thank the informants, Mrs. Vesna Čavar, MD, the Director of the Primorje-Gorski Kotar County Red Cross Society and her collaborator Mrs. Branka Marečić for their affability to participate in an interview and for providing the documentation related to the »Migrants RI 2017« exercise.

---

[26] Čavar, personal communication (Note 12).

*Prerna Thaker and Ravi Rao*

# Challenges faced by refugees to access health care in Germany

Abstract
The number of refugees seeking protection in Germany has increased significantly since 2015. This has created an additional burden on the health care system of Germany. Migrant populations have different health care needs from the host population; however, they face barriers using health services. A systematic review was conducted in order to evaluate such barriers in Germany. The database search yielded 4.223 records. A final of 8 articles were included in the narrative synthesis. Our findings show that access to health care in the study population of the included articles widely followed the principles of horizontal equity in health care as far as educational attainment is concerned, but showed a social gradient with respect to subjective social status. Barriers faced by asylum seekers towards comprehensive primary care (e.g., language discordance with GPs) might also be exacerbated by policy restrictions, which create obstacles to access unless conditions are acute, painful or emergencies.

## 1. Introduction

The number of refugees seeking protection in Germany from war, persecution and natural disasters has increased significantly since 2015. This has created an additional burden on the health care system of Germany. Like most other EU countries, Germany too lacks the data for a clear picture of asylum seekers' and refugees' health and healthcare needs.[1] Refugees and asylum-seekers are granted access to medical care services by international humanitarian law and, in the case of Germany, also by European Union directives and the German

[1] Laura Frank, Rahsan Yesil-Jürgens, Oliver Razum, Kayvan Bozorgmehr, Liane Schenk, Andreas Gilsdorf, Alexander Rommel, Thomas Lampert: Health and healthcare provision to asylum seekers and refugees in Germany. In: Journal of Health Monitoring 2 (2017), pp. 22–42.

Constitution. However, as migrants come from many countries belonging to various cultures, they face different problem regarding health care access. Migrant populations may have different health care needs, preferences and expectations or face barriers in use of health services. The aim of this systematic review is to review the challenges faced by migrants in Germany. The challenges will be classified by the socio-economic model (SEM).

The SEM follows the assumption that individual decisions and behaviors are determined by reciprocal interactions within and between the social and physical environment of individuals and are interdependent in nature. At the same time, individuals also contribute to their social ecology in terms of constructing norms, beliefs and culture across multiple macro-systems.[2] Consequently, micro systems feed into macro systems and vice-versa.

This model recognizes the importance of social environmental and biological factors that may foster or inhibit individual attitudes and behaviors.[3] Since the 1980s, SEM has been applied to understand health behaviors. Barriers to health services utilization have been conceptualized in McLeroy et al.[4] adaption of the SEM. This acts as a framework to explore the determinants of health behavior in the dynamic interplay between individuals and their environment.[5]

[2] Dawn Henderson, Tiffany Baffour: Applying a Socio-Ecological Framework to Thematic Analysis Using a Statewide Assessment of Disproportionate Minority Contact in the United States. In: The Qualitative Report 20 (2005), pp. 1960–1973.

[3] Jun Sung Hong, Gabriel J. Merrin, Shantel Crosby, Debra M. Hernandez Jozefowicz, Jeoung Min Lee, Paula Allen-Meares: Individual and Contextual Factors Associated with Immigrant Youth Feeling Unsafe in School: A Social-Ecological Analysis. In: Journal of Immigrant and Minority Health 18 (2016), pp. 996–1006.

[4] Kenneth McLeroy, Daniel Bibeau, Allan Steckleret, Karen Glanz: An Ecology Perspective on Health Promotion Programs. In: Health Education Quarterly 15 (1988), pp. 351–377.

[5] Wendy Sword: A socio-ecological approach to understanding barriers to prenatal care for women of low income. In: Journal of Advanced Nursing 29 (1999), pp. 1170–1177.

## 2. Levels of the SEM

### *2.1 Intrapersonal Level*

The intrapersonal level consists of the individual-level factors that determine and affect health services utilization behavior. These include demographic factors (for example, socio- economic standing, gender, and age), personal history, and personal beliefs and knowledge about healthcare utilization. Specific factors, which have been identified in the literature on refugee populations include stressors, such as history of organized deliberate violence and oppression,[6] post migration stressors such as acculturation stressors[7] and a lack of knowledge about available health care services.[8]

---

[6] Patricia J. Shannon, Elisabeth Wieling, Jennifer Simmelink-McCleary, Emily Becher: Beyond stigma: Barriers to discussing mental health in refugee populations. In: Journal of Loss and Trauma 20 (2015), pp. 281–296; Ghayda Hassan, Peter Ventevogel, Hussam Jefee-Bahloul, Laurence J. Kirmayer: Mental health and psychosocial wellbeing of Syrians affected by armed conflict. In: Epidemiology and Psychiatric Sciences 25 (2016), pp. 129–141.

[7] Ramin Asgary, Nora Segar: Barriers to Health Care Access among Refugee Asylum Seekers. In: Journal of Health Care for the Poor and Underserved 22 (2011), pp. 506–522; Ida Kaplan, Hardy Stow, Josef Szwarc: Responding to the Challenges of Providing Mental Health Services to Refugees: An Australian Case Report. In: Journal of Health Care for the Poor and Underserved 27 (2016), pp. 1159–1170; Sara Shishehgar, Leila Gholizadeh, Michelle DiGiacomo, Anna Green, Patricia M. Davidson: Health and Socio-Cultural Experiences of Refugee Women: An Integrative Review. In: Journal of Immigrant and Minority Health 19 (2017), pp. 959–973.

[8] Asgary, Segar: Barriers to Health Care Access (Note 7); Kaplan, Stow, Szwarc: Responding to the Challenges (Note 7); Shishehgar et al.: Health and Socio-Cultural Experiences (Note 7); Miriam Posselt, Karalyn McDonald, Nicholas Procter, Charlotte de Crespigny, Cherrie Galletly: Improving the provision of services to young people from refugee backgrounds with comorbid mental health and substance use problems: addressing the barriers. In: BMC Public Health 17 (2017), p. 280; Bukola Salami, Jordana Salma, Kathleen Hegadoren: Access and utilization of mental health services for immigrants and refugees: Perspectives of immigrant service providers. In: International Journal of Mental Health Nursing 28 (2019), pp. 152–161; Marit Sijbrandij, Ceren Acarturk, Martha Bird, Richard A. Bryant, Sebastian Burchert, Kenneth Carswell, Joop de Jong, Cecilie Dinesen, Katie S. Dawson, Rabih El Chammay, Linde van Ittersum, Mark Jordans, Christine Knaevelsrud, David McDaid, Kenneth Miller, Naser Morina, A-La Park, Bayard Roberts, Yvette van Son, Egbert Sondorp, Monique C. Pfaltz, Leontien Ruttenberg, Matthis Schick, Ulrich Schnyder, Mark van Ommeren, Peter Ventevogel, Inka Weissbecker, Erica Weitz, Nana Wiedemann, Claire Whitney, Pim Cuijpers: Strengthening mental health care systems for Syrian refugees in Europe and the Middle East: integrating scalable psychological interventions in eight

## 2.2 *Interpersonal Level*

On the interpersonal level, health care encounters in McLeroy's et al. model is seen as being influenced by groups, such as social networks and social supports. These social networks and supports are provided by family, friends, neighbors, acquaintances and co-workers.[9]

Furthermore, the relationship between the physician and the service user inherently affects health care encounters.[10] Specific interpersonal barriers in health care encounters include language barriers between migrants and healthcare providers.[11] Other interpersonal determinants, which may affect the relationship between the healthcare provider and the service user include agency characteristics, skills, knowledge and attitudes and philosophy of health service providers, and financial resources.[12] This was identified to be particularly the case with barriers connected to intercultural communication between migrants and native health care professionals.[13]

---

countries. In: European Journal of Psychotraumatology 8 (2017), doi: 10.1080/20008198.2017.1388102.

[9] McLeroy et al.: An Ecology Perspective (Note 4).

[10] Sword: A socio-ecological approach (Note 5).

[11] Asgary, Segar: Barriers to Health Care Access (Note 7); Tam Truong Donnelly, Jihye J. Hwang, Dave Este, Carol Ewashen, Carol Adair, Michael Clinton: If I was going to kill myself, I wouldn't be calling you. I am asking for help: Challenges influencing immigrant and refugee women's mental health. In: Issues in Mental Health Nursing 32 (2011), pp. 279–290; Hassan et al.: Mental health and psychosocial wellbeing (Note 6); Natasja Jensen, Marie Norredam, Stefan Priebe, Allan Krasnik: How do general practitioners experience providing care to refugees with mental health problems? A qualitative study from Denmark. In: BMC Family Practice 14 (2013), p. 17; Kaplan, Stow, Szwarc: Responding to the Challenges (Note 7); Joyce M. O'Mahony, Tam Donnelly: Health care providers' perspectives of the gender influences on migrant women's mental health care experiences. In: Issues in Mental Health Nursing 28 (2007), pp. 1171–1188; Posselt et al.: Improving the provision of services (Note 8); Salami, Salma, Hegadoren: Access and utilization of mental health services (Note 8); Meryam Schouler-Ocak: Providing care for migrants and refugees. In: European Psychiatry 41 (2017), doi: 10.1016/j.eurpsy.2017.01.165; Helena D. Dow: Migrants' Mental Health Perceptions and Barriers to Receiving Mental Health Services. In: Home Health Care Management & Practice 23 (2011), pp. 176–185; McLeroy et al.: An Ecology Perspective on Health (Note 9).

[12] Sword: A socio-ecological approach (Note 5).

[13] Asgary, Segar: Barriers to Health Care Access (Note 7); McLeroy et al.: An Ecology Perspective on Health (Note 9); Kaplan, Stow, Szwarc: Responding to the challenges (Note 7); Schouler-Ocak: Providing care for migrants (Note 11).

### 2.3 *Organizational Level*

The organizational level in McLeroy et al.'s model focuses away from inter- and intrapersonal factors and looks more towards environmental determinants of behavior and how organizational characteristics inform health care encounters.[14]

### 2.4 *Community Level*

In McLeroy et al.'s, SEM community is defined as face-to-face primary groups to which individuals belong or relationships within a defined geographical or political area, which implies that community is characterized by certain power structures within these areas.[15] In the context of health care encounters, the most predominant community level factor shaping access is the stigmatization of illness amongst refugee populations.[16]

### 2.5 *Policy Level*

On the policy level of McLeroy et al.'s model is the use of regulatory policies, procedures and laws to protect the health care of the community. Such policies and procedures also regulate mental health care access for refugees and may promote or prohibit access through eligibility criteria and entitlements according to national law and provisions. It has been identified in various pieces of literature, that healthcare entitlements may be one of the most prominent barriers for refugees.[17]

---

[14] McLeroy et al.: An Ecology Perspective on Health (Note 9).

[15] McLeroy et al.: An Ecology Perspective on Health (Note 9).

[16] Asgary, Segar: Barriers to Health Care Access (Note 7); McLeroy et al.: An Ecology Perspective on Health (Note 9); Hassan et al.: Mental health and psychosocial wellbeing (Note 11); Posselt et al.: Improving the provision of services (Note 8).

[17] Asgary, Segar: Barriers to Health Care Access (Note 7); Dow: Migrants' Mental Health Perceptions (Note 11); Schouler-Ocak: Providing care for migrants (Note 11); Yvonne Wohler, Jaya Dantas: Barriers Accessing Mental Health Services Among Culturally and Linguistically Diverse (CALD) Immigrant Women in Australia: Policy Implications. In: Journal of Immigrant and Minority Health 19 (2017), pp. 697–701.

## 3. Methodology

A systematic review of the literature was undertaken to identify publications that examine the challenges faced by migrants. For this systematic review, we searched the PubMed, EMBASE & EBSCO databases in Citavi 6 in January 2019 for peer-reviewed studies published between January 2000 and January 2019 and written in English. Search strings included the main search keywords were combined with the Boolean operators AND and OR to expand and narrow search terms in order to include different versions of the word and search strings.

### *2.1 Search Strategy*

This systematic review applies methodological standards established by Cochrane and PRISMA. The screening and selection phases of the systematic review were carried out jointly for the objective.

### *2.2 Review Questions*

The following objectives, questions, populations and settings were defined for the systematic review on the challenges faced by migrants accessing health care in Germany

**Challenges faced by migrants accessing health care**

| | |
|---|---|
| P | Temporary labor migrants<br>Highly skilled and business migrants<br>Irregular migrants<br>Refugees<br>Asylum seekers<br>Forced migrants |
| C | Comparison between the different migrant groups |
| O | Qualitative Outcome –<br>Challenges faced by migrants |

Tab. 1: PICO – evidence based search strategy (Patient/Population, Intervention, Comparison and Outcome) for challenges faced by migrants accessing health care

### 2.3 *Search Strings*

In order to find relevant articles for the specific objectives in PubMed, EMBASE, EBSCO search strings were developed for each of the following concepts Migrants, challenges and health care. In PubMed, EBSCO and EMBASE search string #1 was combined using ›AND‹ with each of the specific search strings (i.e. #1 AND (#2)). For Cochrane Library one generic search using the terms for migrants was used to search for all relevant systematic reviews.

### 2.4 *Search limits*

The search limit that was applied for this systematic review is a time limit: literature was searched in PubMed, EMBASE and EBSCO from 2000 onwards for all the three specific objectives. In Cochrane Library, systematic reviews were searched for all three specific objectives. Language was limited to English. However, geographical limits were not applied in the search phase.

### 2.5 *Running the literature search*

The final searches in PubMed, EMBASE, EBSCO and Cochrane Library were run. Due to overlap between the two specific objectives, the search strings were combined in a single search. The relevant full text publications were subdivided into these two specific objectives during the screening of full article phase. PubMed, EMBASE, EBSCO and Cochrane Library output, including all indexed fields per hit (e.g. title, abstract), were exported to Citavi and saved in separate folders per database. Duplicate articles were removed through automatic and manual duplicate removal.

Peer reviewed literature selection

From the articles retrieved from PubMed, EMBASE, EBSCO and Cochrane Library the relevant references will be selected by a two-phase selection procedure, based on:

- Screening of title and abstract (first selection phase): in this phase, titles of publications were screened based on the inclusion and exclusion criteria. If the title was inconclusive, the abstract was read. Articles with titles and abstracts that suggest that they did not contain information relevant to the review objectives were not selected for full text assessment (no reason for exclusion documented per article). In case of doubt, the article was checked using full-text in the second selection step. Articles that were excluded during screening of title and abstract were stored in an indexed folder in Citavi 6.

- Screening of full article (second selection phase): the articles selected during the first phase were assessed in full text. PDF-files of the original articles were downloaded and stored. Articles were included if the reported information was relevant and of sufficient quality.

| | **Inclusion** | **Exclusion** |
|---|---|---|
| Study Design/ Type | • Randomized controlled trials (RCTs) Prospective observational studies (e. g. cohort studies)<br>• Retrospective observational studies (e. g. case-control studies)<br>• Cross-sectional studies | Meta-analysis or systematic review<br>• Narrative review<br>• Case reports<br>• Non-pertinent publication types (e. g. expert opinions, letters to the Editor, editorials, comments, |
| | | conference abstract/poster, news, consensus document, chapter)<br>• Animal studies<br>• Genetic studies, biochemistry or molecular studies<br>• Outbreak studies (except<br>• when data on contact tracing for challenges were reported) |
| Study Quality | Study Duration (2000–2019) | Insufficient methodological quality (both inherent methodology as well as insufficient description of inherent methodology provided; based on quality checklists) |

| | **Inclusion** | **Exclusion** |
|---|---|---|
| Study Population | Temporary Labor Migrants<br>Highly skilled and business migrants<br>Irregular migrants<br>Refugees<br>Asylum seekers<br>Forced migrants | Homeless population Prisoners<br>Other types of vulnerable population |
| Study Population | Temporary Labor Migrants<br>Highly skilled and business migrants<br>Irregular migrants<br>Refugees<br>Asylum seekers<br>Forced migrants | Homeless population Prisoners<br>Other types of vulnerable population |
| Geographical Areas | Germany | |
| Study Comparison | Comparison between the subgroups of migrant population | Study Comparison |
| Outcomes | Qualitative Outcomes | Outcomes |

Tab. 2: Inclusion and Exclusion criteria for peer-reviewed literature

## 2.6 *Types of studies*

Studies to be included in this systematic review are cohort studies, case-control studies, cross-sectional studies, randomized controlled trials and quasi-randomized trials. Systematic reviews will be used to consult their references.

## 2.7 *Types of participants*

The study population in this systematic review will include all groups of migrants, refugees and asylum seekers. According to UNESCO a migrant is one »as covering all cases where the decision to migrate is taken freely by the individual concerned, for reasons of ›personal convenience‹ and without intervention of an external compelling factor.«[18] The various categories of migrants, which are included in this systematic review, are:

1) temporary labor migrants: Men and women who migrate for a limited period.[19]
2) highly skilled and business migrants: People with qualification seeking employment in country different from their country of origin.
3) irregular migrants: People who try to enter a country without proper documentations and permits.[20]
4) refugees: According to the 1951 United Nations Convention relating to the Status Of Refugees, a refugee is a person residing outside his or her country of nationality who is unable or unwilling to return because of a well-founded fear of prosecution on account of race, religion, nationality, membership in a particular social group of political opinion.[21]
5) asylum seekers: People who move across borders in search of protection but who may not fulfill the strict criteria laid down by the 1951 convention.[22]
6) forced migration: this includes refugees and asylum seekers but also people forced to move by environmental catastrophes or developmental projects.[23]

Review team members Prerna Thaker and Ravi Rao alternated review duties for each paper. Both reviewers independently screened titles and abstracts, retrieved full texts of potentially relevant articles and assessed article eligibility for inclusion and exclusion criteria, while discrepancies were resolved by discussion.

To identify the challenges towards health care access for migrants in Germany, the socio- ecological model (SEM) was used as an organizing framework to situate the barriers on the various SEM layers

---

[18] Commission on Human Rights: Report on the fifty-fourth session. https://www.ohchr.org/EN/HRBodies/CHR/54/Documents/E.1998.23_EN.pdf (accessed 9/24/2019).
[19] Stephen Castles: International Migration at the Beginning of the Twenty-First Century: Global Trends and Issues. In: International Social Science Journal 52(2005), pp. 269–281.
[20] Castles: International Migration at the Beginning (Note 19).
[21] Castles: International Migration at the Beginning (Note 19).
[22] Castles: International Migration at the Beginning (Note 19).
[23] Castles: International Migration at the Beginning (Note 19).

spanning from individual to policy level. In this study, McLeroy et al.'s adaptation of the SEM was used, which is geared specifically towards explaining how different individual and environmental factors determine health seeking behavior in individuals.

### *2.8 Statistical Analysis*

Review team members extracted the data and assessed risk of bias of included papers. Extracted data included data regarding names of author, date of publication, journal name, state in which the study was conducted, type of study, study duration and major themes of challenges, which have been reported in the study.

Narrative approach syntheses of all the studies, which have been included, was conducted. Sensitivity analyses were done to test the robustness of overall findings by excluding studies with high risk of bias and to explore heterogeneity of challenges by excluding specific migrant population.

## 3. Results

The database search yielded 4223 records. After removal of 5 duplicates, 4118 record were included and scanned by reading abstracts. 4110 records were excluded by duration, language or study design, location or population. A final of 8 articles were included in the narrative synthesis. All included studies were done in Germany and examined, at least in part, the challenges faced by migrants to access health care. Detailed information is provided in the PRISMA flow diagram in Fig. 1. Information extracted from the selected studies includes: first author and publication date, net sample size, area, year of data collection, classification of migrant population analyzed, state in which the study was conducted, study design, study period, sample size, theme under which the challenges can classified under the SEM model and the challenges reported (Table 1).

The themes under which the challenges identified are as under-Intrapersonal Barrier-Subjective Social Status, Health status, Female sex- Socio economic status is traditionally composed of education, income and profession. Bozorgmehr et al. have reported that utilization of health services was significantly and positively associated with increased need for health services adjusted for SES variables, language and place.[24]

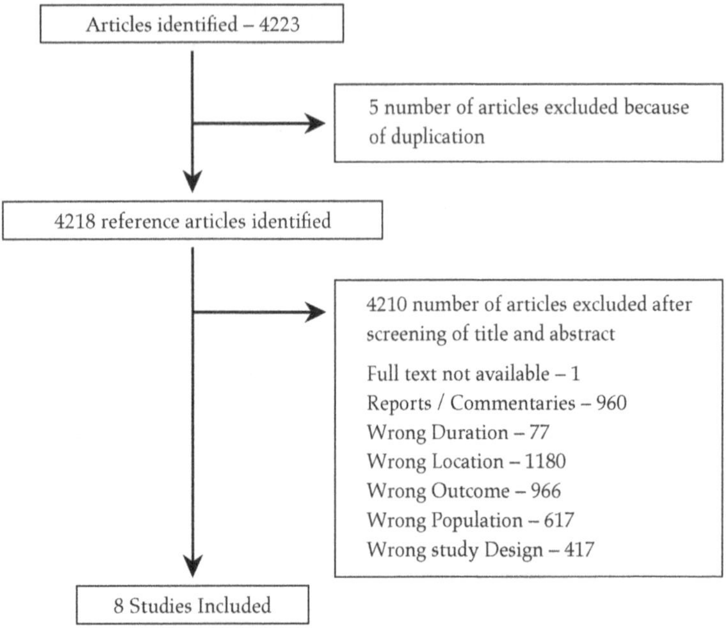


Fig. 1: PRISMA flow diagram

Bozorgmehr et al. performed a secondary exploratory analysis on cross-sectional data obtained from a population-based questionnaire survey among all asylum-seekers registered in three districts in Germany. They have reported that utilization of health services was significantly and positively associated with increased need for health services adjusted for SES variables, language and place. However, health care access was not significantly associated with subjective social status after controlling for age, sex, language and general health status.[24] Place of residence, which indicates that access to health care, measured by utilization of hospital and specialist services met the principles of vertical equity.

[24] Kavyan Bozorgmehr, Christine Schneider, Stefaine Joos: Equity in access to health care among asylum seekers in Germany: evidence from an exploratory population-based cross-sectional study. In: BMC Health Services Research 15 (2015), pp. 1–12.

Age: Bozorgmehr et al. and Fakoya et al. have reported an increase odds ratio with increase in age of migrants, however the results are not statically significant. Bozorgmehr et al. found that the unadjusted simple regression estimates obtained from bivariate models showed statistically significant positive associations between age, a negative health status and utilization of any type of physician. Fakoya et al. conducted a web-based survey (available in multiple languages) to all people living outside their country of birth in the World Health Organization (WHO) European area. They found that age was not significantly associated with health care access ($p = 0.79$).[25]

Altered Identity and double home experience: A novel theme was reported by Paal et al about altered identity having an effect on health care access. This was reported mainly due to the feeling of been alienated in Germany. Many reasons were attributed to this like language, culture etc.

### *Interpersonal Barriers*

Language: Many studies suggested that language is one of the most pronounced barriers for asylum seekers.[26] In Germany, language is a

---

[25] Bozorgmehr, Schneider, Joos: Equity in access to health care (Note 24); Ibidun Fakoya, Debora Álvarez-del Arco, Andrew Copas, Bryan Teixeira, Koen Block, Anne-Francoise Gennotte, Alain Volny-Anne, Janneke P. Bil, Giota Touloumi, Julia del Amo, Fiona M. Burns: Factors Associated With Access to HIV Testing and Primary Care Among Migrants Living in Europe: Cross-Sectional Survey. In: JMIR Public Health and Surveillance 3 (2017), doi: 10.2196/publichealth.7741.

[26] Kevin Claassen, Pia Jäger: Impact of the Introduction of the Electronic Health Insurance Card on the Use of Medical Services by Asylum Seekers in Germany. In: International Journal of Environmental Research and Public Health 15 (2018), doi: 10.3390/ijerph15050856; Arnd Giese, Muebrra Uyar, Halil Uslucan, Stefan Becker, Bernhard F. Henning: How do hospitalised patients with Turkish migration background estimate their language skills and their comprehension of medical information – a prospective cross-sectional study and comparison to native patients in Germany to assess the language barrier and the need for translation. In: BMC Health Services Research 13 (2013), pp. 1–9; Daniel Huhn, Florian Junne, Stephan Zipfel, Roman Duelli, Franz Resch, Wolfgang Herzog, Christoph Nikendei: International medical students – a survey of perceived challenges and established support services at medical faculties. In: GMS Zeitschrift für Medizinische Ausbildung 32 (2015), doi:10.3205/zma000951; Piret Paal, Johannes Bükki: »If I had stayed back home, I would not be alive any more …« – Exploring end-of-life preferences in patients with migration background. In: PLOS ONE 12 (2017), doi: 10.1371/journal.pone.0175314.

particular barrier as health care professionals often do not speak other languages or do not feel confident enough to provide therapeutic services in a foreign language and refugees often times may only speak English, if they speak any foreign language at all. The language barrier is therefore directly connected to whether interpreters are arranged for by health care providers and much influenced in state provided services by interpreter entitlements depending on the migration status, as detailed in barriers to health care access on the policy level. Classen et al. surveyed 260 asylum seekers in the three municipalities Bochum, Datteln and Herne in North Rhine Westphalia, Germany. These were chosen because Bochum is one of the municipalities, which have introduced the EHIC for asylum seekers as soon as possible.

They found that language was not significantly associated with consultation of a physician ($p = 0.50$). Giese et al. have conducted a cross sectional study on Turkish patients and found that although the majority of patients with Turkish migration background have spent most of their lives in Germany a large part of this population has limited German language skills and difficulties obtaining information related to treatment when hospitalized. Huhn et al. carried out telephone interviews with deans of medical faculties. They have stated that the most frequently reported problem by far is the perceived lack of language skills of foreign students. Un-known physicians and fear of the doctor: Schbeider et al. obtained cross-sectional data on the resident population taken from the German Health Interview and the European Union Statistics on Income and Living Conditions. It was stated that a major holdback for immigrants to access health care were unknown physicians.[27]

Patients Silence: In the qualitative study conducted by Dilger et al., it has been reported that patients were not confident whether what they wanted to convey was correct.[27]

---

[27] Hansjorg Dilger, Linn Leissner, Lenka Bosanska, Christina Lampe, Ursula Plöckinger: Illness Perception and Clinical Treatment Experiences in Patients with M. Maroteaux-Lamy (Mucopolysaccharidosis Type VI) and a Turkish Migration Background in Germany. In: PLoS ONE 8 (2013), doi: 10.1371/journal.pone.0066804; Christine Schneider, Stefanie Joos, Kayvan Bozorgmehr: Disparities in health and access to healthcare between asylum seekers and residents in Germany: a population-based cross-sectional feasibility study. In: BMJ Open 5 (2015), doi: doi:10.1136/bmjopen-2015-008784.

*Organizational Barriers*

Possession of EHIC (European health insurance card) / No health care vouchers: Within the group of asylum seekers studied by Claassen et al. who had used both the EHIC and healthcare-vouchers (n = 93), it was found that after receiving the EHIC, there was also a significant intra-individual increase of the consultation rate ($\Delta = 0.27$, $p < 0.01$).[28] It was also found that asylum seekers in Germany who were in possession of the EHIC visited their ambulant doctors significantly ($p = 0.00$) more often, as compared to the rest of the asylum seekers who had to ask the authorities for healthcare-vouchers. In the study done by Bozorgmehr et al., 16 % of their population reported inability to access health care because of lack health care vouchers.[29]

Waiting lists: In the study done by Bozorgmehr et al. they have shown that a majority of their sample population (32 %) could not access health care because of the long waiting periods.[30]

Financial Barriers: Indirect costs have shown an adverse effect on accessibility to health care.[31] Long distance, lack of time: Other organizational factors affecting access to health care by Bozorgmehr et al.[32]

*Policy Barriers*

Legal Restrictions: Bozorgmehr et al. have reported migrant-specific access barriers to comprehensive health care might be exacerbated by legal restrictions, which create obstacles to access unless conditions are acute, painful or emergencies.[33]

## 4. Discussion

The purpose of this study was to identify challenges to health care access for asylum seekers in Germany. Both the literature review

[28] Claassen, Jäger: Impact of the Introduction (Note 26).
[29] Bozorgmehr, Schneider, Joos: Equity in access to health care (Note 24).
[30] Bozorgmehr, Schneider, Joos: Equity in access to health care (Note 24).
[31] Bozorgmehr, Schneider, Joos: Equity in access to health care (Note 24).
[32] Bozorgmehr, Schneider, Joos: Equity in access to health care (Note 24).
[33] Bozorgmehr, Schneider, Joos: Equity in access to health care (Note 24).

| | Author | Study Design, Study Period | Sample Size and Population | Theme | Context |
|---|---|---|---|---|---|
| 1. | Bozorgmehr, Schneider, Joos | Cross Sectional study, 10/2014 and 2/2015 | 1017 Asylum-Seekers | Intrapersonal and Organizational barriers, Policy barriers | Subjective social status, higher age, legal restrictions |
| 2. | Claassen, Jäger | Cross Sectional study, 10/2016 and 10/2017 | 260 Asylum-Seekers | Organizational and Interpersonal barriers | Possession of the EHIC, Language |
| 3. | Dilger et al. | Ethnographic study, 5/2011 to 9/2011 | 10 Migrants | Inter-Personal barriers | Patient Silence |
| 4. | Fakoya et al. | Cross Sectional study | 3794 Migrants | Intrapersonal and Organizational barriers, Policy Barriers | Age, Poverty, Immigration status |
| 5. | Giese et al. | Prospective study, 7/2011 and 3/2012 | 121 Migrants | Interpersonal barriers | Language barrier |
| 6. | Huhn et al. | Cross Sectional study, 4/2013 to 10/2013 | International medical students | Interpersonal barrier | Language barrier |
| 7. | Paal, Bükki | Cross Sectional study, 2/2016 to 10/2016 | 37 Migrant | Intrapersonal and Interpersonal barriers | Altered identity and language use on practical and emotional levels, provision of narratives of ›double home‹ experience |
| 8. | Schneider, Joos, Bozorgmehr | Cross-sectional feasibility study, 10/2014 and 2/2015 | 1017 Asylum Seekers | Intrapersonal and Interpersonal barriers, Organizational barriers, Policy barriers | Financial barrier, waiting for improvement of symptoms, waiting lists, un-known physician, fear of doctors, no healthcare vouchers, long distance, lack of time, other reasons |

Tab. 3: Summary of findings

and thematic analysis used the socio-ecological model to demonstrate the complex nature of health care access. In our study, we found that 6 out of 16 German states were under-review in the included articles. Our findings show that access to health care in the study population of the included articles widely followed the principles of horizontal equity in health care as far as educational attainment is concerned, but showed a social gradient with respect to subjective social status. Barriers faced by asylum seekers towards comprehensive primary care (e. g., language discordance with GPs) might also be exacerbated by policy restrictions, which create obstacles to access unless conditions are acute, painful or emergencies. Improving this equity in access to primary care could also help to reduce hospital admissions for those with higher needs.[34] It is also seen that asylum seekers in possession of the EHIC are significantly more likely to seek ambulant medical care than those receiving healthcare-vouchers. On the contrary, it can also be seen that demanding for healthcare-vouchers at the social security office could be a barrier for asylum seekers.[35] Barriers, such as foreign language and difficulties understanding the legal rights to accessing healthcare, presented a problem for 20 to 25 % of participants who experienced difficulties, although this finding is likely to have been underestimated in the study done by Fakoya et al. Language barriers lead to poor health literacy among patients and consequently impact the treatment of HIV as well as potentially facilitating onward transmission of the disease.[36] Language has been a recurrent interpersonal theme, which has come up in this review. Apart from the already mentioned studies, Giese et al. and Huhn et al. have also shown language as a major challenge for migrants in Germany.[37] However, it may be noted that Hunh et al. studied the students at a medical facility in Germany.[38] These students may vary from the asylum seekers, which have been studied by others, nevertheless language has been felt as a barrier to access health care by them too. Studies have also shown that fear of deportation has prevented individuals from seeking care.[39] In Germany, language is a

[34] Claassen, Jäger: Impact of the Introduction (Note 26).

[35] Claassen, Jäger: Impact of the Introduction (Note 26).

[36] Fakoya et al.: Factors Associated With Access (Note 25).

[37] Giese et al.: How do hospitalised patients with Turkish migration (Note 26); Huhn et al.: International medical students (Note 26).

[38] Huhn et al.: International medical students (Note 26).

[39] Fakoya et al.: Factors Associated With Access (Note 25).

particular barrier as health care professionals often do not speak other languages or do not feel confident enough to provide therapeutic services in a foreign language and refugees often times may only speak English, if they speak any foreign language at all. The language barrier is therefore directly connected to whether interpreters are arranged for by health care providers and much influenced in state provided services by interpreter entitlements depending on the migration status, as detailed in barriers to health care access on the policy level.[46] Studies have also shown that poverty or financial situation may influence access to health care, with a substantial proportion of all groups reporting missing clinic appointments due to travel expenses and delaying or foregoing medication due to cost of the drugs.[40] Paal et al. have hypothesized that asylum seekers are stuck between their German home (e.g. for medical reasons) and their home elsewhere. A simple question such as »Besides this country, is there another place where you feel at home?« may help in sensitively screening complex issues related to migrant, which require an adequate response by health care. This is required to understand culture-based presumptions, which need to be challenged in order to deliver high quality care to all patients regardless of their background.[41] The most frequent reasons for unmet health needs stated by Schneider et al. were financial barriers (66 %), the decision to wait for an improvement of symptoms (38 %) and long waiting lists (32 %). Unmet needs due to lack of a health voucher were reported in 16 %.[42]

## 5. Conclusion

This comprehensive review covers a plethora of factors involved in creating barriers for the migrant population accessing health care in Germany. To improve access a flexible response is required to meet health needs of newly arrived refugees, which are both feasible and necessary. Access to the German regular health care system must be increased. The development of a more mobile and pre-structured doc-

[40] Fakoya et al.: Factors Associated With Access (Note 25); Schneider, Joos, Bozorgmehr: Disparities in health (Note 27).
[41] Paal, Bükki: »If I had stayed back home …« (Note 26).
[42] Schneider, Joos, Bozorgmehr: Disparities in health (Note 27).

umentation system for the asylum seekers should be promoted. One possibility could be a digital documentation in the OPD supplemented by a uniform health book that stays with the patient. This would help to easily identify conditions by the providers. Instead of teaching the whole language to new asylum seekers, certain key words to describe their conditions can be made familiar to them so that they can better relate their illness. The legal circumstances of health care access and the cost-bearing responsibilities must be reconsidered. The medical workers can also be introduced to the field of migration health and review of intercultural understandings of health and illness.

*Tarek Mahjoub*

# What it takes to fit in: an opinion piece on the integration of adolescent refugee migrants in Germany

Abstract
Waves of migration have been a part of human history since the beginning of time, simply due to availability of basic survival resources. However recently, migration issues and so-called crises have found themselves at the center of economic and geopolitical concerns. These concerns do not hinder the waves of migration but do seem to have significant effects on the subsequent social implications that are brought along. In this opinion piece, I will be focusing on the different aspects concerning the integration of adolescent refugee migrants in Germany. Namely, I will be mentioning the magnitude of the issue, the concept of social well-being, and how the issue of integration is intermingled with the social, economic, and geopolitical state of the countries involved. I will also be giving an overview of my research on the topic along with literature findings. Finally, I will be mentioning recommendations and potential policies for involved stakeholders.

## 1. Introduction

With an unprecedented increase in refugee numbers, one must question the reason behind these numbers and the various implications that come with them. 65.6 million refugees were counted for by 2016, 51 % of which were minors under 18 years of age.[1] To provide these children and adolescents with their rights to education, they must be registered with local schools, but their journey does not end there. The children still have to face different obstacles in their daily lives, which determine and are determined by how well they adapt to the host culture. They will need to integrate along with the host society in order to fit in, which can be very challenging considering that

[1] UNHCR: Global Trends 2016. Forced Displacements in 2016. https://www.unhcr.org/globaltrends2016/ (accessed 9/24/2019).

there are underlying ethical, cultural, social, geo-political, and even economic factors that influence that process.

In order to provide the optimal environment with all the influencing factors put into consideration, a clear, well-described picture of the understanding of integration should be available for all. Furthermore, the benefits and obstacles should be clear to all stakeholders involved. Frequently, policymakers seem to use a top-down technique when determining what is and is not important to implement within a project to help in the process of integration. The perspective of the child or adolescent if often disregarded or included as an annex. There will not be a full understanding of integration and how to facilitate it if the perspective of the children or adolescent is not fully explored as a main pillar of the process. Attaining the personal experience and perspectives of the children or adolescents along with the understanding what the social systems can provide can allow policymakers to find optimal solutions that satisfy all stakeholders.

## 2. Integration

Integration in the context of migration and refugees is a continuous and multi-dimensional process. If facilitated, it provides social and economic benefits to the new communities to which the migrants are moving. Given, however, that a welcoming and enabling environment must be provided to the migrants and refugees in order to help them become functioning and productive members of a truly integrated new community.[2]

Social well-being is one of the three pillars of health, according to the World Health Organization's definition, besides mental and physical well-being.[3] Due to an innate sense of belonging in humans, integration is part of social well-being. Maintaining social health is connected with maintaining physiological and psychological well-being.[4] Hence, enabling social well-being through integration that

[2] UNHCR: Global Trends 2017. Forced Displacements in 2017. https://www.unhcr.org/globaltrends2017/ (accessed 9/24/2019).

[3] International Health Conference: Constitution of the World Health Organisation. UN, New York 1946.

[4] Jana Nikitin, Alexandra M. Freund: Feeling Loved and Integrated or Lonely and Rejected in Everyday Life: The Role of Age and Social Motivation. In: American Psychological Association 54 (2018), pp. 1186–1198.

might enable the creation of a more inclusive environment for all involved and have a positive economic impact by enabling the productivity and high functioning of all members of society, and reducing the ultimate burden on the GDP per capita spent on the health sector.

In the presence of immigrant and host communities, the process of integration becomes a responsibility of both, as it is not a one-sided affair. Building a societal bridge requires intensive work from both ends in order for them to meet in the middle. In this situation, communication, cooperation and compromise by both the host community and the immigrant community is key. This is why all parties involved should be heard, and their experiences and opinions documented, in order to abstract categories and themes to what seems to be a main issue and what all communities think should be the focus.

Resilience is another substantial factor to be considered in the overall equation of social integration. While a specific definition is still to be agreed upon; resilience is usually described as a dynamic positive development in response to different adverse and stressful situations. It is an up and coming topic that has been suggested by many researchers to be taken as a pivotal area when researching vulnerable populations, namely refugees and children or adolescents.[5] The integration of adolescent migrants and refugees will also depend on their resilience; therefore, more research should focus on influencing that characteristic of growth of the individual and the group.

The adolescent age is where the child starts learning about their physicality and their social position within their communities, so it is a crucial age, in which many personal traits are set. In addition, the adolescents of refugee and migrant families often go through stressful, if not traumatic experiences pre-arrival and post-arrival to their new place of residence. Pre-arrival factors are the ones, which cause the family to flee in search of a better life in a country or city that could be completely strange and foreign to their own, away from friends, and sometimes family, be it safety from wars, economic instability, or discrimination due to their identity. Post-arrival factors that determine how the adolescents find themselves within their new communities depend on their identifying individuality, their sur-

[5] Marieke Sleijpen, Niels van der Aa, Trudy Mooren, Cornelis J. Laban, Rolf J. Kleber: The Moderating Role of Individual Resilience in Refugee and Dutch Adolescents After Trauma. In: Psychological Trauma 11 (2019), pp. 732–742.

rounding environment being their direct family, friends, and teachers, and the system in which the individual and their proximal relationship interact together and within each other.

Therefore, these adolescents are especially vulnerable and require a high resilience to all they are subjected to. It would be in the best interest of all parties involved to learn about their experiences, opinions, and feelings in order to provide the optimum environment for them as they strive for social, mental and physical equality.

## 3. Statistics

To understand the magnitude of the problem, a wide look at the numbers should be taken; specifically, the number of refugees, who are registered in Germany, under 18 and registered in a school system. Moreover, the GDP of the country spent on refugees, and on education should be inspected, that way it can be estimated how much is being invested in the education of the adolescent refugees as it is the education system that provides the means of integration to them through integration and language courses, productive skill learning and vocational training, and higher education that can contribute into the country's economy in the future.

The UNHCR Global Trends 2017 report provided the total number of forcibly displaced people worldwide, which was 68.5 million people, of which 40 million (58.4 %) were considered internally displaced and 3.1 million (4.5 %) were considered asylum seekers with pending statuses. The remaining 25.4 million (37 %) are international refugees in different countries than their own. The UNHCR also estimates that out of the 25.4 million refugees, half are under 18 years of age. The report also showed that in the ranking of countries with the most refugees hosted, Germany takes the sixth rank. 970.400 people were being hosted as refugees; the majority of them originate from Syria, Iraq, Afghanistan, Eritrea, and the Islamic Republic of Iran, in descending order. It is important to know where the majority of the refugees come from if efficient and fair representation and support for the refugees is to be provided, considering that each country has its own set of languages, dialects, and cultural norms that should be taken into consideration during the process of integration. Moreover, it is worth mentioning that even though the number of refugees and asylum seekers seem to be large in Germany, one must consider the German population and the percentage that the refugees represent. In 2017, Germany's population was 82.79 million people, meaning that the refugees amounted to only 1.2 % of the whole population. The number of refugees under 18 years of age in Germany is estimated to be 485.200, considering the proportion of refugees under 18 years of age worldwide.[6]

As one of the signatories to the 1951 Convention Relating to the Status of Refugees and its 1967 protocol, Germany has done its part in respecting and abiding by the rights and responsibilities towards the asylum seekers and refugees that come into Germany.[7] Every country that hosts any number of refugees has the responsibility of investing into the refugees' health and wellbeing. To do that, a certain percentage of the national GDP will have to be allocated into caring for the social security of these refugees, medical care, housing, and integration courses. The country should assess its priorities in order to determine how much of the GDP it can allocate to the hosting and integration of refugees. However, with proper and efficient GDP investment and suitable allocation, there is more often a bigger return and positive feedback on the country's economy. Refugees that flee their countries are usually looking for a new life and have a proactive demeanor. If provided with a supporting environment, while initially depending on government aid to get up on their feet, the refugees may be able of becoming productive members of society by attaining high and low-skilled jobs and filling gaps in the market.

A report from the Organization for Economic Co-operation and Development (OECD) in 2017 showed that Germany had spent 16 billion Euros during the peak of the refugee crisis in 2015, hosting about 900.000 refugees by the end of the year. While it seems like a lot of money, the cost of housing, social protection and education for refugees only amounted to 0.5 % of the country's GDP that year.[8] In addition, the Federal Ministry of Finance in Germany have made 25 million Euros available for integration programs for newly arriving refugees in 2015. Germany has also spent 4.2 % of the total GDP

[6] UNHCR: Forced Displacements in 2017 (Note 2).

[7] UNHCR: Convention and Protocol Relating to the Status of Refugees. United Nations General Assembly, Geneva (1967).

[8] OECD: Who bears the cost of integrating refugees? In: Migration Policy Debates (2017). https://www.oecd.org/els/mig/migration-policy-debates-13.pdf (accessed 9/24/2019).

in 2015 on its education, less than the European Union average (4.9 %).[9]

Estimating the number of refugees that arrived in 2015 and estimating the fraction of the GDP that is spent on the education and integration of refugees in 2015, it seems somewhat insufficient. The data seems to also show that the GDP invested in the refugees does bring out an eventual positive return in productivity. The OECD report in 2015 also shows that, on average, annual expenditure per refugee seem to decrease with the increase of time of their stay.[10] Moreover, a later report by the OECD in 2016 showed that the average employment rate in immigrants who arrive to European OECD countries under international protection starts off at about 19 % within the first year and substantially and regularly increases to more than 70 % with the subsequent years.[11] Investing in the integration of immigrants will only speed up the process in which they become more productive members of society.

## 4. Racism and Discrimination

After showing the raw information and data, it might seem simple to fix through investing more into refugees that arrive and will bring more economic return in the future. However, there is a geopolitical side to the issue. Many political parties are now expressing their view on migration, as it is a new and upcoming topic in the midst of a migration and refugee crisis. The conservative and right-wing politicians openly express that they do not welcome the immigrants flowing in illegal ways, while the liberal and left-wing politicians try to show an open-arms approach to all immigrants flowing in. Since 2015, right wing and conservative politicians are gaining more popularity, which is providing a platform for discriminatory speech in the

[9] Eurostat: How much do Member States spend on education (8/28/2017). https://ec.europa.eu/eurostat/web/products-eurostat-news/-/DDN-20170828-1 (accessed 9/24/2019).

[10] OECD: How will the refugee surge affect the European economy? In: Migration Policy Debates (2015). https://www.oecd.org/migration/How-will-the-refugee-surge-affect-the-European-economy.pdf (accessed 9/24/2019).

[11] OECD: Making Integration Work. Refugees and others in need of protection, doi: 10.1787/9789264251236-en.

media. It is thus becoming increasingly accepted to be openly discriminant or even racist towards immigrants.[12]

Racism is defined as the exercise of power against a racial or ethnical group that are deemed inferior by individuals and/or institutions with the occasional cultural support. Individual racism or racial discrimination is the belief that one person's race is superior to another race of people and the person acts upon the said belief and, in doing so, behaves in a certain way towards other so-called inferior races. Institutional racism is deeply rooted within the laws and the system in a country and the corporations within the country. It is the restricted access to the rights and opportunities to citizens that are of a minority race in comparison to the general public. This is the level where segregation and incarcerations happen. Cultural racism is an intergenerational belief in superiority that is ingrained into the culture through institutional means, ideological beliefs, negative stereotyping, and omission of important historical contributions related to the minority group.[13]

These three classifications are not independent of each other, and cultural racism seems to be the main driving factor affecting individual and institutional behaviors. Ultimately, the institutional discrimination is often supported by many politicians who voice their opinions so that individual racism becomes increasingly accepted, especially in the media. Media is a powerful and influencing tool that can create prejudices and stereotypes in order to easily persuade the audience. This can create an intolerant environment that makes it more difficult to create harmonious and accepting environments within local communities. Additionally, these politicians are facilitating the institutional discrimination that could make it harder to fund and implement programs in schools and refugee camps that are targeted towards the inclusion and integration of refugee and migrant populations.

An example of media being utilized to instill emotions of fear, hate, and prejudice towards migrants is the media reporting on crime

---

[12] Carl C. Berning, Elmar Schlueter: The dynamics of radical right-wing populist party preferences and perceived group threat: A comparative panel analysis of three competing hypotheses in the Netherlands and Germany. In: Social Science Research 55 (2016), pp. 83–93.

[13] Enrique W. Neblett Jr.: Racism and Health: Challenges and Future Directions in Behavioral and Psychological Research. In: American Psychological Association 25 (2019), pp. 12–20.

rates, specifically performed by people who are migrants or of migrant backgrounds. According to the BBC news the far-right political party Alternative für Deutschland *(AfD)* had claimed that 447 killings and murders were committed by illegal immigrants in Germany in 2017.[14] The numbers claimed were not accurate as there were only 27 cases of committed or attempted murder by illegal immigrants in Germany. Refugees and immigrants make up about 2 % of the current German population. Given that, the Bundeskriminalamt (BKA) has shown that a mere 7.9 % of all crimes have been linked to at least one Non-European immigrant, including refugees, legal and illegal asylum seekers. On the other hand, legal migrants and citizens with a German, Schengen, or EU passport were responsible for the remaining 92 % of the crimes committed in Germany in 2017.[15]

Despite the low percentage of the incidents that include immigrants and illegal asylum seekers as suspects, it is often the case that they get the most attention in local papers and media. The far-right media often uses the incidents to prosecute and create a negative image for immigrants, so that reasoning could be given to the unwelcoming demeanor, almost as if all refugees, asylum seekers, and immigrants, whether legal or otherwise, are expected to be the ideal citizens with a collective clean criminal record. The media disregards the social pressures, limitations, discrimination, and incarcerations that refugees are subject to, focusing on criminal acts to justify why they do not belong in the host communities. That is not to say that any given crime rate is acceptable by any certain population, but it is only ethical to observe and weigh these numbers fairly and regardless of the racial background of the suspects involved.

## 5. The Urge to Fit In: Societal Factors that affect the integration of Adolescent Arab Migrants in Freiburg, Germany; A Qualitative Study

As a student of the Master of Science in Global Urban Health at the Albert-Ludwig-Universität in Freiburg, I have decided to investigate

---

[14] Reality Check team: Are migrants driving crime in Germany? In: BBC News (9/13/2018). https://www.bbc.com/news/world-europe-45419466 (accessed 9/24/2019).

[15] Bundeskriminalamt: General information on police crime statistics. In: Police Crime Rates (2017).

the issue of integration within young adolescents and children with migrant backgrounds. I have found plenty of research that focused on the parents, the father as the breadwinner of the family, and the mother as either a partner or a single mother. I came across articles about the integration of adolescents in the sense of numbers of mental illnesses and difficulties the adolescents have harbored through their journeys to their host countries. Therefore, I believe it is important to give a voice to the children and young adolescents, their teachers, and their families through a qualitative research in order to learn about their experience and their opinions on the process of integration that they have to go through.

To be able to do so, I based the framework of my thesis on the Bioecological Systems Theory developed by Urie Bronfenbrenner in 1979,[16] a socio-environmental framework where a child's development will depend on the circles they interact with. At the center of the circle lies the child and the layers on top consist of different direct and indirect parties with whom the child interacts with and in which these parties interact within each other.

I have focused my research on the center, the individuality of the children, and the two layers above. The first layer is the microsystem where all the parties in which the individual interacts with is directly located, including the parents at home and the teachers at school. The second layer of the framework is the mesosystem. This is the system where all the parties in the microsystem interact with the individual and with each other, so in observing these interactions we can understand more about the integration of these children.

Using grounded theory, the data was collected from the teachers, parents, and children through a series of focus group discussions and in-depth interviews. Afterwards, recordings were transcribed and translated from Arabic to English. The whole text was put through a data analysis that defines the grounded theory, where it was coded initially into meaning units, then run through a focused coding process, which cross-checked the formed meaning units with the initial coding and the translated transcriptions. The meaning units were abstracted further into categories and then themes. At that point, theories were deduced from the themes that are abstracted.

As grounded theory is being used as the tool for data analysis, it is hard to predict any expected results. However, the study provided a

---

[16] John W. Santrock: Life-span Development. 9th Edition. New York 2010.

wider scope on what it means to be an Arab refugee or migrant child in the German school system. It also provided a deeper look into the balance and struggle of these children with their parents as they try to find their place between their family's culture and the new culture they are forced to adopt to. The study also showed the opinions of the teachers who try to work towards a harmonious existence between all their pupils, regardless of their background. In addition, the study took a glimpse into the mental well-being and coping mechanisms of the participants and their families, when there appeared to be any.

Expected were new results in the data abstraction stage. As the grounded theory is quite a dynamic tool, different themes that were thought to be unimportant had made themselves apparent. Care was given to stray away from any bias and open up to new ideas, no matter how unexpected the resulting theories might be.

The study ultimately found three themes: The language barrier and culture difference were the two most common themes to be brought up by the adults involved within the study. Many misunderstandings happened mostly between the teachers and the parents due to language barriers. However, this barrier seemed to only be a problem between the parents and teachers, while the children seemed to only suffer for some months before they actually picked up the new language. The teachers attempted to overcome the language barrier by providing translators at the parent-teacher meetings, but the teachers had struggled to reach out to the parents to set a time and date for an appointment. This might not affect the integration of the child directly, but rather indirectly, when the parents do not put enough effort to integrate themselves and their families. That could negatively affect the child's process through missed school materials and events. Another issue brought up by the study was how the weight of the responsibility of the integration was distributed on the family environment and the school system. It showed that the parties responsible for the child's development and integration did not have a clear-cut working definition on integration, or a proposed structure of distribution of responsibilities that would facilitate the integration of migrant children in school and at home. These discrepancies with culture, language, and communication ultimately affected the child's process negatively. Providing integration and language courses to the parents is approaching the issue from a single side. Teachers in schools with immigrants should be provided with training on how to handle the cultural differences. Working on creating an accepting environment from both sides might have an impact on future generations where the differences are bridged through early exposure of local schoolchildren to different cultures and people with different backgrounds. It might humanize the insecurities and fears that are created by these differences, which may lead to different forms of discrimination.[17]

The third finding was a rather surprising and positive one. The study found social sports, and football in particular, are the key to integration for these children. When the children take part in these sports, the language barrier is no longer a problem. Students attain a sense of belonging and self-development as they start playing in teams with different groups. Sports as a humanitarian development tool has been discussed in many conventions that have stressed on the importance and simplicity of the tool. Many conventions urge sports organizations, the private sector, and the governmental sector to work together to develop strategies that offer safe spaces where young talents can be developed without prejudice or threat to their social well-being.[18]

## 6. Conclusion, Recommendations, and Potential Policies

Humans have always migrated in the search for better resources and opportunities. Representing only 3.4 % of the population of the world,[19] international migrants including refugees will all have to go through a process of adapting to change. They all have to learn new languages, cultural norms, and adapt to new living spaces. Integration is the process that entails that adaptation. However, integration is not the responsibility of the migrants alone; the host communities are

---

[17] Laurier Fortin, Marc Bigras: Risk Factors Exposing Young Children to Behaviour Problems. In: Emotional and Behavioural Difficulties 2 (1997), pp. 2–14.

[18] Elizabeth Cheung-Gaffney: Sports and Humanitarian Development: A Look at Sports Programming in the Refugee Crisis Through a Case Study of KickStart Joy Soccer Project at the Zaatari Refugee Camp. In: Journal of Legal Aspects of Sport 28 (2018), pp. 208–221.

[19] United Nations, Department of Economic and Social Affairs, Population Division: The 2017 revision. In: Trends in International Migrant Stock (2017). https://www.un.org/en/development/desa/population/migration/data/estimates2/docs/MigrationStockDocumentation_2017.pdf (accessed 9/24/2019).

also responsible for facilitating the process of integration by providing opportunities of language and culture learning programs, education, and career building. This is especially the case for younger adults, adolescents and children, who can be reached more easily through the school education system.

The younger migrant population goes through a uniquely tough experience as they start understanding their place within society as well as the added pressure of fitting into their new communities. Therefore, their integration depends on how accepting and supportive the system they are in is willing to be.

Moreover, it shows that investing in rehabilitation and integration programs does propagate a positive economic growth with time. The money spent by the state per migrant person decreases with the increase of number of years that the person resides in the country. The average employment rate also increases with time. Ergo, the productivity of the migrant is proportional to the amount of effort and money invested into providing them with the initial steppingstones in the form of integration programs, language courses, and equal access to opportunities.

However, the process of integration is hindered by individual, institutional, and cultural discrimination. Right wing and conservative politicians and decision-making stakeholders are gaining increasing popularity. These stakeholders usually have an unwelcoming and sometimes prejudiced view on migration and refugees.

Proper integration will need communities where the vast majority has a welcoming and realistic view on the issue of migration. Discrimination can be diminished only when it is fixed at the level of cultural racism. Tackling individual racism is a good starting point to eventually reach through to institutional and cultural racism. A promising strategy is to try to reach out to the communities and involve them in social events that include members of migrant populations, like cooking events or cultural evenings where both communities can join together, get to know each other, and learn about one another, so there is less prejudice held by any party. It is also a good way to tackle negative stereotypes that some might use as a generalization towards a certain race or group of people, whether that mentality is held by people from the host communities or the migrants.

A good potential policy would be introducing education to all the registered refugees and asylum seekers, regardless of their final residency status. Asylum seekers are temporarily hosted in arrival centers until their papers go through the bureaucratic process and afterwards, they receive a final decision on their refugee status. During that time most adult asylum seekers do not have the right to seek education or jobs. They become stressed and might fall into depression due to the uncertainty of their status. Investing more money in language courses and vocational training shortens the time that the asylum seekers need to take to start to integrate and find jobs when they are allowed to do so, making them productive members of society much sooner. Moreover, it gives asylum seekers some activity to look forward to and fill their time and give them a sense of purpose. Additionally, the skills learned will come in handy for them even if they end up being rejected from a refugee status in Germany. They will be able to use their newly acquired skills in any country they move to, which brings international development.

Schools should be considered a vantage point where most integration programs can be implemented. In Germany, every child has the right to education. Every child registered will eventually go to a school and their parents will have to be involved with the school in one way or the other. Introducing school events and sporting programs that are directed towards joining all the community together could be easier to implement where the students and the parents of both communities and their teachers could take part in school events together. By exposing the different communities to each other, they no longer are strange or unknown to each other. They may start humanizing the other group by creating personal relationships and acquaintanceships. This might erase the fear of the different or the unknown and bridge the gap between different cultures.

Another important factor to keep in mind is the segregation of migrants and local communities that usually happens by building affordable housing in areas further away from the center, where most local communities would be situated. That causes the formation of so-called ghetto areas with a predominant migrant population. This segregation can become a barrier to the process of integration, as the communities will have less chances of mixing. One recommendation would be to implement the events within the different schools of the city or even different cities.

When more individuals start becoming tolerant, more of them may become involved in the public awareness demonstrations against racism and hate. More people might speak up against any form of discrimination. More citizens may start to vote for liberal and tolerant leaders and politicians. Slowly but surely this might decrease the institutional racism drastically. Eventually, this might create a community with open-minded individuals and institutions that treat everyone with impartiality. This may facilitate the integration of the migrant population as they will not feel like they are unwelcomed in their new homes, accelerating the process of becoming functional members of society that give back to the country's economy, social diversity, and all in all prosperity.

*Iva Rinčić and Amir Muzur*

# Migrants' health and European culture: strengthening ties for better understanding. The case of Rijeka 2020 European Capital of Culture

Abstract
In last few years, Europe has faced one of the biggest migration crisis in the history, influencing different aspects of (post)migration experiences and life. Migrants' health is a challenging concept, formed of objective and subjective dimensions (legal regulation, personal moral values, previous experiences, literacy, religious norms, cultural impact, etc.). Despite great need for better understanding, migrants' health as a complex phenomenon is often neglected, remaining on the margins of mainstream migration-related research and professional interest. The aim of this article is to address migrants' health in relation toward European cultural policies, the European capital of culture program, ECOC. Being one of the European most influential cultural programs, ECOC is deeply involved in promotion of cultural diversity and multiculturality. However, migrants' culture is seen mainly in the terms of music and food, omitting culture – health boundaries, while more reflective approach might be a key for a better understanding of migrants' health. A short review of the ECOC program database related to migrations is offered, including main points needing re-evaluation. Specially, the Rijeka ECOC 2020 project will be critically analyzed, having migration as one of key topics within the program for the next year.

## 1. Introduction

Migrations are not new phenomena. On the contrary, people move because of economic, social, political, religious, and cultural reasons from ancient times, changing their own place of living, but also being affected, both positively and negatively, by the host country. However, despite the centuries of experiences, as a process of moving, either across an international border, or within a State. Encompassing any kind of movement of people, whatever its length, composition and causes; it includes refugees, displaced persons, uprooted people, and economic migrants,[1] claiming migrations are an easily understandable one-sided story, would be incorrect. So far, no unified theory on migration has emerged,[2] making migrations persist as a constant challenge for various academic disciplines, policy makers, and other stakeholders (social groups, institutions, authorities, media, individuals, etc.). Numerous experts are involved in different phases of migration process, trying not only to help, but to grasp and comprehend critical differences between historical »individual relocation« actions and global migration processes we are facing nowadays.[3] Beside this structural shift going on within the last few decades, many other changes might be observed as well – traditional sectors addressed by historical migration waves (security, work and labor, social and humanitarian aid, etc.), recently upgraded through a broad cross-structural approach (especially in Europe, since 2015), encompassing education, health care, science and research, media, and culture. This is not surprising; confronted with rising numbers, needs, rights, and often (but now always) positive public expectations, »migration advocates« have headed a broad campaign of welcoming migrants, using all available political and public resources in reaching the goal.

It is no novelty using and implementing culture as a tool of the promotion of dialogue between different social groups, of achieving better community relations, and overcoming multicultural challenges. Some might claim that the recent migration crisis put on stake the role and mission of modern culture itself, mainly cultural institutions, which should revise their operation and vision, so as »to address the needs of society that is culturally more diverse than the one they were established for.«[4] There is no doubt, modern societies are in need for culture that might help to better navigate new challenges, includ-

---

[1] Richard Perruchoud, Jillyanne Redpath-Cross (Eds.): Glossary on Migration. International Migration Law 25. Geneva 2011. https://publications.iom.int/system/files/pdf/iml25_1.pdf (accessed 6/17/2019).

[2] Carmen Boghean: The phenomenon of migration. Opportunities and challenges. In: The USV Annals of Economics and Public Administration 16 (2016), pp. 14–20, here p. 14.

[3] Aristide R. Zolberg: The Next Waves: Migration Theory for a Changing World. In: The International Migration Review 23 (1989), pp. 403–430.

[4] European Agenda for Culture. Work Plan for Culture 2011–2014. Report on the role of public arts and cultural institutions in the promotion of cultural diversity and intercultural dialogue. Working group of EU member state experts, 2014. http://ec.europa.eu/assets/eac/culture/library/reports/201405-omc-diversity-dialogue_en.pdf (accessed 9/24/2019).

ing migration. However, the question that remains here is how this should be done and which are known cultural structures, policies, platforms, and tools already used in promoting new post-migrant European societies. Beside this mainstream culture, is there a need and place for promoting hidden parts of migrants' culture, and if so, what are the main aspects of this approach? Having all this in mind, our main intention here is to overcome the framework of migrants' culture, by introducing a new momentum, the one of migrants' health.

## 2. Europe and migrations 2015–2019: some numbers and observations

Modern Europe is facing new 21$^{st}$-century migrations phenomena, and how the European future is going to look like depends in a great manner on the readiness to re-think its migration policies and roles, but also some other social and cultural patterns and myths.

Throughout history, the European continent was often exposed to migration. Even before most recent movements, great migration processes and variations occurred many times (Roman period, Middle Age movements, Age of Discovery 15$^{th}$–17$^{th}$ century movements, 19$^{th}$ century labor move, post World Wars I and II migrations etc.), becoming indispensable for the development of many modern states, and shaped social and labor dynamics of the old continent. In his recent 2018 document, in the chapter on Post-war European transition, Hass recognizes four main periods: 1) 1945–1970s, 2) mid-1970s–mid-1990s, 3) mid-1990s–2008 and 4) 2008–ongoing.[5] Although all periods of the middle and the second half of the 20th century in Europe have been marked by thousands of displaced people, refugees, people leaving communist regimes in East Central Europe, or coming from ex-colonies, it is only the last migration crisis (since 2014) that has attracted such a level of interest, both political/public and scholar.

In 2015, EU+ (including 28 EU countries, Norway, and Switzerland) reported the number of 1.255,649 first-time asylum applicants, a 123 % rise compared to year before (562.280). The highest number (441.800) was in Germany, but in relative terms (according to the

5 Hein de Haas: European Migrations: Dynamics, Drivers, and the Role of Policies. Luxembourg 2018.

number of citizens), the peaks were in Hungary (entering mainly from Serbia) and Sweden. While Finland had a 822 % rise in 2015 compared to 2014, five countries reported a decline in applicants (Croatia, Latvia, Lithuania, Romania, Slovenia). The majority of asylum seekers originated from Syria, representing 29 % of all applications, followed by Afghanistan (14 %), and Iraq (10 %). By the end of 2015, more than 900.000 applications were still pending.[6] The European case was not isolated: the United Nations High Commissioner for Refugees (UNHCR) estimated that there were 59 million individuals displaced worldwide in 2015.[7] In 2016, the total number of asylum seekers in Europe was 1.204,280, falling the year later to 649.855, and in 2018 to 634.600 (with the estimation that 1 out of 10 applications for asylum in EU+ was repeated).[8] Although applicants from Syria, Afghanistan, and Iraq still are lodging the highest numbers (altogether 26 % in 2018), during 2018, authorities reported the rise of application from other countries (Columbia + 210 %, Venezuela + 88 %, Georgia + 72 %, Palestine + 61 %, Turkey + 48 %, etc.). Citizens from the majority of those countries, especially from Latin America and Western Balkans, were able to enter the Schengen zone without visa. The rise of asylum seekers from those countries was 30 % compared to 2017. Europe is still struggling with the consequences of the 2015–2016 crisis, but at the same time already loosing pace with new challenges.

Judging from the numbers of the 2015 migration peak, there is no doubt Europe was faced with serious pressure to act fast and promptly. At the same time, there was a plea for a new regulatory framework agreeable to all member states, addressing urgent short-term needs, but also dealing with some long-term issues. This was preceded by the conclusion that previous coordination, such as Dublin

[6] N.N.: Asylum in the EU Member States: Record number of over 1.2 million first time asylum seekers registered in 2015. Syrians, Afghans and Iraqis: top citizenships, Eurostat Press Office (3/4/2016). https://ec.europa.eu/eurostat/documents/2995521/7203832/3-04032016-AP-EN.pdf/790eba01-381c-4163-bcd2-a54959b99ed6 (accessed 5/19/2019).

[7] Christian Dustmann, Francesco Fasani, Tommaso Frattini, Luigi Minale, Uta Schönberg: On the economics and politics of refugee migration (10/18/2016). https://voxeu.org/article/economics-and-politics-refugee-migration (accessed 9/24/2019).

[8] N.N.: EU+ asylum trends 2018 overview (2/13/2019). https://www.easo.europa.eu/sites/default/files/EASO-2018-EU-Asylum-Trends-Overview.pdf (accessed 9/24/2019).

Convention,[9] should be replaced by more workable alternatives, mainly in the field of coordinated security and asylum policy. Another question stroke the European publicity – the question of how to distribute the burden of refugee migrations across the countries equally. Not all countries were ready and willing to accept this proposal, stating reasons beyond the financial ones, pointing to gaps and shortages in common external and internal politics, decision making processes, and finally, to the non-existence of a common set of European interests and values. Several years later, Europe is far from the migration peak (although migration, especially illegal, is not over), but facing deep structural problems.[10] Moreover, there have been present strong voices claiming that, within the present structure, Europe (EU) has reached the limits of its own framework as defined by the current treaties,[11] urging for some new solutions and overcoming existing policies. One of the reason for such claims is the fact that, for the first time, Europe was entered by the large number of people very different from the host population, »not just in their languages, cultures and identities, but also in their religious beliefs, outlooks, lifestyles and everyday practices.«[12] Their absorption has already revealed more difficulties than the absorption and integration of immigrants more similar to the native population in the past.[13]

---

[9] Regulation (EU) No 604/2013 of the European Parliament and of the Council of 26 June 2013 establishing the criteria and mechanisms for determining the Member State responsible for examining an application for international protection lodged in one of the Member States by a third-country national or a stateless person.

[10] N.N.: As EU stresses the migration ›crisis‹ is over, Italy makes hundreds of migrants homeless. In: The Conversation (3/8/2019). http://theconversation.com/as-eu-stresses-the-migration-crisis-is-over-italy-makes-hundreds-of-migrants-home less-113137 (accessed 9/24/2019).

[11] Maria Demertzis, Jean Pisani-Ferry, André Sapir, Thomas Wieser, Guntram Wolff: One size does not fit all. European integration by differentation. In: The Bruegel (9/19/2018). https://bruegel.org/wp-content/uploads/2018/09/PB-2018_03_final3.pdf (accessed 9/24/2019).

[12] Jan Pakulski, Stefan Markowski: Globalisation, immigration and multiculturalism – the European and Australian experiences. In: Journal of Sociology 50 (2014), pp. 3–9, here p. 4.

[13] Dorota A. Gozdecka, Selen A. Ercan, Magdalena Kmak: From multiculturalism to post-multiculturalism: Trends and paradoxes. In: Journal of Sociology 50 (2014), pp. 51–64.

## 3. Migrants' health: bridge between migration and post-migration studies

The recent crisis in Europe has opened various fields of migration studies. Although those phenomena have previously been present in various historical, economic, social, and political research agendas, the field is still considered fragmented and selective. According to Martiniello,[14] one group of researchers is interested in migrations flow and patterns of mobility, trying to answer the questions why people move, how they do this, where they go, what sources they use, and finally, what policies they face (and encourage) by their behavior. Other groups of researchers, on the other side, are more oriented toward what we could call post-migration studies, or what happens to migrants after the setting in new countries (how they select a country, do they integrate, assimilate, or form a group distinctive from the mainstream society; how other citizens treat them, what rights they have, etc.). No matter how migrations flow or how later integration goes on, those are inseparable phenomena, but what is often at stake is a sharp distinction between what we could determine as migration and post-migration studies.

Such a divided approach has many consequences, but it is crucial especially in one aspect – that it relates to migrants' health, immanent for migrant population before, during, and after the migration process. »Migrants are likely to experience specific challenge in relation toward health due to the nature of being migrant.«[15] As a consequence of that, research topics might greatly vary: from how different routes and migration forms influence health – at both individual and population levels – to the issue in what way pre-migration health status affects decisions to migrate and shapes post-migration experience, and to classic post-migration questions (such as different types of migrant and health experience.[16] Although in the last few years, migration experience has increasingly been recognized as a determinant of migrants' health,

[14] Marco Martiniello: Comparisons in Migration Studies. In: Comparative Migration Studies 1 (2013), pp. 7–22, here p. 18–19.

[15] Anita A. Davies, Anna Basten, Chiara Frattini: Migration: A Social Determinant of the Health of Migrants. Geneva 2006.

[16] N.N.: Harmful, unfounded myths about migration and health have become accepted, used to justify policies of exclusion. In: Science Daily (12/8/2018). https://www.sciencedaily.com/releases/2018/12/181205232658.htm (accessed 9/24/2019).

bidirectional relationship between migration and health remains poorly understood, and action on migration and health remains limited, negatively impacting not only those who migrate but also sending, receiving, and ›left-behind‹ communities.[17]

Public health is very much present in research of migrant's health, stressing social determinants of health approach, »such as structural factors, aside from medical care, that are determined by social and economic policies and inequalities and have important effects on health.«[18] At the same time, there are numerous studies following different patterns, using migration experience as a crucial determination for migrant's health, but most of them focus on only one set of factors: behavioral, structural, economic, cultural, etc. Each set recognizes and explores one selected aspect relevant for migrants' health, leaving other influences and traits outside of scope, and making full (or hopefully more advanced?) understanding of migrants' health unattainable. This is probably one of the reasons why results or evidence of migrants' health research are in disparity, sometimes even being contradictory. According to the latest studies and reports, being migrant at the same time might be a trigger for a higher risk of developing illness.[19]

While contemplating on how to ameliorate the health conditions of migrants, there is probably a set of reasons standing behind the existing gap between reality of migrants' health and what is considered relevant in understanding this complex issue. A comprehensive research on this topic has already been done,[20] but with limited suc-

---

[17] Heide Castañeda, Seth M. Holmes, Daniel S. Madrigal, Maria-Elena DeTrinidad Young, Naomi Beyler, James Quesada: Immigration as a social determinant of health. In: Annual Review of Public Health 36 (2015), pp. 375–392.

[18] Paula Braveman, Susan Egerter, David R. Williams: The social determinants of health: coming of age. In: The Annual Review of Public Health 32 (2011), pp. 381–398.

[19] N.N.: Migrants and refugees at higher risk of developing ill health than host populations, reveals first-ever WHO report on the health of displaced people in Europe (1/21/2019). http://www.euro.who.int/en/media-centre/sections/press-releases/2019/migrants-and-refugees-at-higher-risk-of-developing-ill-health-than-host-populations-reveals-first-ever-who-report-on-the-health-of-displaced-people-in-europe (accessed 9/24/2019); Mathieu Ichou, Matthew Wallace: The Healthy Immigrant Effect: The role of educational selectivity in the good health of migrants. In: Demographic Research 40 (2019), pp. 60–94.

[20] Kolitha Wickramage, Jo Vearey, Anthony B. Zwi, Courtland Robinson, Michael Knipper: Migration and health: a global public health research priority. In: BMC Pub-

cess in changing structural background of the problem. Before going further, it is important to stress the difficulties in understanding that health complexity is not a migrants' exclusive; sociologists of health have spent the last few decades trying to answer this question. Many remarkable findings came out,[21] but the totality of the health concept remains unfathomable, scampering our skills, knowledge, tolerance, and understanding. »Why is that so« is one of the crucial questions in the field of humanities and social sciences research of life and health, trying to overcome the existing body-mind-spirit (and culture) partition, the dominance of the so-called biomedical health paradigm, and exclusivity of evidence-based medicine. Despite the fact our behavior is deeply culturally informed, culture as a key in understanding health is still deeply neglected and »there is no other variable used so poorly in understanding health«[22] ceding in front of a measurable, universal, and standardized approach. Another problem is even more troublesome – not only culture is often neglected as important in understanding society phenomena (including migrants' health), but it is often seen superficially and selective, urging for more relevant, applicable and responsible cultural experience. »We say the neglect of culture is the single biggest barrier to advancing the highest attainable standards of health worldwide.«[23]

Having in mind diversity occurring within migrants' population, in relation toward pre-migration, migration, and post-migration processes, toward family left in original country and local population in the host country, it is obvious that we are dealing with robust matter. Recognizing the uncertainty of current social reality of the migrants' health is just a first step. No statement claiming such decisions would be wrong, but there is strong evidence many of them have been done

---

lic Health 18 (2018), pp. 1–9; H. G. Virupaksha, Ashok Kumar, Bergai Parthsarathy Nirmala: Migration and mental health: An interface. In: Journal of Natural Science, Biology and Medicine 5 (2014), pp. 233–239.

[21] Mrjorie Kagawa Singer, Annalyz Valdez Dadia, Mimi C. Yu, Antonella Surbone: Cancer, Culture, and Health Disparities: Time to Chart a New Course? In: A Cancer Journal for Clinicians 60 (2010), pp. 12–39.

[22] Mrjorie Kagawa Singer, William Dressler, Sheba George, The NIH Expert Panel: Culture: The missing link in health research. In: Social Science and Medicine 170 (2016), pp. 237–246. http://dx.doi.org/10.1016/j.socscimed.2016.07.015 (accessed 9/24/2019).

[23] David Holmes, David Napier: Cultivating the Role of Culture in Health. In: The Lancet 384 (2014), pp. 1607.

without having in mind long-term consequences, omitting the needed preparations and maybe (just maybe) unadvisedly.

Europe is globally known as a continent of many cultures: culture in Europe is beyond invisible routine, it is the way of living, policy, and politics, and, after all, a great business opportunity. Faced with recent migrations trends, it was expected that (multi)culture related sectors will rise and expand. And they did, leaving many questions open, such as: Whose culture was introduced? What aspects of migrants' culture did Europe perceive, recognize, and promote? Did such culture promotion in any aspect add value to migrants' health puzzle?

## 4. European Capital of Culture as a model for promoting culture in Europe – what does migration have to do with it?

The term culture has a remarkable widespread and variations of (mis) use in everyday life. There are literally countless definitions and theories related to culture, but the basic sociological explanation treats culture as an overarching system of meaning. Many ideas in the sociology of culture have changed during the last few decades, replacing Talcott Parson's holistic view of culture during 1970's by more fine-grained approaches to the cultural process in everyday life.[24] However, the main position on culture as a dominating social phenomenon has remained vivid until today, representing culture in different aspects. Last century's debate on culture has continued in this century as well, tackling sensitive questions related to cultural and national identities, processes of economic globalization, and in Europe, having specific implications for the understanding of the integration process.[25]

In Europe, there are numerous ways of cultural promotion, but probably one of the most famous is the European Capital of Culture title (ECOC; until 2001, European City of Culture). The first ECOC title was awarded in 1985, as an intergovernmental initiative promoted by the then Greek Minister of Culture Melina Mercouri

[24] John R. Hall, Marshall Battani, Mary Jo Neitz: Sociology of Culture. London and New York, Routledge 2003.

[25] Andrea Mihaela Nita: Cultural phenomena and processes in contemporary society – determinants of cultural policies. In: Challenges of the Knowledge Society 2 (2012), pp. 1768–1774.

(1920–1994), as an extra exertion to the political unification of Europe. Since 1999, ECOC has been a title awarded to cities by European Union (EU) for one calendar year – the time period of preparation and organization of series of cultural events with a strong European dimension. Until 1999, each year one city was awarded; in 2000, nine European cities were awarded; since 2001, each year there are two Capitals, but from 2021 on, every third year one city in a candidate country, a potential candidate, or a country which is part of the European Free Trade Association/European Economic Area will be awarded the title as well. The impact of the European Capital of Culture is remarkable, going beyond cultural sphere and spreading into social, educational, urban-planning, economic, and regional dimensions. The true aim of engagement is to reach more diverse audiences – particularly in parts of a city or segments of its population that do not represent the usual audience for cultural events.

Over time, the political message behind the European Capital of Culture has also changed. According to the initial document from 1985,[26]

> the intention was to use the new concept to stimulate the expression of a culture, which (…) is characterized by having both elements and a richness born in diversity (…). To help bring the peoples of the Member States closer together (…). The event should open up to the European policy particular aspects of the culture of the city, region or country concerned.

Celebrating the 25th anniversary of the European Capital of Culture (ECOC) program in 2010, the European Commission also noted a lack of Europe in the program and a need for »bringing European added values«

> A lot of past capitals have … struggled with the European dimension of the event and there was considerable discussion on whether it should be further defined (…). It seemed to be agreed in the end that there were limits to how far the European dimension should be pre-defined as each city had its own European narrative depending on its geographical location and its history, its past and present populations (…). In some cases, the cities did in fact have a good European dimension in their projects, but did not make it visible enough in their communication material.[27]

---

[26] Resoultion of the Ministers responsible for Cultural Affairs, meeting within the Council, of 13 June 1985, concerning the annual event ›European City of Culture‹ (85/C 153/02), Official Journal of the European Communities No C 153/2.

[27] Summary of the European Commission conference: Celebrating 25 years of Eur-

Such change of perspective opened some old, but also new questions, such as how much Europe has changed in the last four decades. Is there a (rising) gap in understanding European values? Are communication and visibility more important than artistic freedom and integrity, politics more than culture? What are the messages ECOC and all Europe want to send? What and whose culture they stand for? Are there changes to be introduced in ECOC due to the change of Europe? How did (recent) migrations reflect within the ECOC program? If culture in European Capital of Culture stands for the way of living and goes beyond artistic messages, should health as a cultural issue also be present? Does the triangle of migration, culture, and health represent a socially recognizable matrix, worthy of discussion, analysis, and promotion?

For some period already, the migration topic has been relevant to the European Capital of Culture agenda: the most famous example is the Istanbul 2010 movie project The Immigrants – Towards a Common Future, or other notable cases such as labor daily migration phenomena in Essen-Ruhr (Istanbul partner city), and migration and exile case in Copenhagen (1996).

Being of interest to the media, ECOC is very much devoted to regular tracking of the capital's experiences and background behind the main program. At the request of the European Commission, a few years ago, two documents (Palmer Report I and II) were prepared in order to analyze intentions, priorities, and performances of the Capitals of Culture during the period 1994–2004, concluding that »All ECOCs reported that they experienced problems with regard to the planning and delivery of the European dimension of their program.«[28] Quantitative content analysis of the Palmer Report – searching for the frequency of certain keywords in different ECOC applications – brings interesting observations and further conclusions with regard to the European dimension. As one would expect, the main keywords in the Palmer Report are: city, culture, Europe, capital, tourists, visitors, region, funding, infrastructure, and success; but »[s]ubjects such as interculturality and immigrant culture are also high on

---

opean Capitals of Culture, Brussels, 3/23–24/2010. https://ec.europa.eu/programmes/creative-europe/sites/creative-europe/files/library/capitals-culture-25-years-conclusions_en.pdf (accessed 9/24/2019).

[28] Robert Palmer: European Cities and Capitals of Culture: Study Prepared for the European Commission. Brussels 2004.

the agenda.«[29] According to Palmer, in the period 1994–2004, Europe has hardly been connected to interculturality or diversity, no matter how high they are at the EU cultural policy agenda. Additional examples of multiculturalism and multilingualism were present in the Luxembourg case, the interfaith dialogue in Graz, and finally, the migration and exile in Copenhagen, while some terms were almost never mentioned (interculturalism, ethnicity).

As one would anticipate, some cities pay more attention to migrations as part of culture, mainly due to historical, social, or economic reasons, recognizable in their ECOC application. Good example of such a case is Rijeka (Croatia), to which the title was awarded for 2020 under the name »Rijeka: Port of Diversity. Water, Work, Migrations.«[30] It is not surprising that migration is one of the selected topic in Rijeka's bid book, since Rijeka had long ago been mapped as a relevant port in European e/immigration history. Currently, Rijeka is preparing for the third visit of European Expert Panel, scheduled for autumn 2019,[31] with many expectations and challenges on how the proposed program will be realized. In Rijeka 2020, the case of migration has been covered by the program of Kitchen of Diversity. In the explanatory text, available on the web page, ambitious ideas are listed:

> Impulse: Millions are on the move. Wars, natural disasters, poverty and political oppression are forcing them on the road, but some are also motivated by curiosity and a desire for adventure. Employment, family and educational opportunities are the main reasons for migrations, the most powerful factors in our unstable geopolitical environment. Food is an important instrument of culture, the beginning of sharing. The KITCHEN thus becomes an open workshop for exchanging ideas, habits and opinions.
>
> An informal impulse that connects people and brings them together. It functions as a platform for confronting experiences regarding migrations from other parts of Europe.
>
> (…)
>
> We need the kitchen because contemporary Europe is faced with the trauma of migration which presents a challenge for the Union. We must

[29] Nicole Immler, Hans Sakkers: (Re)Programming Europe: European Capitals of Culture: Rethinking the role of culture. In: Journal of European Studies 44 (2014), pp. 3–29, here p. 10.

[30] N.N.: Rijeka bid book fro European Capital of Culture 2020 (2/24/2016). https://rijeka2020.eu/tag/bid-book/ (accessed 9/24/2019).

[31] N.N.: Rijeka European Capital of Culture 2020: Second Monitoring Meeting Report by the Expert Panel, European Commission 2018. https://rijeka2020.eu/wp-content/uploads/2018/08/2nd-Monitoring-Meeting.pdf (accessed 9/24/2019).

build the capacities to learn how to ethically and efficiently manage the migration waves flowing into European cities. Culture is the true response for the challenge of migrations because it allows us to contemplate the issue from different perspectives – nomadic, cosmopolitan, subcultural, as well as ethnic and religious.[32]

If we take a more careful look into the Kitchen of Diversity program, the activities are mainly devoted to the topics of food and music of different migration groups:[33] Porto Etno (festival combining music and gastronomy of national minorities of Rijeka and the Primorje-Gorski Kotar County – Bosnia nad Hercegovina, Macedonia, Hungary, Somalia, Senegal, Italy, Mexico, Brasil, Slovenia, Croatia) and Furioza Cycle (education and cultural workshops, music festival, etc.). Instead of courage, readiness, and responsibility to use ECOC as a platform for more socially relevant exploration of migration cultures (including migrants' health), once again, the stage has been narrowed down, politically correct but at the same time socially irrelevant, lacking critically needed European voice and message. Invisible aspects of culture (including values, beliefs, communications, behavior, family relations, interpersonal relations, modesty, notion of space and time, and finally, health) again are neglected, due to the recognition and promotion of culture mainly through popular lenses of food, music, and clothes, omitting real cultural experiences, and finally, jeopardizing the way for a better integration of migrants into a new society. »Migrants often move with their culture and traditional norms which often differ from host community.«[34] Reducing those differences to exotic experiences of different cuisine and music might seem good for a city promotion strategy but is miles away from the real need of modern European societies.

## 5. Conclusion

Although it is not unexpected that health is completely related to culture, such position is often neglected, mainly due to the impact

---

[32] N.N.: Kitchen of Diversity: Centre for creative migrations. https://rijeka2020.eu/en/program/kitchen/#info (accessed 9/24/2019).
[33] Douglas Murray: The Strange Death of Europe: Immigration, Identity, Islam. London 2018.
[34] Migration: A Social Determinant of the Health of Migrants, Geneva 2006.

and influence of the dominant biomedical paradigm. In such a framework, health as a part of cultural context remains out of the public and scholarly scope. One of those scopes is the migrants' health and culture, both introducing complex and variant implications that considerably vary across the migrant groups and from person to person. As culture is often seen as separate, health is mainly developed within typical medical indicators, recently enriched with new technologies. But what is missing is a deep culture-health migrant-post migration study. Let us not forget that being a migrant means to deal with a concept of »inherited vulnerability.«[35]

According to Castañeda et al., the cultural framework is mainly used in relation to topics and outcomes such as acculturation, mental health, chronic disease, health care access, maternal and child health, substance use, physical activity and obesity and social capital, with presumption that cultural or ethnic group »becomes a major – even primary – determinant of health-related individual behaviors and tends to assume that the responsibility for adopting healthy cultural practices lies with individuals.«[36] This could be true in some aspects, but does not promote the complex picture of a cultural framework.

One of the main sins of modern Europe is to be superficial when facing the problem of migrations. In this chapter, we have stressed only a few arguments of abundant challenges related to the phenomenon of recent migration waves from the perspective of cultural theory and sociology of health. In particular, we analyzed the case of the title awarded to the city of Rijeka, Croatia, European Capital of Culture in 2020, and its inadequate approach to the issue of migrations: even if Rijeka has historically been the scene of a major migration wave from Europe to the United States at the beginning of the 20th century, it missed the opportunity to reveal the complexness of the problems of the migrants' health and culture, ceding to the more popular aspects of migrant cuisine and music. In this way, European culture has chosen one more time to close its eyes in front of an urging issue and orient toward a safer and more pleasant hedonist enjoyment.

---

[35] Sue Le Mesurier: The phenomenon of migrations. Its significance or meaning in human societies throughout history. International Federation of Red Cross and Red Crescent Societies (speech at the Seminar on Current Migration Phenomena, Spanish Red Cross, Seville) (3/16/2012). https://www.ifrc.org/PageFiles/89397/the%20phenomenon%20of%20migration_TYPEFI_final_En.pdf, p. 3. (accessed 9/24/2019).

[36] Castañeda et al.: Immigration as a social determinant (Note 17), p. 380.

## Acknowledgments

This work has been supported by University of Rijeka projects Bioethical standards of urbanity: framing city for the life ethics (with special emphasis to Rijeka) (uniri-human-18–49–1179) and New trends in bioethics of Middle and South-East Europe: researching and networking the resources (uniri-human-18–4–1130).

*Wielant Machleidt*

# The importance of strangeness experiences for ego-constitution and society

Abstract
Migration means transgression of national and cultural borders and coping with the experience of strangeness. People with lack of basic trust develop aversive feelings towards strangers resulting in xenophobia. This significantly affects the mental health of migrants. A positive attitude toward strangers requires migrants and natives to take a developmental step, a cultural adolescence that contributes to the management of foreign experiences, the consolidation of ego-constitution, and the development of tolerance in multi-cultural societies. Mutual trust through intercultural communication prevents social exclusion and separation processes (»parallel societies«) and paves the way for social integration.

## 1. Introduction

The postmodern project of global migration and cultural change has proven as vulnerable to worldwide fears of strangers, hate and populism. Globally, people from different cultures come into contact with one another, whenever they are searching for better living and development conditions in the long term. Many of them are possibly fleeing persecution, wars or natural catastrophes or, alternately, encounters occur on a short-term basis in the context of trade relationships, travel or international education. These are the everyday phenomena of globalization. Migration sciences analyze the changes of people and societies in the course of migration. They examine to what extent and under which conditions and opportunities social behavior, culturally based practices, and mutual expectations and values change for the people or groups involved within the scope and course of intercultural encounters.[1] On the one hand, this can lead to adaptive processes, but

[1] Andreas Zick: Psychologie der Akkulturation: Neufassung eines Forschungsbereichs. Wiesbaden 2010.

it can also result in conflicts, which provide essential incentives for the transformation of modern pluralist societies and their individual citizens, as well as changes within the day to day realities of interpersonal coexistence. More intensive analysis of the psychological and social processes of migration began in the second half of the 20th century, with comparative studies of possible acculturation strategies and their relationship to the psychological and social consequences associated with stress and cultural change in the affected societies.[2] Last but not least, the frequently difficult underlying psychosocial conditions of migration have a compounding impact on the requisite integrative processes in the host country. At the same time, there is increasing evidence that successful acculturation is directly associated with psychological stability and mental health of the individuals and the host societies at the same time.[3] But the migrants as well as the societies have to cope with challenges on the way of their development to global and cultural change.

The article analyzes the individual psychological and social contexts of the success of dealing with experiences of strangeness. In particular, considered are situations that exceed limits and the extent of xenophobia and hatred or limits of acceptance and tolerance towards strangers. Described in detail are the social conditions for tolerating and successfully integrating strangers in the host societies while avoiding spin-off processes (parallel societies).

## 2. Borders and experiences of strangeness

Formative for migration is borderline crossing and neither the immigrants themselves nor the locals of the host country can escape the accompanying experience of strangeness. Borders serve to separate and differentiate between belonging, self and stranger, from economics, from the cultural and the religious, and in the consciousness of social communities, they do not only have a territorial regulatory function. They are also an experienced symbolic space in which peo-

---

[2] Wielant Machleidt: Die Angst vor Flüchtlingen in Politik und Gesellschaft. Lecture at the Lindauer Psychotherapie Wochen, June 2017.

[3] Wielant Machleidt, Iris Tatjana Graef-Calliess: Mental Health and Approaches to Treatment among Refugees and Migrants. In: Gerhard Besier, Katarzyna Stokłosa (Eds.): How to deal with refugees? Europe as a Continent of Dreams. Vienna, Zurich 2018, pp. 247–269.

ple come to know identity, continuity, security, and safety. So, what makes the experiences of strangeness that accompany the border crossings so threatening that uncertainties and fears, shame, envy, hatred, anger, and violence arise?

Migration always has a utopian moment. This utopian moment lies in the ambivalence between the Elysian expectation of salvation and the fear of deadly apocalypse. Between these poles of ambivalence, the experience of alienation moves in principle as an essential egocentric and social constitutive field of tension. Because of this ambivalent character, experiences of strangeness constitute hardly bearable experiences and easily lead to mental upheaval in all involved. Feelings of curiosity about the stranger(s) and the fear of the stranger(s) alternate with each other and characterize this ambivalence as a fluctuation of emotions. Refugees are »the messengers of misfortune« says Brecht. They are received with paranoid fears of impending disaster, fear of material disadvantage and alienation or as »saviors in distress« with soaring expectations in the form of liberation and redemption fantasies. A reduction in fear and expectation through mutual understanding and confidence building is then essential.

For this, helpful are the finding of commonality(s) and consensus(s) as a bridging function as well as explanations of one's own cultural background with diverse descriptions, comparisons, and references to shared contexts of understanding. The strangeness between two people is a definition of a relationship and in this sense the stranger is always the stranger in the self of the involved individual. The »stranger« or the »strangeness«, which remains foreign, is only when all attempts of reference have failed, the »otherness«, to which in the communication situation no understanding access can be won – and thus a potential fear factor! Understanding does not succeed without limits. The global present time has become too complex for that. Non-understanding, misunderstanding and speechlessness mark border situations in intercultural understanding access with the danger of a break in a relationship. All parties involved must then demand the enduring of non-understanding through otherness as an intercultural social and political practice. Many politicians have understood that precisely in case of misunderstandings and speechlessness of conflicts, dialog must be conducted.

## 3. Territorial reflex and projective fear

It is a well-known fact that locals compete with migrants for material livelihoods. Group egoism and xenophobia occur regularly as a kind of »territorial reflex« and are something of an anthropological constant. The resulting stereotypical rejection of strangers can be understood as the result of actual social conflicts. However, these conflicts do not explain how it is that an inversely proportional relationship between migrants' densities and xenophobia can be observed. Obviously, an irrational element, which arises in the imagination of humans, plays a significant role. Analogous to the Adorno's remark of an »anti-Semitism without Jews« there is something like a »xenophobia without a stranger«.[4]

Whether people are more likely to experience positive or negative effects in encountering strangers has a lot to do with their individual development. Anyone who has developed a secure bond with their parents, who has experienced safety and basic trust, is already active in infancy with exploring curiosity about strangers. Therefore, Bohleber states: »There is a reciprocal relationship between basic trust and xenophobia«.[5] A disturbed basic trust finds its projective expression in a fear of social disadvantages and descent, of struggles for self-assertion, fears of becoming victims of sociopolitical upheavals, of threats to moral and cultural order, etc. All of these are threat phantasies with a vague, at best, reality character.

*Summary:* The emotional character of the life experience accumulated before the biographical background predisposes for dealing with strangers. If this is predominantly positive, then it opens up the chance to get from the strangers everything that their own family, group, society, economy, culture, science etc. could not provide.

---

[4] Hans-Jürgen Wirth: Fremdenhass und Gewalt als familiäre und psychosoziale Krankheit. In: Psyche – Zeitschrift für Psychoanalyse 55 (2001), pp. 1217–1244.

[5] Werner Bohleber: Ethnische Homogenität und Gewalt. Zur Psychoanalyse von Ethnozentrismus, Fremdenhass und Antisemitismus. In: Klaus Ahlheim (Eds.): Die Gewalt des Vorurteils. Schwalbach 2007, pp. 225–240.

## 4. Theories on fear of strangers and xenophobia

### *4.1 Xenophobia*

In the case of xenophobia, which is characterized by aggressive emotions, an underlying narcissistic disorder with hostility, self-insecurity, and megalomaniacal fantasies is assumed. As a result of the narcissistic structure, mere presence of strangers stimulates insult and aggressive impulses. These are aimed at the stranger, there persecuted and punished with the aim of annihilation. The demonization of the opponent justifies one's own hatred and counter-aggression. Linked to regressive ethnic fantasies of purity and a strong need for a merging (»ethnic«) community, the narcissistic dynamic for xenophobia and violence emerges in the far-right and populist world of thought. Let's take a closer look at this xenophobia.

The English writer A. L. Kennedy says: »In a hateful society, the self-esteem of a nation at some point depends on who it despises«.[6] Xenophobia is also referred to as »negative peak emotion« (»negativer Spitzenaffekt«). It is composed of different base emotions like fear and aggressive emotions like resentment, anger and rage. These form the hostile attitude and are associated with arrogance, an increase in the sense of oneself, and devaluation of migrants. Hatred arises in appropriately disposed persons (for example, narcissistic) not only in case of actual but already in case of fantasized threat and injury and is therefore prone to populism and racism. Xenophobia is contagious. This contagion of emotions causes splitting of the people through hatred. It brings each other at a distance. The hater does not tolerate the stranger anymore! On the other hand, the hater is hated by the stranger. »To live in hate and experience hate« – this is the »double meaning of the existence of the stranger«, pointed by Kristeva.[7] The constant hatred alters the stranger, who complies to rejection, cowers oneself anxiously and hides guiltily. Hatred has for the local population the function of identity saver through splitting and demarcation. It predefines what we are not and who we do not want to be. Uncertain people are therefore as susceptible as addressees of hate-driven

---

[6] A. L. Kennedy: In einer hasserfüllten Gesellschaft. In: Süddeutsche Zeitung (25/10/2015).

[7] Julia Kristeva: Fremde sind wir uns selbst. Frankfurt am Main 2013, pp. 199–210.

identity requirements. Hate conceals their own »weaknesses« and seeks such in others in order to fight them there.

### *4.2 Empathy versus prejudice*

In sociological studies it could be shown that such a thing as individual prejudices exists.[8] Such people are more prone to adopting xenophobic slogans than people without this property (pre-imprint). It has also been shown that a reciprocal relationship between racism/hatred and empathy can be assumed. The more hatred someone feels the less able he is to empathize. Here is a scientific example: Neurobiological studies have shown that people who imagine or see pain in another person activate their own corresponding brain areas for pain perception (MRI). This is interpreted as a neurophysiological correlate for an empathic reaction. In a study by Alessio Avenanti et al. at the University of Bologna, compared were on the basis of a pain experiment empathic reactions between Italians and black Africans living in Italy. Subjects were shown film clips showing white or black hands, either pricked with a needle or stroked with a cotton swab. Meanwhile, the scientists measured the brain activity of the subjects (MRI). Looking at black and white hands injured with a needle, normal black Africans and Italians had the same central nervous activity in the pain sensory brain areas. So, they reacted fully empathic. However, when racist black Africans and Italians were shown hands with a foreign skin color being stung, the central nervous responses failed to appear and were seen as a sign of lack of empathy. If black and white hands were dyed with violet color, also racist set subjects showed central nervous reactivity, reacting empathically. Therefore, it can be stated that socio-culturally transmitted racial prejudices and stereotypes find a psychobiological imprint in the neural networks and displace specifically empathetic experiences.

*Conclusion:* If one starts from this empirical background of individual readiness for xenophobia, it seems to me that the expedient discussion is less about innate but rather about the biographically and socio-culturally mediated dispositions. The option is then to neutralize previously communicated hate attitudes by psychoeducation and to regenerate the ability for empathy.

---

[8] Klaus Ahlheim (Ed.): Die Gewalt des Vorurteils. Schwalbach 2007, pp. 263–264.

## 5. Integration as a form of cultural adolescence

What does transition actually mean for the newcomers? As far as the integration of migrants and refugees in the host country is concerned, the newcomers essentially need to establish and develop a new life focus in a space somewhere between each of the cultures. In a developmental psychology respect, this complex task is comparable with normative adolescence, where creative powers and resources become available for the process of active self-development.[9] The change of the cultural and social context caused by migration is a powerful stimulus for personal development, and so it is reasonable to describe this as a form of »cultural adolescence«.[10] The similarities between normative and cultural adolescence can be seen in the way that, just as adolescents assume certain tasks and roles as they grow into adults in society, migrants also need to assume these tasks and roles once again, no matter what their age, as they grow into the host society. In this respect, migrants need to detach themselves from their »parental substitutes« in the form of the country of origin and the representatives of state and society, and cope with first hand experiences of unfamiliarity or strangeness, acquire a new language, as well as form relationships and connections within a socially and culturally new environment. In addition, the incoming migrant needs to establish professional and educational qualifications, seek work in order to survive, restructure family and gender relationships, to mourn that which has been lost and, not least, to develop a new bi-cultural identity. This development process – like all phases of individuation – goes hand in hand with an increased vulnerability to psychological aberrations. In order to accomplish a successful integration into the host country, it is necessary to shape a new positive interplay of individual components from the two cultural frameworks. If this is to be achieved, favorable social conditions and parental substitutes by means of sponsorships, integration facilitators and volunteer helpers form the best guarantee for success.

---

[9] Peter Blos: On Adolescence. A Psychoanalytic Interpretation. New York 1962.

[10] Wielant Machleidt: Migration, Kultur und psychische Gesundheit. Kohlhammer 2013.

## 6. Development of Identity in a Foreign Land

In connection with the development of identity in a foreign country, the particularly crucial question is the extent of transformation an individual may undergo without becoming a complete stranger to him or herself. Cultural identity is essential for an individual's feeling of self-worth. The construct of cultural identity is at the heart of intercultural psychotherapy for migrants. This concerns the restoration of social acceptance and a sense of belonging, and a balancing out of certainties and ambiguities relating to ethnic-cultural interferences. (Re-)construction of identity is more than just a simple coping strategy, it is an existential challenge for the individual in a foreign country, and a therapeutic task accompanying the acculturation processes.

## 7. Mental Health, Migration and Acculturation

Today, it is assumed that the critical life event of migration, the »cultural adolescence« and implicit development of identity, correlate with a heightened psychological vulnerability, but do not per se represent a psychopathological event.[11] It is far more often the case that social contextual factors and risk constellations that accompany migration are pivotal for the in part increased incidence of mental disorders among migrants and their descendants. Such factors might include social class, work and living conditions, experiences of discrimination, social exclusion and uncertain residency status, as well as particularly traumatic life experiences among refugees, whether prior to, during, or after their escape.[12]

---

[11] Jan Ilhan Kizilhan: Psychologie der Migration. In: Wielant Machleidt, Ulrike Kluge, Marcel Sieberer, Andreas Heinz (Eds.): Praxis der interkulturellen Psychiatrie und Psychotherapie. Migration und psychische Gesundheit. 2nd Edition. Munich 2018, pp. 67–75; Wielant Machleidt, Andreas Heinz: Dynamische Modelle der Migration. In: Wielant Machleidt, Ulrike Kluge, Marcel Sieberer, Andreas Heinz (Eds.): Praxis der interkulturellen Psychiatrie und Psychotherapie. Migration und psychische Gesundheit. 2nd Edition. Munich 2018, pp. 31–41.

[12] Laurence J. Kirmayer, Lavanya Narasiah, Marie Munoz, Meb Rashid, Andrew G. Ryder, Jaswant Guzder, Ghayda Hassan, Cecilie Rousseau, Kevin Pottie: Common mental health problems in immigrants and refugees: General approach to the patient in primary care. In: Canadian Medical Association Journal 183 (2011), p. 12; Dinesh

Contextual factors such as hostility towards foreigners, and racism (as a form of subjectively perceived discrimination), were identified as being highly significant in the higher rate of emotional distress with depressive and anxiety symptoms among migrants.[13] In this context, comparable lack of language skills can contribute to the depressive symptom as was seen in a group of late re-settlers with German heritage coming from former Soviet Union states.[14] There are interesting correlations between acculturation and psychological stress: characteristics of a lower general level of acculturation, or more limited linguistic acculturation, go hand in hand with increased psychological stress, especially depression. Alternately, successful acculturation can protect the individual from emotional distress.[15]

However, although these relationships have been demonstrated repeatedly, migrants cannot and should not generally be seen as somehow more susceptible to mental illness than non-migrants. In the international, often heated, debate, there are no effective linear casual factors to be identified that connect the stresses in the migration process with mental illnesses. It is far more likely that an interplay of various psycho-social, stress-related issues, as well as culturally and migration-linked adverse factors can be surmised. In the context of the vulnerable life experience of migration, these factors are likely to facilitate the emergence of a mental illness in the subject. A more consistent connection between the stress situation and a mental disorder can more likely be shown, if at all, in the sense of a higher probability of mental illness following severe experiences of trauma (see below). Just as much as stressful factors, individual migration and culturally specific salutogenetic factors and resources, with all their consequences, need to be included in any discussion of pathological

Bhugra: Mental health for nations. In: International Review of Psychiatry 28 (2016), pp. 342–374.

13 Ulrike Igel, Elmar Brähler, Gesine Grande: Der Einfluss von Diskriminierungserfahrungen auf die Gesundheit von MigrantInnen. In: Psychiatrische Praxis 37 (2010), pp. 183–190; Saffron Karlsen, James Y. Nazroo: Relation Between Racial Discrimination, Social Class, and Health Among Ethnic Minority Groups. In: American Journal of Public Health 92 (2002), pp. 624–631.

14 Hongliu Ding, Lee Hargraves: Stress-associated poor health among adult immigrants with a language barrier, in the United States. In: Journal of Immigrant Minorities Health 11 (2009), pp. 446–452.

15 Wielant Machleidt, Marcel Sieberer: From Kraepelin to a modern and integrative scientific discipline: The development of transcultural psychiatry in Germany. In: Transcultural Psychiatry, 50 (2013), pp. 817–840.

factors, in order to avoid a one-sided pathography in the understanding of the processes of migration.

## 8. Social development and the strangeness

The strangeness is an important stimulus for individual and social developments. Societies grow in their dealings with foreign countries and cultures, just as was shown in the example of cultural adolescence for the individual migrant. However, there are serious indications from sociological research that suggest limitations on manageable immigration. The social trust in a community or democracy has a sensitive internal connection to its functioning. A certain degree of social trust is »an indispensable prerequisite for a vibrant civil society and a functioning democracy«.[16] This also means that »self-governing political organizations (municipalities, democracies) can only receive and integrate a limited number of strangers without losing the social trust that is indispensable for them«.[17] Conversely, this means that the critical limit to the capacity of a society to absorb strangers is marked by the resilience of social trust among themselves. The British researchers Alexander Betts and Paul Collier have explained the background to this, they say: »The more immigrants live in a community, the lower the trust is not only between the different groups, but also within the groups«.[18] As a result, a high proportion of immigrants also leads to various forms of reduced cooperation among each other. That means, in plain language, that the abilities of the local people to cope with experiences of foreignness caused by migrants are the most important resources for the integration and at the same time the limit! Where too many newcomers arrive, the resources of the locals are not enough to handle their foreign experiences sufficiently well and the limit is reached. Then, the society requires increased investment in the production of social trust. Such activities can be initiated by the communities or by the citizens in the civic voluntary work, as is often done today.

These are important background insights not only for legitimacy,

---

[16] Cited in: Herfried Münkler, Marina Münkler: Die neuen Deutschen. Berlin 2016, p. 72.

[17] Münkler, Münkler: Die neuen (Note 16).

[18] Alexander Betts, Paul Collier: Gestrandet. Munich 2017.

but also for the need to publicly express individual feelings and perceptions in the migration society. These are to be understood as indications of the quality and resilience of social trust. Both the fears of citizens as well as the euphoric feelings of an individual can be interpreted as a social signal about the available social trust resources. They are something like seismographic perceptions of the social constitution of the community. In a liberal democracy, as the political theorist Hannah Arendt points out, the functioning of »public space« plays a crucial role as a regulator of social trust.

## 9. The public space

Hannah Arendt presented in detail in her main work »Vita activa or the active life« the function and meaning of »public space«.[19] In this space, everyone is visible to the public and audible for the widest possible public in a common world. The entry of people, of migrants and refugees into the public space is of great importance for the diversity and development of this public space, because it serves as a stage on which they become visible and tangible. They do not have to and should not hide. The strangers as part of the public space give themselves and the locals the opportunity to perform the necessary work of de-alienation/confidence building and to regulate their coexistence again and again. The ability of this public space to function is a constituent feature of liberal democracies, especially in critical times such as the current refugee movements.

The discourses in public space are linked to the inherent option and chance of collective consensus or compromise formation between the social groups and have an identity and self-reinforcing function for the individual citizen, especially in times of crisis. A public debate on the »how« to cope with immigration can have a socio-integrative function that reduces frightening fears by providing orientation. Public space, in a liberal democracy, has the task of creating social confidence in immigrants and facilitating their integration into society (see press reports on increasing employment of refugees).

---

[19] Hannah Arendt: Vita activa oder vom tätigen Leben. Stuttgart 1958, pp. 62–64.

## 10. Integration into the host society vs. parallel society

What connects an aging affluent civil society with immigrants is the hope of integration. But how can this hope be fulfilled?

Sociologists and psychologists have convincingly drawn attention to the connection between a positive social environment and the psychosocial development of the newcomers. Newcomers and locals are mutually reinforcing or inhibiting mutual development in the process of integration. Indeed, the conditions of integration created for the migrant groups by the host society reflect the degree of acceptance or resistance of a society and directly reflect the integration successes or failures of immigrants. Successful integration is a challenging goal and requires a broad basic consensus in a civil society, coupled with attractive integration conditions and a willingness and ability to integrate among migrants. This requires a departure from the integrative hardships and inconsistencies of previous decades that are reminiscent of archaic initiation rituals. Favorable integration conditions minimize the formation of so-called »parallel societies«, as ethnically homogenous segregation areas (»Little Istanbul«) panicky feared by the natives as breeding grounds of dissociality, crime, and terror. However, the more a migrant-dependent society refuses to allow migrants to find their way into their midst, the more important replacement spaces such as migrant communities become, where migrants receive advice and support from their ethnic peers. The migrant communities serve as bridgeheads in the integration and as passageways into the host society. Where this useful transit function is blocked by resistance from the receiving society, accumulations of migrants in ghettos or parallel societies arise as a substitute homeland. With their resistance to integration, xenophobic societies produce exactly what they fear most: the formation of migrant ghettos and »parallel societies« as quasi »extraterritorial segregation spaces« whose inhabitants live in a juxtaposition rather than coexistence with indigenous society.

The debate on integration in Germany is essentially shaped by two motives: on the one hand, the panic fear of parallel societies and demarcating ethnic groups and, on the other, the need for social reproduction (population growth) and economic and cultural gains through integration. In the latter motive lies the hope for the success of the vision of a civil society »in which people from different regions of origin and with different religious confessions live together«.[20] Integration is far from »charity« in this respect, but is driven by self-interest, with the expectation that migrants will profitably use the »social capital« they have acquired through investment in their skills and thereby prevent the danger of their being drifted into segregation areas. Integration becomes understood as a promising social experiment and as prevention prophylaxis by confidence building and capture of the strangeness into the own.

12 principles (imperatives) have been developed for a systematic and forward-looking integration policy.[21] These include, in particular, offering women work and social participation, exemplifying and practicing integration in schools, under the conditions of balanced relations between natives and migrants (30 %), as well as taking active action against discrimination in urban districts, developing opportunities for life planning for young people, keeping open the education and training system and an early labor market integration, and not least and indispensable, the reference to the Basic Law. This includes parting with yesterday's migration policies and a self-confident liberal democracy that has agreed on what immigration targets are and how it wants to achieve them.

## 11. Parting with yesterday

Integration of migrants requires a postmodern civil society with skills in managing strangeness experiences and with good caregiving skills. This postmodern civil society must identify with itself and with its societal long-term perspectives. Its citizens should bring along »a good dose of tolerance for frustration« and not be easily disturbed or discouraged. Then a modern immigration society is on the right path.

[20] Münkler, Münkler: Die neuen (Note 16), p. 185.
[21] Münkler, Münkler: Die neuen (Note 16), pp. 227–278.

# Addresses for correspondence:

Sylvia Agbih, M.A.
Bielefeld University
Department of Philosophy
Universitätsstr. 25
D-33615 Bielefeld
sylvia.agbih@uni-bielefeld.de

Dr. Robert Doričić
University of Rijeka
Faculty of Medicine, Department of Social Sciences and Medical Humanities
Braće Branchetta 20
HR-51000 Rijeka
robert.doricic@medri.uniri.hr

Dr. Katharina Fürholzer
University of Pennsylvania
Comparative Literature & Literary Theory
720 Williams Hall
US-Philadelphia, PA 19104
kfuer@sas.upenn.edu

Dr. Frank Kressing
Ulm University
Institute of the History, Philosophy and Ethics of Medicine
Parkstraße 11
D-89073 Ulm
frank.kressing@uni-ulm.de

Prof. Dr. Wielant Machleidt
Kaiser-Wilhelm-Str. 18
D-30559 Hannover
wielant.machleidt@t-online.de

Tarek Mahjoub, M.Sc.
Zentrum für Medizin und Gesellschaft
Albert-Ludwig-Universität Freiburg
Bugginger Straße 43
D-79114 Freiburg im Breisgau
tarek.mahjoub92@gmail.com

Full Prof. Dr. Amir Muzur
University of Rijeka
Faculty of Medicine and Faculty of Health Studies
Braće Branchetta 20
HR-51000 Rijeka
amir.muzur@medri.uniri.hr

Dr. Marcin Orzechowski
Ulm University
Institute of the History, Philosophy and Ethics of Medicine
Parkstraße 11
D-89073 Ulm
marcin.orzechowski@uni-ulm.de

Associate Prof. Dr. Iva Rinčić
University of Rijeka
Faculty of Medicine and Faculty of Health Studies
Braće Branchetta 20
HR-51000 Rijeka
iva.rincic@medri.uniri.hr

Dr. Ravi Rao
4th T, Block, Jayanagar
Bengaluru
IN-560 041 Karnataka
dr.ravirao.j@gmail.com

Dr. Giovanni Rubeis
Heidelberg University
Institute of History and Ethics of Medicine
Im Neuenheimer Feld 327
D-69120 Heidelberg
giovanni.rubeis@histmed.uni-heidelberg.de

Pranab Rudra
Ulm University
Institute of the History, Philosophy and Ethics of Medicine
Parkstraße 11
D-89073 Ulm
rudrapranab@gmail.com

PD Dr. Maximilian Schochow
Ulm University
Institute of the History, Philosophy and Ethics of Medicine
Parkstraße 11
D-89073 Ulm
maximilian.schochow@uni-ulm.de

Tamara Schwertel, M.A.
Siegen University
Department of Social Sciences
Adolf-Reichwein-Straße 2a
D-57076 Siegen
tamara.schwertel@uni-siegen.de

Professor Dr. Florian Steger
Ulm University
Institute of the History, Philosophy and Ethics of Medicine
Parkstraße 11
D-89073 Ulm
florian.steger@uni-ulm.de

Prerna Thaker
University of Freiburg
Fahnenbergplatz
D-79085 Freiburg im Breisgau
thaker_prerna@yahoo.com

Associate Prof. Dr. Ivana Tucak
University of Josip Juraj Strossmayer of Osijek
Faculty of Law
Stjepana Radića 13
HR-31000 Osijek
itucak@pravos.hr

Dr. A. Katarina Weilert, LL.M.
Forschungsstätte der Evangelischen Studiengemeinschaft e. V. (FEST)
Institute for Interdisciplinary Studies
Schmeilweg 5
D-69118 Heidelberg
katarina.weilert@fest-heidelberg.de

Dr. Pedro Alejandro Villarreal Lizárraga
Max Planck Institute for Comparative Public Law and
International Law
Im Neuenheimer Feld 535
D-69120 Heidelberg
villarreal@mpil.de

Vera Vogel
Düsseldorf University
LVR Clinic for Psychosomatic Medicine and Psychotherapy
Bergische Landstraße 2
D-40629 Düsseldorf
vera.vogel@hhu.de

Assistant Prof. Dr. Ivana Zagorac
University of Zagreb
Faculty of Humanities and Social Sciences
Ivana Lucica 3
HR-10000 Zagreb
izagorac@ffzg.hr